T0314046

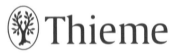

Orthodontic Aligner Treatment

A Review of Materials, Clinical Management, and Evidence

Theodore Eliades, DDS, MS, Dr Med Sci, PhD, DSc, FIMMM, FRSC, FInstP
Professor and Director
Clinic of Orthodontics and Pediatric Dentistry;
Director of Research and Interim Director, Institute of Oral Biology
Center of Dental Medicine, Faculty of Medicine
University of Zurich
Zurich, Switzerland

Athanasios E. Athanasiou, DDS, MSD, Dr Dent
Executive Dean and Professor of Orthodontics
Department of Dentistry
School of Medicine
European University Cyprus
Nicosia, Cyprus;
Honorary Professor of Orthodontics
Hamdan Bin Mohammed College of Dental Medicine
Mohammed Bin Rashid University of Medicine and Health Sciences
Dubai, United Arab Emirates

239 illustrations

Thieme
Stuttgart • New York • Delhi • Rio de Janeiro

Library of Congress Cataloging-in-Publication Data is available from the publisher

© 2021. Thieme. All rights reserved.

Georg Thieme Verlag KG
Rüdigerstrasse 14, 70469 Stuttgart, Germany
+49 [0]711 8931 421, customerservice@thieme.de

Thieme Publishers New York
333 Seventh Avenue, New York, NY 10001 USA
+1 800 782 3488, customerservice@thieme.com

Thieme Publishers Delhi
A-12, Second Floor, Sector-2, Noida-201301
Uttar Pradesh, India
+91 120 45 566 00, customerservice@thieme.in

Thieme Publishers Rio, Thieme Publicações Ltda.
Edifício Rodolpho de Paoli, 25º andar
Av. Nilo Peçanha, 50 - Sala 2508
Rio de Janeiro 20020-906 Brasil
+55 21 3172 2297 / +55 21 3172 1896

Cover design: Thieme Publishing Group
Cover illustration: Guido Pedroli
Typesetting by DiTech Process Solutions, India

Printed in Germany by Beltz Grafische Betriebe 5 4 3 2

ISBN 978-3-13-241148-7

Also available as an e-book:
eISBN 978-3-13-241149-4

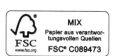

Contents

Section I Introduction: Types and Material Properties

1 Aligner Treatment: An Overview 2

Lauren Teske†, T. Gerard Bradley, and Sarandeep S. Huja

2 Material Properties of Aligners 9

Iosif Sifakakis, Spiros Zinelis, and Theodore Eliades

Section II Clinical Management

3 Early Treatment in Preteens and Teenagers Using Aligners 18

Eugene K. Chan and M. Ali Darendelile

Contents

14 Biological Properties of Aligners 170

Shaima Rashid Al Naqbi, Harris Pratsinis, Dimitris Kletsas, Athanasios E. Athanasiou, and Theodore Eliades

15 Aligner Treatment from the Patient Perspective 177

Eleftherios G. Kaklamanos, Theodore Eliades, and Athanasios E. Athanasiou

Foreword

Over time, changes in the armamentarium of orthodontics are "invented" and offered up to the profession. Some of these changes are described as new and improved; some are also termed "game changers" and are broadly disseminated and widely advertised in that tone. However, many of these changes in the appliances and strategies of orthodontics are not new at all, they do not produce a significant improvement that can be demonstrated, and most of these advancements do not endure. On the other hand, some changes do improve our knowledge and patient care, and they result in an important, obvious, and enduring change. For example, one of the last big changes that has occurred in orthodontics was confirmed by the disappearance of the dark room; everyone had one and now they are being repurposed or disappearing from the typical office design. Of course, this affect was produced by the real change—improvements in patient imaging.

This book highlights another invention that has and is changing orthodontics, and that is well appreciated by all of orthodontics: treatment with a series of plastic aligners. This development is not new at all in that it was first discussed by Kesling in the 1940s. He suggested that a series of removable rubber-like "positioners" could be used to treat a malocclusion to a planned result. Perhaps, due to patient or practitioner resistance, his efforts did not produce the desired change in orthodontics, but his ideas continued. Fast forward in time, through inquiry to refinement by the likes of Sheridan, Hilliard, Nahoum, Ponitz, McNamara, Rinchuse, Boyd, and many others, include developments in materials (importantly thermoforming plastics), technical advancements in computer hardware and software notably intraoral scanners and computer-aided design/computer-aided manufacturing (CAD/CAM), and the bedrock for a significant change in orthodontic treatment had been laid.

So, as the century turned, Chishti and Wirth (former orthodontic patients) began the planning and development of a new and clear aligner approach and in 2000 started marketing the Invisalign System. Through a computerized model, a plan was constructed that intended to move teeth from the initial malocclusion to the desired result via a series of clear aligners. But, because this approach was clearly different from traditional orthodontic approaches, practitioners resisted aligner treatment at first. Likewise, educational institutions did not hasten to teach this new technique; in some schools, it was banned. Practitioners who did adopt the technique and presented their experiences were severely criticized. Also, academics that performed research on the approach were sometimes ostracized.

So, now two decades later, one could ask "Where are we now?" First of all, there are many more companies that offer aligners. Most schools teach the technique, many practitioners have incorporated the technique in their practices, and individuals who have knowledge and experience with aligners are popular speakers and teachers. But, best of all, the public is very interested and they seek it out in this form of orthodontic treatment.

At this point, one can conclude that aligner treatments are here to stay and will continue to be of interest to all of orthodontics as the technique continues to improve and mature. Better information regarding aligner treatment will continue to increase through proper research and via presentations, journals, and textbooks.

So, what's the next big advancement? To that inquiry, I would argue that this book answers the question; it is the next advancement. Sure, there are already some books on aligner treatment, but for the most part those books are "How To" books; few, if any, describe aligner treatment as does this book. In this book, the topic at hand is discussed on the basis of experience and evidence, and that is its strength.

The book itself is logically separated into chapters that address the main topics of the subject, and the authors represent a global perspective and in many ways demonstrate their area of inquiry and depth of experience and expertise. The authors are knowledgeable, honest, and accurate, and it is clear that they respect the scientific perspective.

The chapter topics are important and cover the subject as it is known and appreciated at the present time. They address the benefits and drawbacks of aligner treatment, the materials involved, case selection, limitations by age and type of malocclusion, and patient reaction to the treatment. But there is much more—as you will find out.

Clinicians must have an understanding of biomechanics, materials, biology, periodontal response, occlusion, etc., to properly use this treatment. And, as always is the case, the practitioner's ability to formulate a high-quality diagnosis and treatment plan is paramount. But, if clinicians do possess these characteristics when using aligners, orthodontic knowledge increases, treatment improves, and patients are better served.

What's next? Sooner rather than eventually the teeth will be scanned in the orthodontist's office, digital tooth movement planning will be accomplished in the orthodontist's office, and the necessary aligners will be printed in the orthodontist's office. Many practitioners are not far from this now. We will all notice these things are occurring as time goes on. But, like the disappearance of the dark room, we may notice something ancillary as well—like the disappearance of alginate or a constriction in many companies that manufacture aligners.

The cost of this book and the time necessary to read it will be an excellent investment in terms of increasing your knowledge, ability, skills, and service to others. Pay attention to this book; you will not regret it.

Rolf G. Behrents, DDS, MS, PhD, Phd (Hon)
Professor Emeritus
Graduate Orthodontic Program
Center for Advanced Dental Education
Saint Louis University
Saint Louis, Missouri, USA;
Editor-in-Chief, The American Journal of
Orthodontics and Dentofacial Orthopedics
Editor-in-Chief, AJO-DO Clinical Companion

Preface

With the expansion of adult orthodontic treatment in the 1980s, the use of minimally visible appliances became a high priority, which could not be satisfied by ceramic or plastic brackets. The need to develop clear or "invisible" orthodontic appliances led to the development of removable, thermoplastically formed appliances which apply forces to teeth based on a predetermined strain. As result of this development, new treatment philosophy and technique of the clear aligner was introduced, stretching the functional ability of these appliances to their limits by incorporating more treatment types in managing different malocclusions of various age groups.

The initial systems featured a case planning and execution of a planned series of orthodontic tooth movements outside the control of the clinician. This made the orthodontic community skeptical about the generalized, large-scale application of these systems to routine practices but, on the other hand, boosted the treatment provided by nonspecialist practitioners. With the commercial patents expiring, the systems made available by different companies to clinicians expanded and a wide spectrum of aligner types are currently available, with some allowing for an in-office management of treatment planning and aligner fabrication.

The attractiveness of aligners to the esthetically conscious adult and adolescent patients expanded their use. As a result, orthodontic postgraduate programs gradually incorporated these systems in their curricula to cover a gap of training for the graduating specialists who previously had to rely largely on the educational material and instructions of dental industry to cover their needs on this technique. This, in turn, initiated the need to depart from the previously followed substantiation of treatment through a series of case presentations, anecdotal evidence, expert opinions, and other low-quality scientific evidence and include robust data analysis from designed studies on the topics of outcome assessment, undesirable effects, and other parameters of treatment such as duration, oral microbiota changes, and forces generated by aligners.

There is a discrepancy between the advanced, rapid pace of developments in the field of clear aligner orthodontic therapy and the status of relevant scientific documentation and evidence. The book reviews the subject from clinical, technical, materials, and treatment outcome perspectives, emphasizing on the principles and evidence of aligner treatment. It also includes a clinical manual, case presentations, and tips on various applications of aligner treatment in adolescents and adults to be used by the reader. As such, it serves as a reference source of the aligner technique with many different systems. It also includes the most recent guidelines on clinical management with aligners and presents the evidence in a variety of fields. This extends from material properties, to assessment of treatment outcome, to forces generated with aligners. This book also provides a detailed list of case planning with aligner systems for a wide spectrum of malocclusions.

Theodore Eliades, DDS, MS, Dr Med Sci,
PhD, DSc, FIMMM, FRSC, FInstP
Athanasios E. Athanasiou, DDS, MSD, Dr Dent

Contributors

Shaima Rashid Al Naqbi, DDS, MSc (Ortho)
Orthodontic Specialist
Fujairah Specialized Dental Center
Ministry of Health and Prevention
Fujairah, United Arab Emirates

Athanasios E. Athanasiou, DDS, MSD, Dr Dent
Executive Dean and Professor of Orthodontics
Department of Dentistry
School of Medicine
European University Cyprus
Nicosia, Cyprus;
Honorary Professor of Orthodontics
Hamdan Bin Mohammed College of Dental
    Medicine
Mohammed Bin Rashid University of Medicine and
    Health Sciences
Dubai, United Arab Emirates

Haylea Louise Blundell, BHsc (Dent), M Dent
Orthodontic Resident
School of Dentistry
University of Queensland
Brisbane, Queensland, Australia

T. Gerard Bradley, BDS, MS, Dr Med Dent
Professor of Orthodontics and Dean
School of Dentistry
Health Sciences Center
University of Louisville
Louisville, Kentucky, USA

**Eugene Chan, BDS, MDsc (Ortho), MOrth RCSEd,
    MRACDS, PhD**
Honorary Associate
Department of Orthodontics
Sydney Dental Hospital
University of Sydney
Sydney, New South Wales, Australia

**Ali M. Darendeliler, BDS, PhD, Dip Orth,
    Certif Ortho, Priv Doc, MRACDS (Ortho), FICD**
Professor and Chair
Discipline of Orthodontics
Faculty of Dentistry
University of Sydney;
Head
Department of Orthodontics
Sydney Dental Hospital
University of Sydney
Sydney, New South Wales, Australia

**Theodore Eliades, DDS, MS, Dr Med Sci, PhD,
    DSc, FIMMM, FRSC, FInstP**
Professor and Director
Clinic of Orthodontics and Pediatric
    Dentistry;
Director of Research and Interim Director,
    Institute of Oral Biology
Center of Dental Medicine, Faculty of
    Medicine
University of Zurich
Zurich, Switzerland

Raj Gaddam, BDS
Orthodontic Resident
School of Dentistry
University of Queensland
Brisbane, Queensland, Australia

Sarandeep S. Huja, DDS, PhD
Professor of Orthodontics and Dean
James B. Edwards College of Dental Medicine
Medical University of South Carolina
Charleston, South Carolina, USA

Anna Iliadi, DDS, MSc, Dr Med Dent
Research Associate
Department of Biomaterials
School of Dentistry
National and Kapodistrian University of Athens
Athens, Greece

**Eleftherios G. Kaklamanos, DDS, Cert,
    MSc (Ortho), MA, Dr Dent**
Associate Professor
Department of Orthodontics
Hamdan Bin Mohammed College of Dental
    Medicine
Mohammed Bin Rashid University of Medicine and
    Health Sciences
Dubai, United Arab Emirates

Dimitris Kletsas, PhD
Research Director
Director of the Institute of Biosciences and
    Applications
National Center of Scientific Research "Demokritos"
Athens, Greece

Dimitrios Kloukos, DDS, Dr Med Dent, MAS Ortho, MSc LSHTM
Senior Lecturer/Research Associate
Department of Orthodontics and Dentofacial Orthopedics
Center of Dental Medicine
Faculty of Medicine
University of Bern
Bern, Switzerland

Despina Koletsi, DDS, MSc, Dr Med Dent, MSc DLSHTM
Research Associate and Clinical Instructor
Department of Orthodontics
School of Dentistry
National and Kapodistrian University of Athens
Athens, Greece;
Visiting Scientist
Clinic of Orthodontics and Pediatric Dentistry
Center of Dental Medicine
University of Zurich
Zurich, Switzerland

Simon J. Littlewood, BDS, FDSRCPS, MDSc, MOrthRCSEd, FDSRCSEng
Consultant Orthodontist
St. Luke's Hospital
Bradford, UK

Amesha Maree, BDS
Orthodontic Resident
School of Dentistry
University of Queensland
Brisbane, Queensland, Australia

Spyridon N. Papageorgiou, DDS, Dr Med Dent
Senior Teaching and Research Assistant
Clinic of Orthodontics and Pediatric Dentistry
Center of Dental Medicine
University of Zurich
Zurich, Switzerland

William Papaioannou, DDS, MScD, PhD
Associate Professor
Department of Preventive and Community Dentistry
School of Dentistry
National and Kapodistrian University of Athens
Athens, Greece

Raphael Patcas, Dr Med Dent, Priv Doc, PhD
Head of Academic Unit
Clinic of Orthodontics and Pediatric Dentistry
Center of Dental Medicine
University of Zurich
Zurich, Switzerland

Harris Pratsinis, PhD
Senior Researcher
Institute of Biosciences and Applications
National Center of Scientific Research "Demokritos"
Athens, Greece

Marc Schätzle, Dr Med Dent, Odont Dr, MOrtho RCSEd
Senior Research Scientist
Clinic of Orthodonitcs and Pediatric Dentistry
Center of Dental Medicine
University of Zurich
Zurich, Switzerland

Phil Scheurer, Dr Med Dent
Specialist in Orthodontics
Private Practice
Fribourg, Switzerland

Iosif Sifakakis, DDS, MSc, Dr Dent
Assistant Professor
Department of Orthodontics
School of Dentistry
National and Kapodistrian University of Athens
Athens, Greece

Lauren Teske[†], BS, DDS, MS
Orthodontic Specialist
Green Bay, Wisconsin, USA

Tony Weir, BDSc, MDS (Ortho)
Honorary Clinical Senior Lecturer
Department of Orthodontics
School of Dentistry
University of Adelaide
Adelaide, South Australia, Australia

Anastasios A. Zafeiriadis, DDS, MSc, Dr Dent
Research Associate
Department of Orthodontics
Faculty of Dentistry
School of Health Sciences
Aristotle University of Thessaloniki
Thessaloniki, Greece

Spiros Zinelis, PhD
Associate Professor
Department of Biomaterials
School of Dentistry
National and Kapodistrian University of Athens
Athens, Greece

Section I

Introduction: Types and Material Properties

I

1 Aligner Treatment: An Overview*

Lauren Teske†, T. Gerard Bradley, and Sarandeep S. Huja

Summary

For almost 20 years, clear aligners have been used with growing popularity in addressing with success patients' demands for esthetic orthodontic treatment. Many companies all over the world have developed methods of fabricating custom-made clear aligners designed to gradually and sequentially move teeth to their desired positions. Treatment efficacy with clear aligners has been reported to be good but further investigation of the various aspects of this kind of orthodontic treatment modality is needed for scientific evidence and further clinical improvement. This chapter presents an overview of the patients' esthetic treatment demands, which led to the popularity of this modality of orthodontic therapy, as well as important aspects of the clear aligner method, the orthodontic tooth movement with clear aligners, and the material properties of clear aligners. Clear aligner material efficiency and effectiveness should continue to be studied, as a better understanding of the material properties and treatment outcomes could lead to better sequencing of tooth movement and more efficient treatment.

Keywords: orthodontic aligners, orthodontic treatment, malocclusion, patients' esthetic treatment demands, orthodontic tooth movement, clear aligners material properties

1.1 Introduction

Patients' demands for esthetic orthodontic treatments have grown to include esthetic appliances, such as ceramic brackets, lingual orthodontics, and clear aligner therapy.[1,2,3] If patients' orthodontic treatment motivations are esthetically driven, they may prefer a more attractive appliance as well. More Invisalign patients reported seeking treatment to improve their appearance (85 vs. 67% for fixed appliance patients), whereas more fixed appliance patients reported seeking treatment because their dentist referred them (26 vs. 3% for Invisalign patients).[4]

Companies including Align Technology (Santa Clara, California, United States), Allesee Orthodontic Appliances (Sturtevant, Wisconsin, United States), and Smile Direct (Nashville, Tennessee, United States) have developed a method of fabricating custom-made clear aligners designed to gradually and sequentially move teeth to their desired positions.[5] The short-term chemical and physical changes, as well as the structural conformation and leaching before and after use, have been previously studied on Invisalign (Align Technology).[6,7,8] Invisalign changed in 2013 the material that was used in making their aligners to SmartTrack aligner material, which continues to be a polyurethane-based material but has been claimed to have increased elasticity and a more precise fit.[9] To date, no studies have investigated the mechanical properties of the clear aligners manufactured by Allesee Orthodontic Appliances, including Simpli5 and Red, White and Blue, or that of Smile Direct. The latter is a relatively recent entry to the market place with no evidence in the scientific literature to verify its claims of efficacy and efficiency in treatment.

Treatment efficacy with clear aligners has been reported to be 41 to 59%, but further investigation in material behavior is needed for improvement.[10–12] The force delivery properties of aligners are influenced by both the direction of displacement and the stiffness of the material used.[13,14] A more recent study has found that the orthodontic force produced by a thermoplastic material is strongly correlated with its hardness and elastic modulus. Therefore, any significant differences in the properties of clear aligners may have an impact on what aligner system the practitioner chooses to use.[15] Material properties may even affect the treatment outcome, as it was found that patients wearing a harder aligner material for a 2-week activation time showed the best results in all measurements of occlusal and alignment improvement, although the difference was not statistically significant.[16]

It is also important to determine if the material's properties change after use, as biofilm modification and oral environmental conditions may have

---

*This chapter is dedicated to the memory of Dr. Lauren Teske, a colleague, mother, and friend.

effects on the hardness and viscoelasticity of the material.[17] Previous studies have detected changes in the Invisalign material after use, including increased hardness, decreased mechanical properties, abraded cusp tips, integument adsorption, biofilm calcification, microcracks, delamination, and loss of transparency.[6,7,8]

1.2 Esthetic Treatment Demands

Patients' demands for esthetic orthodontic treatment have grown to include any type of esthetic appliances which are minimally visible.[1,2,3] The appearance of orthodontic appliances plays a significant role in patients' decisions to receive orthodontic treatment. A survey found that 33% of young adults would be unwilling to wear visible braces if needed.[18] Another study noted that while traditional metal brackets were found to be esthetically acceptable to only 55% of adults, clear aligners were acceptable to over 90%.[1] Furthermore, they showed no difference in acceptability ratings when considering the appliances for their own treatment or for their children's treatment, and they were willing to pay more for appliances they deemed more esthetic. Clear aligner preference extends to adolescents as well, as surveyed 15- to 17-year-olds rated clear aligners most acceptable and attractive over ceramic, self-ligating, traditional, and shaped brackets.[19]

As more adults are seeking orthodontic treatment, esthetic improvements of appliances may be a major factor in the increase of acceptability of orthodontic treatment in this group of patients. Perceived personal characteristics of adults may be influenced by their dental appearance and orthodontic appliance design: greater perceived intellectual ability was associated with the appearance of no appliance or aligner appliances compared to steel or ceramic appliances.[3]

This could likely influence the patient's orthodontic appliance choice. If their treatment motivation is esthetically driven, they may prefer a more esthetic appliance as well.

1.3 Clear Aligner Therapy

Companies including Align Technology and Allesee Orthodontic Appliances have developed a method of fabricating custom-made clear aligners designed to gradually and sequentially move teeth to their desired positions (▶ Fig. 1.1).[5] The short-term chemical and physical changes, as well as the structural conformation and leaching before and after use have been previously studied on Invisalign (Align Technology).[6,7] However, Invisalign has recently changed the material that was used in making the aligners to Smart-Track aligner material, which continues to be a polyurethane-based material.[9] Align Technology states that the SmartTrack material delivers a lower initial insertion force for improved patient comfort, while maintaining more constant force over the 2-week wear. Additionally, it is claimed to have higher elasticity and a more precise fit. This is beneficial in that it improves tracking and control of tooth movements.[20] No studies to date have investigated the mechanical properties of the clear aligners manufactured by Allesee Orthodontic Appliances, including Simpli5 and Red, White and Blue. Both systems use the company's highly esthetic proprietary material and are designed to treat minor to intermediate anterior misalignment, only differing in the number of aligners the patient has to wear to correct the misalignment.[21]

The aligner manufacturing process differs for the two companies. Align Technology uses stereolithography technology to create plastic resin models from photoactivated polymer.[5] The patient's polyvinyl siloxane (PVS) impressions are scanned and converted into three-dimensional electronic

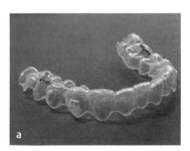
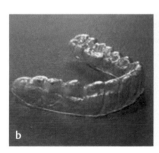

Fig. 1.1 **(a)** Unused Invisalign and **(b)** Simpli5 mandibular aligners.

a

b

models, where the teeth are electronically separated and moved by a technician. Alternatively, the models can be fabricated directly from the patient's intraoral scan.[22] Each stage of treatment is converted into a physical model with a stereolithography apparatus, and an automated aligner system heats, forms, and laser-marks sheet plastic over each model.[5] Ridges from the model formed by stereolithography can be seen in the finished aligner material, and the tray is scalloped along the gingival margin (▶Fig. 1.2). Conversely, Allesee Orthodontic Appliances fabricates their aligners from stone models where the individual teeth are manually sectioned by lab technicians and repositioned with wax.[23,24] The finished product is highly transparent with a straight-line finish instead of scalloping the gingival margins (▶Fig. 1.2). Each system produces clear aligners from the models, each corresponding to a 2- to 3-week interval of treatment. Progressive alignment of 0.25 to 0.5 mm is designed into each aligner.[25] Aligner systems including ClearSmile and Raintree Essix allow more displacement in each aligner (0.5–1 mm) compared to the Invisalign system (0.25–0.33 mm).[25,26]

Benefits of clear aligner therapy include esthetics, comfort, oral hygiene improvement, and reduced chair time.[27] Adult Invisalign patients have reported less pain and fewer negative impacts on their lives than those with fixed appliances.[4,28] Those with fixed appliances took more pain medication during the first week of orthodontic treatment than the Invisalign patients.[4] Adolescents also have positive attitude to aligners. The vast majority did not limit foods, avoid communication, or feel self-conscious while wearing the aligners.[29] After 3 months, 70% had seldom or never experienced discomfort, and 80% had seldom or never

used pain relievers. As treatment progressed, the patients reported even less discomfort.[29] In addition to improved comfort, clear aligners also show favorable consequences for periodontal health compared to fixed appliance treatment.[30] After 24 months, teenagers using Invisalign Teen aligners had the plaque index decreased by 15.1% in the maxilla and 16.6% in the mandible.[29]

Orthodontic appliances must be selected on the basis of more than appearance, as the appliances must have desirable functional properties and treatment outcomes. A systematic review in 2005 determined that there was not sufficient evidence to adequately evaluate Invisalign treatment effects, and that high-quality clinical evidence was needed.[31] Since then, there have been numerous studies that have looked at the efficacy and treatment outcomes of Invisalign treatment. Treatment efficacy with clear aligners has recently been reported to range from 41 to 59%.[10,11,12] While the reported treatment efficacy numbers are low, case reports have shown successfully completed moderate to difficult orthodontic malocclusions, including open bite, extraction, and surgical cases.[32,33,34,35,36,37] Furthermore, resolving moderately severe anterior crowding can be successfully accomplished with Invisalign.[38]

Treatment outcomes of Invisalign have been compared to fixed appliances using the objective grading system of the American Board of Orthodontics. Compared to traditional braces, Invisalign lost an average of 13 more points and had a 27% lower passing rate.[39] While the strengths of Invisalign included its ability to close spaces and correct anterior rotations and marginal ridge heights, it was deficient in correcting large anteroposterior discrepancies and occlusal contacts.[39] Evaluation of dental casts of patients treated with Invisalign

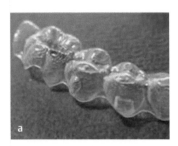
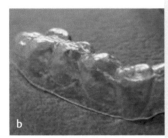

Fig. 1.2 Aligner material. **(a)** Invisalign aligner. Notice the generalized ridges from the stereolithographic manufacturing process, the impression of the attachments on the premolars, and how the aligner is scalloped along the gingival margin. **(b)** Simpli5 aligner. The material appears more translucent in comparison to Invisalign and the edge is trimmed straight across the gingival margins of the teeth.

and their comparison to patients treated with fixed appliances immediately after end of treatment and 3 years posttreatment concluded that patients treated with Invisalign relapsed more than those treated with fixed appliances, particularly in the maxillary anterior region. Even though the Invisalign group relapsed more, the mean alignment was superior to the fixed appliance group before and after the retention phase.[40]

1.4 Orthodontic Tooth Movement with Clear Aligners

The type of desired tooth movement influences the efficacy of treatment with clear aligners. When looking at dental improvements, aligners were most successful in improving anterior alignment, transverse relationships, and overbite.[16] Aligners were least successful at improving buccal occlusion and only moderately successful at improving midline and overjet.[16] One study reports lingual constriction to be the most accurate movement (47.1%) and extrusion to be the least accurate (29.6%).[10] Additionally, it was determined that canine rotation accuracy was significantly lower than for other teeth and lingual crown tip was significantly more accurate than labial crown tip. This study was done without auxiliaries in order to provide a baseline value of what can be achieved with aligners alone. A relatively recent study investigated the efficacy of Invisalign aligners in tooth movements deemed difficult with aligners and analyzed the influence of auxiliaries, including attachments and Power Ridges.[14] It was found that premolar derotation showed the lowest accuracy (40%), while molar distalization was the most effective movement (87%). No statistically significant difference was found with the use of attachments in the efficiency of premolar derotation or molar distalization. Furthermore, no substantial difference was observed if incisor torque (42% mean accuracy) was supported with a horizontal ellipsoid attachment or a Power Ridge. A very recent systematic review looked at 3 randomized clinical trials and 8 prospective and 11 retrospective studies.[41] It concluded that Invisalign aligners is a viable alternative to conventional orthodontic therapy in the correction of mild to moderate malocclusions in nongrowing patients that do not require extraction.[41] This technique is good at levelling, tipping, and derotating some

teeth, but has limited efficacy in arch expansion through bodily movement, extraction space closure, correction of occlusal contacts, and larger anteroposterior and vertical problems.

Other factors can influence orthodontic tooth movement with clear aligners, such as age, gender, root length, and bone levels. A quadratic (U-shaped) relationship between age and tooth movement was found for women, indicating an increase in tooth movement in younger and older women.[11] However, a more linear relationship was found for men, with decreased movement at older ages. This study also found a significant negative correlation between tooth movement and the measurement of the apex to the center of rotation, but bone quality was not correlated with tooth movement.[11] This may account for individual differences in treatment efficacy during clear aligner therapy.

As tooth movement with aligners has been distance-based as opposed to force-based with fixed appliances, recent studies have attempted to quantify the force delivery properties of aligners. Initially, it was determined that median force values for intrusion during rotation of an upper central incisor at the low activation range of ± 0.17 mm were between 0.0 and -0.8 N, with the highest intrusive force being -5.8 N for a rotation of -0.51 mm.[13,14] A few years ago, it has been reported that initial mean moments were 7.3 N mm for maxillary incisor torque, 1.0 N mm for distalization, and 1.2 N mm (without attachments) to 8.8 N mm (with attachments) for premolar rotation.[25] While the recent findings suggest that bodily tooth movements and torque can be performed with aligners since they deliver the necessary force systems, the ideal values (0.35–0.6 N for rotation and tipping, and 0.1–0.2 N for intrusion) were exceeded.[42]

The force delivery properties of aligners are influenced by both the direction of displacement and the stiffness properties of the material used.[13,14] At lower activation ranges, different chemical and physical material properties might be responsible for the different force levels. The local deformations of the material and friction at the contact areas may be of relevance.[13,14]

1.5 Material Properties of Clear Aligners

A better understanding of the material properties could lead to better sequencing of tooth movement and more efficient treatment.[43] It has been found that there is great variety in mechanisms among the initial force systems during clear aligner therapy, as an aligner with high initial force may be followed by an aligner with a low force, resulting in tooth movement that is not constant.[12] Additionally, as the order of sequential aligners increases, aligner strains relating to force delivery increase.[44] A relevant study has found that the orthodontic force produced by a thermoplastic material is strongly correlated with its hardness and elastic modulus; therefore, any significant differences in the properties of clear aligners may have an impact on what aligner system the practitioner chooses to use.[15] Material properties may even affect the treatment outcome, since patients wearing a harder aligner material for a 2-week activation time showed the best results in all measurements of occlusal and alignment improvement, although the difference was not statistically significant.[16]

It is also important to determine if the material's properties change after use, as biofilm modification and oral environmental conditions may have effects on the hardness and viscoelasticity of the material.[17] During the time the aligners are worn, they are exposed to salivary enzymes, byproducts of oral flora, liquids, and trauma caused by swallowing, speech, and bruxism.[6] In vitro testing conditions are unable to simulate the intraoral conditions the aligners are exposed to, including plaque accumulation. Therefore, retrieval analysis obtains critical information since it investigates the material in its intended environment.[17]

Previous studies detected changes in the Invisalign material after use. Differences were found in the surface morphology of aligners after use, including abraded cusp tips, integument adsorption, biofilm calcification, microcracks, delamination, and loss of transparency.[7,9] Delamination of the material can lead to loss of mechanical strength of the aligner.[6] The loss of transparency may be caused by trauma from chewing and bruxism.[6] Additionally, buccal segments showed an increase in hardness and a decrease in mechanical properties, which may be caused by masticatory-induced cold work.[7,8]

Although polyurethane is biocompatible, it is not an inert material, as it is sensitive to heat, humidity, and salivary enzymes.[6] No traceable byproducts were detected after Invisalign aligners were stored in artificial saliva or an ethanol aging solution.[6,7] Furthermore, no evidence of cytotoxicity or estrogenicity was found at various concentrations of aligner eluents.[45] This could be related to the material's structure, as it is composed of polyurethane with added methylene diphenyl diisocyanate and 1,6 hexanediol.[7] The diphenyl structure provides stability and sufficient reactivity to form a polymer free of byproducts.[7] Also, unlike the aromatic rings in bis-GMA, polyurethane has short rigid portions joined by short flexible hinges and long flexible portions.[45] However, the in vitro testing conditions may have underestimated the material's chemical stability.

Past studies have shown that clinical recommendations can be determined from their material study's results. One study found that as the order of sequential aligners increases, aligner strains relating to force delivery increase. It was concluded that final aligners should be thicker or worn for a longer period of time.[44] However, another study determined that thin material (0.508 mm) can deliver higher energy than thick materials (0.762–1.1016 mm), and it, therefore, recommended that thin material be selected to move teeth efficiently.[26]

Other investigations have found changes in the aligner material after use. In the deflection ranges of optimal force delivery (0.2–0.5 mm), the force delivery properties of aligners were different after repeated load cycling, but were not different after thermocycling.[26] Additionally, both thermocycling and load cycling influenced Vickers hardness values. This may be significant because if aligners become hard during use, they may cause discomfort to the patient and induce changes in their force delivery properties. Another study has found that intraoral aging adversely affected the mechanical properties of Invisalign. Contrary to the previous study, used aligners had significantly lower hardness values, with higher elastic index and creep indentation values.[8] The decreased hardness indicates a less wear-resistant material, where the increased elastic index implies the material become more brittle.[8]

While changes in material properties after clinical use have been reported, it has also been found that neither material fatigue nor difference in stiffness plays a significant role in the rate or amount of tooth movement. No significant difference was found in the amount of orthodontic tooth movement between those who wore the same aligner for 2 weeks and those who changed to a new duplicate aligner after 1 week.[43] Another study did not find a substantial difference in the treatment completion rate when comparing hard and soft appliances, with completion rates being 32 and 27%, respectively.[46] However, neither material was the same as the material used by Align Technology. The hard material used was twice as stiff as the commercial material, while the soft material was one-tenth as stiff.

These differing and sometimes contradicting findings suggest that orthodontic tooth movement with clear aligners needs further study. A better understanding of the clear aligner material properties remains pivotal to this ongoing investigation and could potentially lead to better sequencing of tooth movement and more efficient treatment. However, comparisons between studies may be a challenge, as the material used in future studies may not be the same material used in past studies, since the companies continue to evolve the material and its characteristics.

1.6 Conclusion

Patients' survey responses are predominately positive, as all were pleased with the esthetics, comfort, and performance of the aligners. The popularity of aligner as an alternative option to conventional fixed appliances as well as increase in aligner options and sales has grown enormously in the past decade. Clear aligner material efficiency and effectiveness should continue to be studied, as a better understanding of the material properties and treatment outcomes could lead to better sequencing of tooth movement and more efficient treatment.

References

[1] Rosvall MD, Fields HW, Ziuchkovski J, Rosenstiel SF, Johnston WM. Attractiveness, acceptability, and value of orthodontic appliances. Am J Orthod Dentofacial Orthop. 2009;135:276e1–276e12

[2] Ziuchkovski JP, Fields HW, Johnston WM, Lindsey DT. Assessment of perceived orthodontic appliance attractiveness. Am J Orthod Dentofacial Orthop. 2008;133(4, Suppl):S68–S78

[3] Jeremiah HG, Bister D, Newton JT. Social perceptions of adults wearing orthodontic appliances: a cross-sectional study. Eur J Orthod. 2011;33(5):476–482

[4] Miller KB, McGorray SP, Womack R, et al. A comparison of treatment impacts between Invisalign aligner and fixed appliance therapy during the first week of treatment. Am J Orthod Dentofacial Orthop. 2007;131(3):302.e1–302.e9

[5] Kuo E, Miller RJ. Automated custom-manufacturing technology in orthodontics. Am J Orthod Dentofacial Orthop. 2003;123(5):578–581

[6] Gracco A, Mazzoli A, Favoni O, et al. Short-term chemical and physical changes in invisalign appliances. Aust Orthod J. 2009;25(1):34–40

[7] Schuster S, Eliades G, Zinelis S, Eliades T, Bradley TG. Structural conformation and leaching from in vitro aged and retrieved zInvisalign appliances. Am J Orthod Dentofacial Orthop. 2004;126(6):725–728

[8] Gerard Bradley T, Teske L, Eliades G, Zinelis S, Eliades T. Do the mechanical and chemical properties of Invisalign™ appliances change after use? A retrieval analysis. Eur J Orthod. 2016;38(1):27–31

[9] Align Technology, Inc. SmartTrack Aligner Material. [Material safety data sheet]. San Jose, CA: Align Technology, Inc.;2012

[10] Kravitz ND, Kusnoto B, BeGole E, Obrez A, Agran B. How well does Invisalign work? A prospective clinical study evaluating the efficacy of tooth movement with Invisalign. Am J Orthod Dentofacial Orthop. 2009;135(1):27–35

[11] Chisari JR, McGorray SP, Nair M, Wheeler TT. Variables affecting orthodontic tooth movement with clear aligners. Am J Orthod Dentofacial Orthop. 2014;145(4, Suppl):S82–S91

[12] Simon M, Keilig L, Schwarze J, Jung BA, Bourauel C. Treatment outcome and efficacy of an aligner technique—regarding incisor torque, premolar derotation and molar distalization. BMC Oral Health. 2014;14:68

[13] Hahn W, Engelke B, Jung K, et al. Initial forces and moments delivered by removable thermoplastic appliances during rotation of an upper central incisor. Angle Orthod. 2010;80(2):239–246

[14] Hahn W, Zapf A, Dathe H, et al. Torquing an upper central incisor with aligners--acting forces and biomechanical principles. Eur J Orthod. 2010;32(6):607–613

[15] Kohda N, Iijima M, Muguruma T, Brantley WA, Ahluwalia KS, Mizoguchi I. Effects of mechanical properties of thermoplastic materials on the initial force of thermoplastic appliances. Angle Orthod. 2013;83(3):476–483

[16] Clements KM, Bollen AM, Huang G, King G, Hujoel P, Ma T. Activation time and material stiffness of sequential removable orthodontic appliances. Part 2: Dental improvements. Am J Orthod Dentofacial Orthop. 2003;124(5):502–508

[17] Eliades T, Bourauel C. Intraoral aging of orthodontic materials: the picture we miss and its clinical relevance. Am J Orthod Dentofacial Orthop. 2005;127(4):403–412

[18] Bergström K, Halling A, Wilde B. Orthodontic care from the patients' perspective: perceptions of 27-year-olds. Eur J Orthod. 1998;20(3):319–329

[19] Walton DK, Fields HW, Johnston WM, Rosenstiel SF, Firestone AR, Christensen JC. Orthodontic appliance preferences of children and adolescents. Am J Orthod Dentofacial Orthop. 2010;138(6):698.e1–698.e12, discussion 698–699

[20] Align Technology, Inc. SmartTrack Aligner Material. [Brochure]. San Jose, CA: Align Technology, Inc;2013

[21] Allesee Orthodontic Appliances. Aligners. [Brochure]. Sturtevant, WI: Allesee Orthodontic Appliances;n.d

[22] Garino F, Garino B. The iOC intraoral scanner and Invisalign: a new paradigm. J Clin Orthod. 2012;46(2):115–121, quiz 124

[23] McNamara JA, Brudon WL. Orthodontics and Dentofacial Orthopedics. Ann Arbor, MI: Needham Press; 2001:477–479

[24] Kim TW, Echarri P. Clear aligner: an efficient, esthetic, and comfortable option for an adult patient. World J Orthod. 2007;8(1):13–18

[25] Simon M, Keilig L, Schwarze J, Jung BA, Bourauel C. Forces and moments generated by removable thermoplastic aligners: incisor torque, premolar derotation, and molar distalization. Am J Orthod Dentofacial Orthop. 2014;145(6):728–736

[26] Kwon JS, Lee YK, Lim BS, Lim YK. Force delivery properties othermoplastic orthodontic materials. Am J Orthod DentofacialOrthop. 2008;133(2):228–234, quiz 328.e1

[27] Boyd R, Miller RJ, Vlaskalic V. The Invisalign system in adult orthodontics: mild crowding and space closure cases. J Clin Orthod. 2000;34:203–212

[28] Shalish M, Cooper-Kazaz R, Ivgi I, et al. Adult patients' adjustability to orthodontic appliances. Part I: a comparison between Labial, Lingual, and Invisalign™. Eur J Orthod. 2012;34(6):724–730

[29] Tuncay O, Bowman SJ, Amy B, Nicozisis J. Aligner treatment in the teenage patient. J Clin Orthod. 2013;47(2):115–119, quiz 140

[30] Klukowska M, Bader A, Erbe C, et al. Plaque levels of patients with fixed orthodontic appliances measured by digital plaque image analysis. Am J Orthod Dentofacial Orthop. 2011;139(5):e463–e470

[31] Lagravère MO, Flores-Mir C. The treatment effects of Invisalign orthodontic aligners: a systematic review. J Am Dent Assoc. 2005;136(12):1724–1729

[32] Hönn M, Göz G. A premolar extraction case using the Invisalign system. J Orofac Orthop. 2006;67(5):385–394

[33] Womack WR. Four-premolar extraction treatment with Invisalign. J Clin Orthod. 2006;40(8):493–500

[34] Boyd RL. Surgical-orthodontic treatment of two skeletal Class III patients with Invisalign and fixed appliances. J Clin Orthod. 2005;39(4):245–258

[35] Boyd RL. Esthetic orthodontic treatment using the invisalign appliance for moderate to complex malocclusions. J Dent Educ. 2008;72(8):948–967

[36] Marcuzzi E, Galassini G, Procopio O, Castaldo A, Contardo L. Surgical-Invisalign treatment of a patient with Class III malocclusion and multiple missing teeth. J Clin Orthod. 2010;44(6):377–384

[37] Schupp W, Haubrich J, Neumann I. Treatment of anterior open bite with the Invisalign system. J Clin Orthod. 2010;44(8):501–507

[38] Krieger E, Seiferth J, Marinello I, et al. Invisalign® treatment in the anterior region: were the predicted tooth movements achieved? J Orofac Orthop. 2012;73(5):365–376

[39] Djeu G, Shelton C, Maganzini A. Outcome assessment of Invisalign and traditional orthodontic treatment compared with the American Board of Orthodontics objective grading system. Am J Orthod Dentofacial Orthop. 2005;128(3):292–298, discussion 298

[40] Kuncio D, Maganzini A, Shelton C, Freeman K. Invisalign and traditional orthodontic treatment postretention outcomes compared using the American Board of Orthodontics objective grading system. Angle Orthod. 2007;77(5):864–869

[41] Papadimitriou A, Mousoulea S, Gkantidis N, Kloukos D. Clinical effectiveness of Invisalign® orthodontic treatment: a systematic review. Prog Orthod. 2018;19(1):37

[42] Proffit WR, Fields HW, Sarver DM. Contemporary Orthodontics. St. Louis, MO: Mosby Inc.;2013:286–287

[43] Drake CT, McGorray SP, Dolce C, Nair M, Wheeler TT. Orthodontic tooth movement with clear aligners. ISRN Dent. 2012:(e-pub ahead of print)

[44] Vardimon AD, Robbins D, Brosh T. In-vivo von Mises strains during Invisalign treatment. Am J Orthod Dentofacial Orthop. 2010;138(4):399–409

[45] Eliades T, Pratsinis H, Athanasiou AE, Eliades G, Kletsas D. Cytotoxicity and estrogenicity of Invisalign appliances. Am J Orthod Dentofacial Orthop. 2009;136(1):100–103

[46] Bollen AM, Huang G, King G, Hujoel P, Ma T. Activation time and material stiffness of sequential removable orthodontic appliances. Part 1: Ability to complete treatment. Am J Orthod Dentofacial Orthop. 2003;124(5):496–501

2 Material Properties of Aligners

Iosif Sifakakis, Spiros Zinelis, and Theodore Eliades

Summary

This chapter provides information about the composition and physicomechanical properties of contemporary orthodontic aligners. Currently, most aligner manufacturers use polyethylene terephthalate glycol-modified and polyurethane for the manufacturing of these materials. The ideal material for aligners should demonstrate high enough hardness to withstand intraoral wear and low water absorption rate. A high degree of transparency is also required, which should be stable during the 2-week orthodontic treatment periods. In addition, a high modulus of elasticity increases the force delivery capacity of the appliance under constant strain. However, different materials show significant differences in their chemical structure and mechanical properties and, therefore, differences in their clinical behavior are anticipated.

Keywords: aligners, mechanical properties, hardness, water absorption, instrumented indentation testing

2.1 Introduction

Patient demand for orthodontic treatment with aligners has increased, although many clinicians and considerable part of the orthodontic literature remain skeptical about their clinical effectiveness over conventional systems.[1] Part of this skepticism is due to the different material properties of these appliances which affect clinical behavior and tooth movement efficacy. The materials used for the manufacturing of these aligners are viscoelastic, in which the relationship between stress and strain depends on time. In contrast, the materials used for the construction of conventional appliances are metallic and ceramics whose viscoelastic properties are evident only as they near their melting point. Contrary to purely elastic materials, viscous ones demonstrate a time-dependent response during loading. At constant loads, the strain of a viscoelastic material increases over time (a phenomenon known as creep). Creep occurs in metals too, as a result of long-term exposure to high levels of stress that are still below the yield strength of

the material. Another time-dependent response of a viscous material is relaxation, where under constant strain the developed stresses are decreased over time. The extent of this reduction depends on both the magnitude of the load applied and the properties of the material itself.[2] In general, these materials are sensitive to temperature, humidity, time elapsed after insertion, and manufacturing process.[3] Consequently, poor wear resistance and durability along the incisal and occlusal surfaces of thermoplastic retainers is expected after short-term use.[4]

A Google search revealed approximately 27 different aligner products.[5] The Invisalign aligners are still widely used; however, after the expiry of its patent, several aligner systems have been introduced, such as ClearSmile, Clear Aligner, All-In, F22 Aligner, and Orthocaps, which are constructed using computer-aided design/computer-aided manufacturing (CAD/CAM) technology and 3D printing or a stepwise setup model. Nowadays, the clinician may choose between a variety of different scanning technologies, setup software, material, thickness, stiffness, transparency, and finishing quality.[6] Ideally, this choice should be based on the material properties and their clinical performance; however, this is not always feasible. Ideally, an aligner should apply a light and constant force. To exert safe but efficacious forces, the ideal material should exhibit substantial linear elastic behavior with a high yield point, able to ensure that the force is applied within the elastic range. In other words, its relaxation curve should be fairly flat, demonstrating its ability to exert constant and continuous forces over time.[7,8] Moreover, this specific application of these materials should be biocompatible. The aim of this chapter is to review the recent literature on the properties of the materials used for the manufacturing of orthodontic aligners and present an outline of the ideal properties of these aligners.

2.2 Chemical Composition

In general, aligner materials are resin polymers. Currently, aligner manufacturers use polyethylene terephthalate (PET) glycol-modified (PETG), polyurethane (PUR), polypropylene (PP), polycarbonate (PC), thermoplastic polyurethanes (TPU), ethylene vinyl acetate (EVA), polyethylene (PE), and many other materials for the construction of the aligners. Structurally, thermoplastic polymers are divided into either amorphous or semicrystalline.[9] PETG, PC, and copolyester are amorphous polymers, and PP, PE, and EVA are semicrystalline polymers and thus different material properties are anticipated due to these structural differences.[9,10,11] Most of the thermoplastic materials has been extensively used for the construction of orthodontic retainers too.

The new generation of Invisalign aligner material is SmartTrack, a thermoplastic polyurethane with an integrated elastomer. According to the manufacturer, this is highly elastic material that delivers low and constant force to improve control of tooth movements. The urethane-based structure of the new and old generation Invisalign aligners was confirmed by Fourier transform infrared microspectroscopy[3,12] and attenuated total reflectance-Fourier transform infrared spectroscopy analysis (ATR-FTIR).[13,14] A recent study evaluated four different aligner types by ATR-FTIR analysis (▶Fig. 2.1). Identical spectra were obtained from the non-Invisalign thermoplastic materials which matched that of PETG[14] (▶Fig. 2.1).

Blending could be an effective way to develop new polymers with improved performance. A considerable amount of research on polyester blends and optimal blending ratios have been published: PETG/PET, PC/PP, TPU/PP, PETG/liquid crystal polymers, PC/acrylonitrile butadiene styrene, and others.[7,15]

2.3 Material Properties

2.3.1 Mechanical Properties

Orthodontic aligner mechanical properties are strongly influenced by the material of their construction. However, it is impossible to evaluate these properties with the conventional mechanical tests (i.e., tensile, bending, compression, and others) due to the requirement of bulky specimens with predefined dimension which sometimes is impossible to be produced in the determined dimensions. Alternatively to conventional mechanical testing, the development of instrumented indentation testing (IIT) is used to yield a variety of mechanical properties (elastic modulus, creep, relaxation, different expression of hardness, and others), from a simple hardness measurement. This method is based on the continuous recording of time, force, and indentation depth that a Vickers, Berkovich, or other type of indenter is in contact with sample surface and has been already used to characterize the mechanical properties of thermoplastic orthodontic materials and orthodontic adhesives[14,16,17] (▶Table 2.1; see also ▶Fig. 2.2).

Most of the research in hardness deals with thermoplastic materials used for the construction of retainers. The hardness of orthodontic aligners should be high enough to withstand

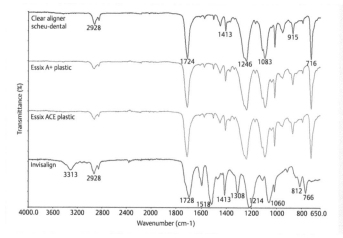

Fig. 2.1 Representative ATR-FTIR spectra from Invisalign aligners and thermoplastic materials.

Table 2.1 Mean values and standard deviations (in parentheses) of indentation modulus (E_{IT}), elastic index (η_{IT}), and indentation creep (C_{IT}) of several materials tested[13,14]

	Essix A+	Essix ACE	Clear Aligner	Invisalign new
E_{IT} (GPa)	2,256 (40)[a]	2,112 (16)[b]	2,374 (4)[c]	2,467 (19)[d]
η_{IT} (%)	35.9 (0.6)[a]	35.7 (0.2)[a]	34.0 (0.1)[b]	40.8 (0.2)[c]
C_{IT} (%)	2.2 (0.3)[a]	2.6 (0.4)[a]	2.7 (0.5)[a]	3.7 (0.3)[b]

Note: Similar superscripts in a row indicate mean values with no statistically significant differences ($p > 0.05$).

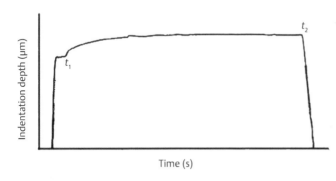

Fig. 2.2 Representative indentation creep curve of a thermoplastic material showing the indentation depth as a function of the time. Indentation creep is measured between t_1 and t_2.

intraoral wear. Significant hardness differences exist between different thermoplastic materials. Invisalign aligners demonstrated higher hardness values compared with the other PETG-tested materials and are expected to demonstrate better wear resistance under clinical conditions.[14] The possible impact of these changes in the mechanotherapy requires further research.[3] Gerard Bradley et al[13] selected Martens hardness against traditional Vickers hardness in order to eliminate the material rebound effect around the indentation, as documented with traditional hardness measurements, thus providing values independent of this experimental complication.

Significant differences were also identified between several PETG thermoplastic materials. These differences might be attributed to two factors: (1) the different molecular weight of the various PETG polymers, and (2) the thermoforming effect on the mechanical properties. Thermoforming may influence the molecular orientation, mean molecular weight, and residual stresses due to rapid cooling of the thermoplastic materials on the stone models.[14]

In vitro studies have reported that PETG materials have higher wear resistance compared with two PP-based materials when subjected to a cyclic wear apparatus with steatite ceramic abraders as an enamel substitute.[18,19] Between three widely used products, Duran and Erkodur, which belong to the PETG family, demonstrated similar values but higher than the values obtained from Hardcast, a PP material.[16]

Further hardness values were obtained from nanoindentation after thermal cycling of Duran (PETG), Hardcast (PP), and three PU materials. Decreases were evident in some of the materials after 500 thermal cycles and in almost all of them after 2,500 thermal cycles[20] (▶ Table 2.2).

The mechanical properties of polymer materials vary according to the degree of crystallinity. The glass transition temperature (T_g) is an important parameter, since the materials soften rapidly on exceeding T_g. As a result, the mechanical properties of polymers with T_g below room temperature may be influenced markedly by changes in temperature. In addition, the properties of the polymers depend strongly on the molecular orientation. Anisotropic materials generally have multiple elastic moduli, i.e., a higher elastic modulus is observed during loading parallel on molecular orientation, in comparison with vertical one.[11,21]

Amorphous polymers have a higher T_g, elastic modulus, and water absorption rate. Most of them are clear due to the passage of visible light through their structure. Semicrystalline polymers have a

Table 2.2 Mean values and standard deviations (in parentheses) of hardness for several thermoplastic materials, intraorally aged or after thermocycling

	Martens hardness (HM) (N/mm²)		Hardness (nanoindentation) (GPa)	
	(13)	(12) Reference and intraorally aged	(15)	(19) As received and after thermocycling (2,500 cycles)
Essix A+	100.0 (0.7)[a]			
Essix ACE	91.8 (0.8)[b]			
Clear Aligner	100.6 (0.6)[a]			
Invisalign	117.8 (1.1)[c]	119 ± 1[a] and 110 ± 6[b]		
Erkodur			0.169[a]	
Duran			0.165[a]	0.18[a] and 0.10[2]
Hardcast			0.099[b]	0.12[a] and 0.01[b]
PUR SMP MM 3520				0.06[a] and 0.01[b]
PUR SMP MM 6520				0.22[a] and 0.20[a]
PUR SMP MM 9520				0.25[a] and 0.19[b]

Note: Similar superscripts in a column indicate mean values with no statistically significant differences ($p > 0.05$).

lower elastic modulus and water absorption rate, while most of them are opaque due to the different refractive indexes of their amorphous and crystalline parts (9–11).

The materials used for the construction of orthodontic aligners should possess a high modulus of elasticity since it increases the force delivery capacity of the appliance under constant strain. As a result, the same force magnitude can be applied by thinner aligners made of materials of higher modulus of elasticity. The values of indentation modulus for Invisalign aligners (E_{IT}) were found within the range (2,000–2,500 MPa) reported for orthodontic thermoplastic appliances[16] and at higher levels compared with the other PETG materials.[14] However, Invisalign aligners demonstrated higher elastic index too, denoting a more brittle material and higher indentation creep, implying that under constant occlusal forces exerted by the opposing dentition, this aligner type is more likely to deform and therefore attenuate the applied orthodontic forces[14] (▶ Table 2.3).

TPU specimens were subjected to tensile test after drying or immersion in distilled water at different temperatures and various exposure durations. Stress–strain curves were created displaying two distinct parts: an initial linear part, used to determine the elastic modulus of the material, and a second part corresponding to the viscoelastic behavior. Drying of unaged TPU introduces an improvement in mechanical properties

Table 2.3 Moduli of elasticity of commercial orthodontic thermoplastic polymers

	Modulus of elasticity
Essix A+, Clear Aligner, Essix ACE, Invisalign	2,100–2,500[13]
Thermoforming Foil Track A (PETG)	Thermoformed: only 743; thermoformed after short- and long-term intraoral exposure: 3,762 and 9,351 (9), respectively
Duran, Erkodur, Hardcast (PETG, PP)	1,500–3,000 (15)
New and intraorally aged Invisalign aligners	2,200–2,500 (12)

due to the elimination of the diffused water molecules in the samples.[22,23]

Specimens from eight dental thermoplastic products were subjected to tensile tests under room temperature or in a simulated intraoral environment. In almost all of the materials, the elastic modulus has changed; however, no significant changes were observed for PUR. Tensile yield stress of the specimens in the simulated intraoral environment decreased in comparison with as received sheets.[11]

Three brands of thermoplastic materials demonstrated a decrease in their modulus and maximum stress after thermoforming and an increase after saliva immersion.[24]

The tear strength of four brands of thermoplastic materials decreased after thermoforming; however, it increased again after 2 weeks of distilled water immersion. The opposite kind of behavior was demonstrated regarding elongation at break: an increase was recorded after thermoforming, which declined after 2 weeks of distilled water immersion.[25]

2.3.2 Water Absorption

Water absorption through humidity in the air, immersion in water, or intraoral application generally causes expansion of the thermoplastic material and induces several physicochemical changes, causing the irreversibly degradation of the mechanical properties of the polymer. Numerous studies indicate water absorption may contribute to the stress relaxation of thermoplastic materials. Therefore, the ideal material for aligners should demonstrate low water absorption rate. Water penetrates the amorphous regions of polymers[26]; however, the crystalline fractions of polymer may also be affected by water addition.[27] The role of water could be explained either by washing out of soluble products or by a chemical reaction.[28] The irreversible plasticizing effect of water can be interpreted considering separately or simultaneously: (1) the rupture of hydrogen bond intrachains and/or interchains in the profit of bond water/polymer and (2) the modification of the free volume of polymer resulting from the water absorption.[22,23]

Water absorption tests include measurements of the weight gain ratio of thermoplastic specimens after the immersion in distilled water. However, these experiments provide insight into water absorption in vitro but the oral environment is much more complicated, regarding chemistry but also usage (periodic removal and reinsertion) of aligners.

During the first 48 hours of immersion, water absorption rate was high for two common PETG products and several PETG/PC/TPU polymer blends. This was followed by a slowdown and a plateau after 2 weeks of immersion, at about 0.5 to 0.8% weight increase. It was demonstrated that the water absorption rate of PETG/PC/TPU blends increased with blending ratio of TPU and that these blends had better performance than the commercial PETG product, regarding dimensional stability.[7]

Water absorption was evaluated in eight commercial thermoplastic products for 2 weeks. Water absorption of all products increased with time and some of them reached a plateau during the measurement period. The PUR product showed the highest water absorption after 1 and 14 days and a high value of 1.50% weight increase. This product did not reach the saturation point within the measurement period. Linear expansion with water absorption ranged from 100.3 to 119.9%. The PE product showed the smallest linear expansion rate. In general, it was shown that the amorphous plastics have higher water absorption rates, while crystalline plastics have lower water absorption rates.[11]

Further research compared the stress relaxation of five commercial orthodontic thermoplastic materials within a water bath and in an atmospheric environment. The stress relaxation curves showed that the residual stress within all materials decreased with time, and that this process was significantly accelerated in the 37°C water bath: the materials delivered only 40 to 65% of their initial forces after immersion in the 3-hour 37°C water bath.[18]

TPU specimens, predried or not, were immersed in distilled water at 70°C for 6 months. During the first 7 hours of immersion, a linear relationship between absorption rate and square root of immersion duration was demonstrated. This behavior corresponded to the diffusion of water in the amorphous zones of polymer. Saturation was reached for the materials after approximately 48 hours and the speed at which the equilibrium plateau was reached depended on the thickness of the sample, the kinetics of diffusion, and the temperature. Diffusion coefficient of water molecules into the immersed samples was higher in the predried samples.[22,23]

Polyethylene glycols grades with molecular weights 4,000 and above are not hygroscopic, i.e., they exhibit minimal moisture uptake when exposed to elevated relative humidity conditions[29]

2.3.3 Transparency

Since this is the main advantage of these appliances, a high degree of transparency is required, which should be stable during the 2-week orthodontic treatment periods. Manufacturers suggest removal of the aligners before eating/drinking;

however, it is not uncommon that the patients do not comply with this suggestion due to social reasons.

The National Bureau of Standards (NBS) system was used to describe levels of perceptible color change upon visual inspection of three commercial aligner products after in vitro staining with coffee, black tea, and red wine. All three types of appliances exhibited relatively color stability after the 12-hour immersion; however, the Invisalign aligners were slightly stained by coffee. After 7 days of immersion, the Invisalign aligners exhibited marked color changes, particularly the specimens that were immersed in coffee. Since the coffee caused the most marked staining, these specimens were further investigated with scanning electron microscopy examination and Fourier transformation infrared analysis. The latter demonstrated that all the tested materials were chemically stable after staining in coffee for 7 days.[30] The transparency of the aligner decreases when the layer thickness increases[31] and in PETG blended with TPU.[15]

The evolution of the various aligner systems is very rapid when compared with the time involved in the clinical data collection and their analysis. As a result, a next generation of the tested aligner system may be commercially released soon after this publication. The optimum choice is further complicated by the inherent limitations of the laboratory analyses. Although the laboratory studies illuminate issues that would have been unethical or highly time-/cost-consuming or even impossible to evaluate in the clinical setting, a lot of clinical variables affecting tooth movement are rather obscure or unknown and, consequently, the clinical environment, regarding saliva, oral function, and microorganism enzymes, cannot be simulated in the laboratory conditions. Further clinical evidences especially on the efficacy of these devices are essential before these devices can reach a worldwide acceptance from the orthodontic community.

References

[1] Zheng M, Liu R, Ni Z, Yu Z. Efficiency, effectiveness and treatment stability of clear aligners: A systematic review and meta-analysis. Orthod Craniofac Res. 2017;20(3):127–133

[2] Lombardo L, Martines E, Mazzanti V, Arreghini A, Mollica F, Siciliani G. Stress relaxation properties of four orthodontic aligner materials: A 24-hour in vitro study. Angle Orthod. 2017;87(1):11–18

[3] Schuster S, Eliades G, Zinelis S, Eliades T, Bradley TG. Structural conformation and leaching from in vitro aged and retrieved Invisalign appliances. Am J Orthod Dentofacial Orthop. 2004;126(6):725–728

[4] Thickett E, Power S. A randomized clinical trial of thermoplastic retainer wear. Eur J Orthod. 2010;32(1):1–5

[5] Weir T. Clear aligners in orthodontic treatment. Aust Dent J. 2017; 62(Suppl 1):58–62

[6] Sifakakis I, Zinelis S, Eliades T. Aligners for orthodontic applications. In: Eliades T, Brantley WA, eds. Orthodontic Application of Biomaterials. Amsterdam: Woodhead Publishing;2017:275–287

[7] Zhang N, Bai Y, Ding X, Zhang Y. Preparation and characterization of thermoplastic materials for invisible orthodontics. Dent Mater J. 2011;30(6):954–959

[8] Lombardo L, Arreghini A, Maccarrone R, Bianchi A, Scalia S, Siciliani G. Optical properties of orthodontic aligners--spectrophotometry analysis of three types before and after aging. Prog Orthod. 2015;16:41

[9] Sawyer LC, Grubb DT, Meyers GF. Polymermicroscopy. 3rd ed. New York, NY: Springer;2008

[10] Ahn HW, Ha HR, Lim HN, Choi S. Effects of aging procedures on the molecular, biochemical, morphological, and mechanical properties of vacuum-formed retainers. J Mech Behav Biomed Mater. 2015;51:356–366

[11] Ryokawa H, Miyazaki Y, Fujishima A, Miyazaki T, Maki K. The mechanical properties of dental thermoplastic materials in a simulated intraoral environment. Orthod Waves. 2006;65:64–72

[12] Gracco A, Mazzoli A, Favoni O, et al. Short-term chemical and physical changes in invisalign appliances. Aust Orthod J. 2009;25(1):34–40

[13] Gerard Bradley T, Teske L, Eliades G, Zinelis S, Eliades T. Do the mechanical and chemical properties of Invisalign™ appliances change after use? A retrieval analysis. Eur J Orthod. 2016;38(1):27–31

[14] Alexandropoulos A, Al Jabbari YS, Zinelis S, Eliades T. Chemical and mechanical characteristics of contemporary thermoplastic orthodontic materials. Aust Orthod J. 2015;31(2):165–170

[15] Ma YS, Fang DY, Zhang N, Ding XJ, Zhang KY, Bai YX. Mechanical properties of orthodontic thermoplastics PETG/ PC2858 after blending. Chin J Dent Res. 2016;19(1):43–48

[16] Kohda N, Iijima M, Muguruma T, Brantley WA, Ahluwalia KS, Mizoguchi I. Effects of mechanical properties of thermoplastic materials on the initial force of thermoplastic appliances. Angle Orthod. 2013;83(3):476–483

[17] Sifakakis I, Zinelis S, Patcas R, Eliades T. Mechanical properties of contemporary orthodontic adhesives used for lingual fixed retention. Biomed Tech (Berl). 2017;62(3):289–294

[18] Fang D, Zhang N, Chen H, Bai Y. Dynamic stress relaxation of orthodontic thermoplastic materials in a simulated oral environment. Dent Mater J. 2013;32(6):946–951

[19] Gardner GD, Dunn WJ, Taloumis L. Wear comparison of thermoplastic materials used for orthodontic retainers. Am J Orthod Dentofacial Orthop. 2003;124(3):294–297

[20] Iijima M, Kohda N, Kawaguchi K, et al. Effects of temperature changes and stress loading on the mechanical and shape memory properties of thermoplastic materials with different glass transition behaviours and crystal structures. Eur J Orthod. 2015;37(6):665–670

[21] Kikutani T, Ito H. Analysis of crystalline orientation by wide-angle X-ray diffraction. J Jpn Soc Polym Process. 2000;12:556–560

[22] Boubakri A, Elleuch K, Guermazi N, Ayedi HF. Investigations on hygrothermal aging of thermoplastic polyurethane material. Mater Des. 2009;30:3958–3965

[23] Boubakri A, Haddar N, Elleuch K, Bienvenu Y. Impact of aging conditions on mechanical properties of thermoplastic polyurethane. Mater Des. 2010;31:4194–4201

[24] Zhang N, Bai YX, Zhang KY. Mechanical properties of thermoplastic materials [in Chinese] Zhonghua Yi Xue Za Zhi. 2010; 90(34):2412–2414

[25] Zhang N, Fang DY, Bai YX, Ding XJ, Zhang Y. A comparative study of mechanical properties of commercialized dental thermoplastic materials [in Chinese] Zhonghua Kou Qiang Yi Xue Za Zhi. 2011;46(9):551–553

[26] Hodge RM, Edward GH, Simon GP. Water absorption and states of water in semicrystalline poly(vinyl alcohol) films. Polymer. 1996;37(8):1371–1376

[27] Iwamoto R, Miya M, Mima S. Determination of crystallinity of swollen poly(vinyl alcohol) by laser Raman spectroscopy. J Polym Sci, B, Polym Phys. 1979;17:1507–1515

[28] Hollande S, Laurent JL. Weight loss during different weathering tests of industrial thermoplastic elastomer polyurethane-coated fabrics. Polym Degrad Stabil. 1998;62:501–505

[29] Price JC. Polyethylene glycol. In: Rowe RC, Sheskey PJ, Owen SC, eds. Handbook of Pharmaceutical Excipients. 5th ed. London/Washington, DC: Pharmaceutical Press/ American Pharmacists Association;2006:545–550

[30] Liu CL, Sun WT, Liao W, et al. Colour stabilities of three types of orthodontic clear aligners exposed to staining agents. Int J Oral Sci. 2016;8(4):246–253

[31] Martorelli M, Gerbino S, Giudice M, Ausiello P. A comparison between customized clear and removable orthodontic appliances manufactured using RP and CNC techniques. Dent Mater. 2013;29(2):e1–e10

Section II

Clinical Management

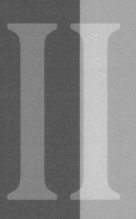

II

3 Early Treatment in Preteens and Teenagers Using Aligners

Eugene K. Chan and M. Ali Darendeliler

Summary

Clear aligner therapy has always been reserved for adults and/or the esthetically conscious patient. Historically, clear aligners did not work well with younger patients, or patients with primary or mixed dentition. The digital platform could not work out the necessary differentiation between the biology of tooth movement between primary and permanent dentition. The constant dental exfoliation and dynamic growth changes may also be harder to track as the case progresses. The lack of compliance in younger patients often led to nonideal clinical finish, prolonged treatment duration, and inefficient treatment. New advances in digital algorithm allowing biomaterials, attachment designs, and optimized velocity of the movement of both primary and permanent teeth within the same subject has opened up a new option for selected young patients. Both early interceptive phase I treatment and full comprehensive orthodontic treatment in children using the clear aligners have become a reality.

Keywords: orthodontics, Invisalign, early treatment, mixed dentition

3.1 Introduction

Patients may be referred early to the orthodontist for interceptive treatment for various reasons. Major reasons include the presence of supernumerary teeth disrupting routine dental eruption, disparity in jaw growth, the presence of parafunctional habits that may have disturbed the equilibrium of dental positioning, missing or early loss of deciduous teeth leading to the early loss of space, or anterior or posterior crossbites that may hinder the symmetry and/or dentoalveolar development. Other reasons may also include trauma, soft-tissue abnormalities, variations in dental anatomy, or transposition of teeth.

Commencing early orthodontic treatment appears logical as it enables the complete or partial correction of many incipient discrepancies or, at least, a reduction in their capacity to become

worse. Interception, or early intervention, employs simple therapeutic techniques that do not strain the limited stores of cooperation young patients can bring to the therapeutic encounter. Its objective is to eliminate or minimize dentoalveolar and skeletal disorders that may interfere with growth, function, esthetics, and the psychological well-being of the child.[1]

For a long time, early interceptive treatment involved various fixed and/or removable appliances such as the headgears, removable or fixed expanders, bite planes, habit breakers, functional appliances such as twin or mono blocks, or fixed partial preadjusted bracket systems.

Recent improvements in aligner therapy have allowed this appliance, historically used for adult esthetic orthodontic treatment, to be considered for such early interceptive treatment.

The success of early interceptive treatment lies within the thorough understanding of the cause of the problem, the knowledge of the patients' potential growth, the deciduous and permanent dentitions' biological response to orthodontic intervention, and good patient compliance. Appliance design in early interceptive orthodontic treatment is rather complex. It has always been varied with many modifications to accommodate for differently timed treatment, targeting different needs and purposes of the interception. The management of the developing dentition is tricky. While early treatment may be indicated dentally, patient maturity and psychological readiness may not be. The window period of treatment in both genders vary quite a fair bit, and also varies within the gender group itself.

Traditional appliances used in interceptive treatment could mostly treat one problem but not the other.

3.2 Fixed Expansion

Transverse expansion required in cases that demonstrate bilateral posterior crossbites (▶Fig. 3.1a) can often be easily corrected with a fixed expansion device. The case shown had the transverse discrepancy corrected in 2 months with

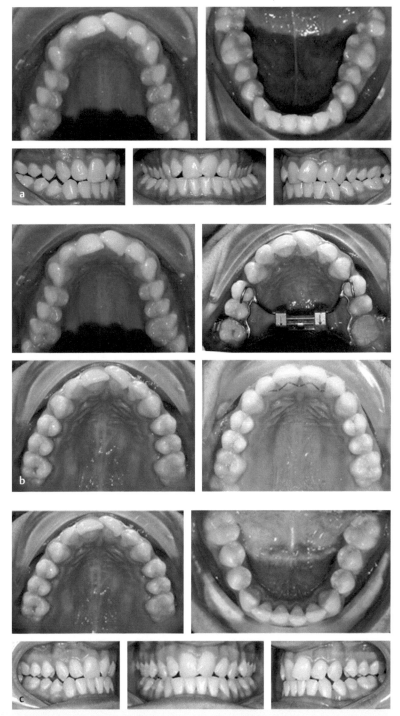

Fig. 3.1 **(a)** A case with bilateral posterior crossbite. **(b)** Posterior crossbites corrected using a Hyrax expander over a period of 2 months, followed by comprehensive orthodontic treatment using the Invisalign appliance. **(c)** Images showing occlusion after immediate Hyrax expansion.

a Hyrax fixed expander (▶Fig. 3.1b). The expander was left in place for a further few months before it was removed to commence a stage II treatment with the Invisalign appliance. This fixed preliminary treatment, although effective in achieving phase I treatment objectives, can only correct the transverse discrepancy. Dental alignment, anteroposterior changes, arch coordination, and dental interdigitation cannot be achieved using this same appliance (▶Fig. 3.1c).

3.3 Removable Anterior Bite Plate Appliance

Increased dental overbites in mixed dentition may lead to increased attrition and wear to the anterior teeth, and may further contribute to a more complex dental malocclusion later (▶Fig. 3.2a). A typical treatment modality is a removable upper anterior bite plane appliance (▶Fig. 3.2b). This appliance is usually worn full time for a period of 6 to 9 months. Incorporating the young patient's vertical dentoalveolar growth, the appliance disocclude the posterior segment and encourages the lower molars to overerupt, hence opening the vertical dimension and correcting the dental overbite (▶Fig. 3.2c). Although other auxiliaries such as screws (for transverse or anteroposterior corrections), finger, and/or Z-springs may be incorporated into these removable appliances, individual tooth movements still cannot be achieved with this appliance unless partial fixed appliances are placed. The patient is usually retained and monitored closely thereafter as they transit into permanent dentition before comprehensive orthodontic treatment may be indicated once again.

3.4 Removable Posterior Bite Plate Appliance

Young patients with a digit sucking habit develops a malocclusion with an anterior open bite, commonly also associated with a constricted upper arch and posterior crossbites (▶Fig. 3.3a). Treatment usually takes about 6 to 9 months with a removable upper dental arch appliance designed with bilateral posterior bite planes. An expansion screw is also incorporated into the palatal aspects of the appliance (▶Fig. 3.3b). The primary

treatment objectives are to allow the canting of the occlusal plane to normalize the occlusion, achieve a positive overbite, and expand the upper dental arch to correct the posterior crossbites (▶Fig. 3.3c). Further dental alignment, arch coordination, and anteroposterior changes were corrected later usually in the permanent dentition using clear aligner therapy (▶Fig. 3.3d).

3.5 Functional Appliance

Early treatment in patients with a Class II malocclusion with skeletal discrepancy needs to be timed well. Monitoring growth parameters such as secondary growth characteristics and charting changes in cervical vertebrae in lateral cephalometric radiographs is useful[2,3] (▶Fig. 3.4a, b). Young patients with a severe skeletal II growth pattern are usually treated just before they hit their growth spurt (▶Fig. 3.5a–c). With good compliance in wearing a functional appliance, the dentofacial discrepancy can usually be corrected within 9 to 12 months (▶Fig. 3.5d–g). The functional appliance used in this case was a Clark twin block. An expansion screw is usually incorporated into this appliance and transverse correction can be achieved together with the anteroposterior discrepancy. After sagittal splinting is achieved, selective grinding of the acrylic of the appliance is done to allow vertical eruption to further correct vertical discrepancies. Despite the ability to correct the dentofacial and malocclusion in all three planes, the typical functional appliance is still not able to individually correct dental alignment problems and complete the case to a high-quality finish with good interdigitation. Fixed appliances or clear aligners are usually necessary to complete the case thereafter.

3.6 Invisalign First

Two-phase treatments using aligners for both phases I and II have not been considered until recently (▶Fig. 3.6). Aligner therapy has always been reserved for the adult, esthetically conscious patient. The fact that they are less visible has that big advantage over conventional fixed appliances, and remains a large drawcard. However, its close to full time, 22-hour daily wear routine has made the patient's compliance of aligner wear paramount in

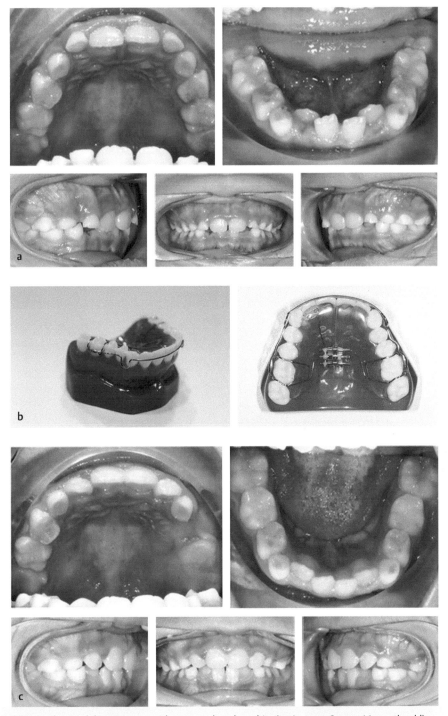

Fig. 3.2 (a) An early mixed dentition case with a severe dental overbite (patient was 9 years 11 months old). (b) Typically corrected using an upper removable appliance with an anterior bite plane and an expansion screw incorporated. (c) Dental overbite corrected in a period of 7 months.

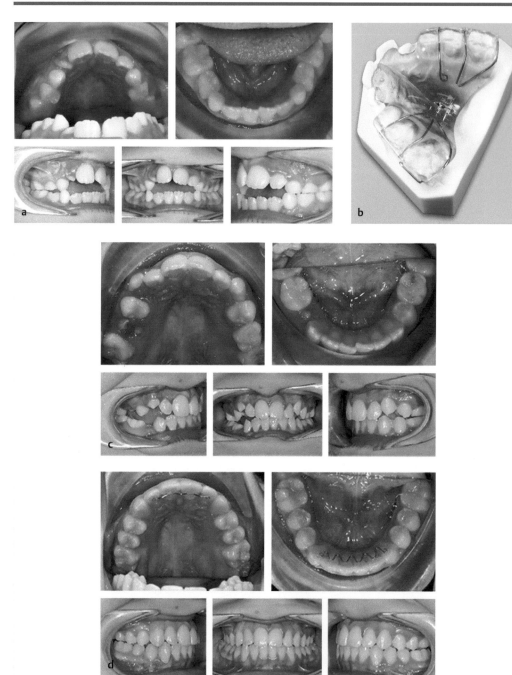

Fig. 3.3 (a) An early mixed dentition case with a severe anterior open bite (patient was 8 years 7 months old). (b) Typically corrected using an upper removable appliance with posterior bite plane or posterior occlusal coverage and expansion screw incorporated. (c) Interceptive treatment corrected over a period of 12 months. (d) Full comprehensive treatment completed using clear aligner therapy.

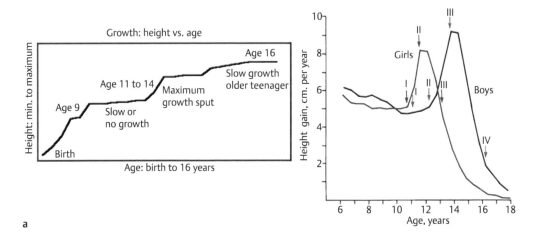

a

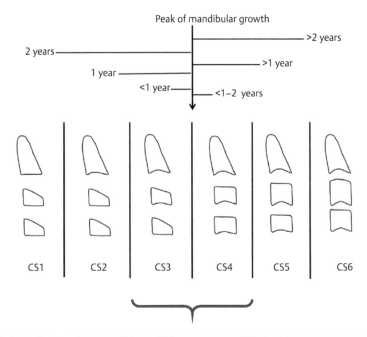

b

Fig. 3.4 **(a)** Physical growth evaluation with leading questions supporting known growth parameters. How rapidly the child has grown recently? Have clothes and shoe sizes changed? At what age did sexual maturation occur in older siblings? What is the child's height–weight when compared with parents/older siblings? **(b)** Timing for orthopedic treatment planned around peak mandibular growth looking at cervical vertebrae.

the success of the orthodontic treatment. Younger patients may not be as responsible or compliant; hence, most parents and clinicians have not considered aligner therapy as their appliance of choice for them.

The recent introduction of new features in aligner therapy has tried to negate such problems. The placement of compliance indicators (▶ Fig. 3.7) on the aligners has given the parent and/or clinician a chance to ensure aligners are

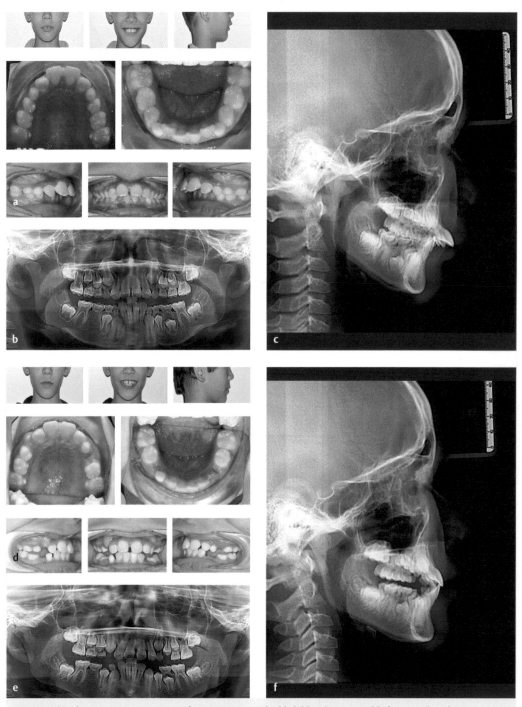

Fig. 3.5 (a) Early interceptive treatment of a 10-year 1-month old child with a removable functional appliance.
(b) Pretreatment panoramic radiograph. (c) Pretreatment lateral cephalometric radiograph. (d) Interceptive
treatment completed in 10 months. (e) Post stage I treatment panoramic radiograph. (f) Post stage I treatment lateral
cephalometric radiograph.

(Continued)

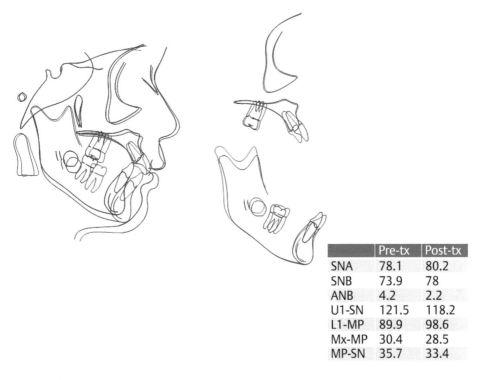

	Pre-tx	Post-tx
SNA	78.1	80.2
SNB	73.9	78
ANB	4.2	2.2
U1-SN	121.5	118.2
L1-MP	89.9	98.6
Mx-MP	30.4	28.5
MP-SN	35.7	33.4

g

Fig. 3.5 (*Continued*) **(g)** Overall and regional superimpositions.

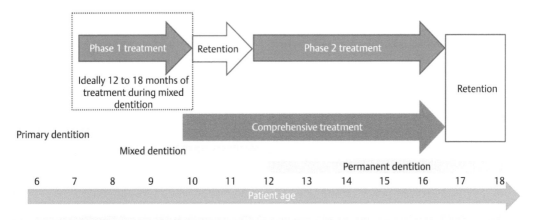

Fig. 3.6 Suggested two-phase treatment protocol with clear aligner therapy.

worn sufficient hours. Optimized attachments designed for deciduous teeth and specifically designed staging protocols for mixed dentition have allowed vertical and transverse dentoalveolar problems to be addressed with aligner treatment, and also precise individual dental movements may be planned. With close monitoring and good patient encouragement, these new features may outweigh the risks of noncompliance and have given the clinician another reason to

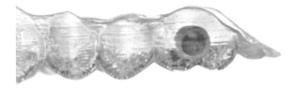

 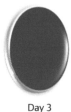 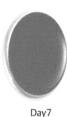

Fig. 3.7 Color changes in the aligner compliance indicator over time.

| Day 1 | Day 3 | Day7 |

consider using aligner therapy for the child with mixed dentition.

Unlimited number of aligners may be ordered over an 18-month period; therefore, quite a variety of cases can be treated using the Invisalign First appliance. The ability to incorporate and maximize these features, such as precision bite ramps, posterior occlusal coverage, individual optimized tooth movements, dental arch expansion, eruption compensators, and anteroposterior correction with elastics, has broadened the treatment aspects of phase I therapy beyond just addressing one or two problems.

Younger patients may not cope well with the procedure of obtaining alginate dental impressions. Overly sensitive gag reflexes have deterred many early orthodontic interventions. With digital intraoral scanner (such as iTero element scanner) getting more popular, the ease of obtaining a digital "impression" of the intraoral hard and soft tissues has made this step a lot more pleasant to both the patient and the clinician. This has enabled the prescription of early treatment more feasible.

The Invisalign First appliance is typically indicated for the early mixed dentition ranging from the age of approximately 6 to 10 years old. However, it is reserved for cases where the permanent first molars have sufficiently erupted, and with at least two incisors that are at least two-thirds erupted (per arch). The case should also have at least two nonmobile primary teeth (C, D, or E),

plus a partially erupted permanent tooth (3, 4, or 5) per quadrant in at least three quadrants.

The default velocity of dental movement within the Invisalign First treatment setup is not differentiated between primary and permanent dentition. However, it is essential for the clinician to understand the biology of tooth movement well. Clinicians should study the current orthopantomogram (OPG) radiographs to identify and recognize the state of resorption of the dental roots of the primary dentition and the anatomy of the roots of the permanent dentition as well as to look at the clinical crown heights and thickness of the dentoalveolus to adjust the velocity of dental movement accordingly.

This treatment modality is applicable for developing the arch form and creating space for erupting dentition. Generically, it can be used to address conditions such as dental arch development, dental expansion, spacing/crowding issues, anteroposterior correction, esthetic alignment, dental protrusions, and/or interferences (including elimination of functional shifts).

The appliance utilizes a default staging pattern for dental arch expansion and movements. The permanent first molars are usually expanded and moved first, followed by the incisors before the deciduous teeth (▶Fig. 3.8). This sequential staging pattern allows the permanent teeth to be well established in the arch before the deciduous teeth are moved. It is logical that with the permanent incisors and molar roots being both wider in

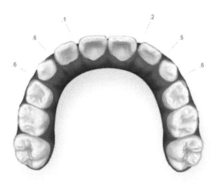

Fig. 3.8 ClinCheck plans showing staging pattern for a typical Invisalign First case.

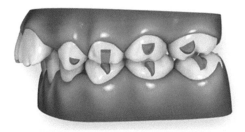

Fig. 3.9 Various types of attachment design on the deciduous and permanent dentition.

girth and longer in length, the resistance to dental movement will be greater. Allowing more aligners and greater pressure expressed on these teeth is necessary to achieve the desired movements. Deciduous teeth have generally shorter clinical crown heights. The propriety software is able to analyze the dental structure, measure the buccal contours and mesiodistal width, understand the direction and type of dental movement required, and design optimized attachments for these primary dentition (▶ Fig. 3.9).

Here are some of the recommended setup preferences:

- Interproximal reduction (IPR) is not recommended for the primary dentition. In general, primary teeth are good space maintainers and therefore IPR in primary teeth is rarely required. During dental arch expansion, both permanent and primary teeth will be buccally expanded. This reflects the phase I treatment goals to develop the arch form and also to maintain or increase space for erupting permanent dentition. Predictable dental arch expansion ranges between 4 and 6 mm per arch.
- The sequential staging pattern allows the movement of the permanent molars before the other teeth; thereafter, simultaneous staging of the other teeth follows. This allows differential anchorage from the other dentition to predictably move the permanent molars.
- If there were any Bolton tooth size discrepancies, the extra spacing will be left mesial and distal to the deciduous canines. This allows sufficient space for the larger permanent canines to erupt uneventfully.

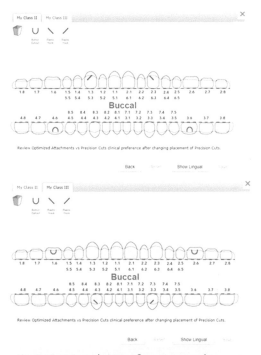

Fig. 3.10 Various elastic configurations may be planned with the Invisalign First treatment plan.

Effective anteroposterior correction can also be incorporated within the Invisalign First appliance. Class II or Class III elastics can be prescribed and designed using a mixed dentition grid during the ClinCheck treatment planning process (▶ Fig. 3.10). Buttons and elastics are readily applied clinically where indicated as well (▶ Fig. 3.11). Attachment design is important using the Invisalign appliance in the mixed dentition. Primary teeth have short clinical crown heights and require attachments to increase the retention of the appliance. In

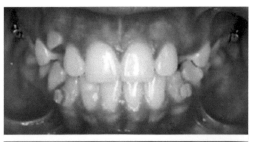

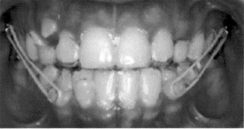

Fig. 3.11 Clinical application of button and elastics.

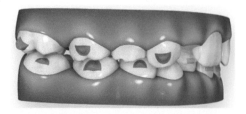

Fig. 3.12 Various types of optimized attachments designed by the software.

the mixed dentition phase, as the child transits into the permanent dentition, there will be a stage where the deciduous teeth have exfoliated, while the permanent teeth are yet to fully erupt. The retention of the appliance on the patient's dentition can be rather challenging during this time. To improve retention on short clinical crowns, optimized retention attachments are automatically placed by the ClinCheck software (▶Fig. 3.12). Hence, primarily, the attachments used in the Invisalign First appliance are for (1) rotation, (2) extrusion, and (3) retention purposes. These attachments can be visualized on the ClinCheck treatment plan and may be modified by the clinician as required. Extrusion and rotation attachments are placed on the permanent teeth by default, whereas the retention attachments are placed on the primary teeth (▶Fig. 3.13).

If the case commences after the exfoliation of the deciduous tooth but before the full eruption of the succedaneous permanent tooth, eruption compensation tabs will be placed. These are visualized as "ghost teeth" on the ClinCheck plans or as a "pontic" clinically (▶Fig. 3.14). The retention of the appliance during this phase is usually compromised—hence, the necessity to time the active treatment well or have a good retention attachment design. As treatment progresses, the permanent tooth/teeth

will erupt into the pontic space. Further in-out and/or rotational corrections will be addressed when new scans or impressions are taken when additional aligners are ordered after the first lot of aligner are exhausted.

Successful phase I treatment usually takes between 12 and 18 months.[4] When conventional removable expansion appliances such as a Hawley expander is prescribed, after the active treatment is completed, the same removable active appliance is usually worn by the patient at night to maintain the correction. The patient is then reviewed 3- to 6-monthly with the periodic trimming of the acrylic of the appliance to accommodate and facilitate the eruption of the permanent dentition. Labial bows and any Adams clasps may also be adjusted accordingly. Periodic panographic radiographs (OPG) may also be taken to assess the need for any other intervention, such as extractions of the deciduous teeth to facilitate the uneventful eruption of the succedaneous permanent teeth. The patient is usually monitored till they are in their permanent dentition, and further phase II treatment will be planned, if indicated.

With the Invisalign First appliance, the aligners cover the occlusal surfaces of the dentition and, therefore, will not serve well as a retention appliance after the active treatment is completed. This is especially so if the phase I treatment has completed early and the permanent teeth do not fully erupt till a few years later. This extended retention period needs to be planned carefully. Exfoliating teeth and their succedaneous dentition are not of the same anatomical shape and size. The eruption of the permanent dentition will be somewhat hindered by the aligners or any vacuum-formed retainers.

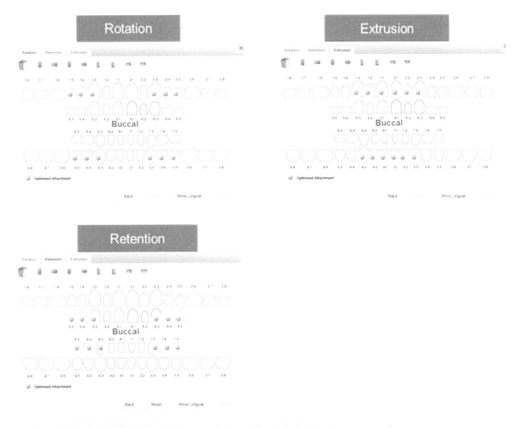

Fig. 3.13 Attachment options for rotation, extrusion, and retention purposes.

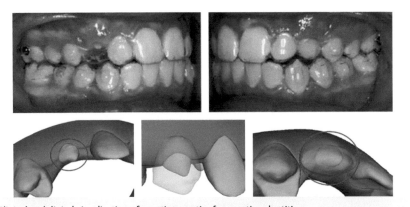

Fig. 3.14 Clinical and digital visualization of eruption pontics for erupting dentition.

Hence, it is advisable to have a fixed retainer placed anteriorly (either upper or lower where applicable; ▶Fig. 3.15a), and a Hawley type retainer designed over it to be worn nightly (▶Fig. 3.15b). Anterior or posterior bite planes can also be added to this retainer to maintain any vertical corrections,

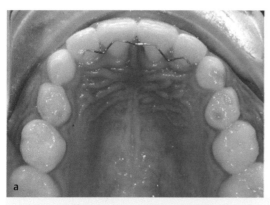 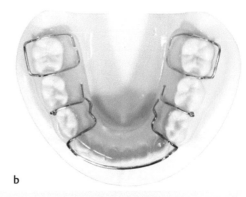

Fig. 3.15 **(a)** A fixed lingual retainer in a completed stage I mixed dentition case. **(b)** A typical Hawley-type removable retainer worn in the mixed dentition.

if necessary. This Hawley retainer can then be trimmed and adjusted accordingly as the patient transits into their permanent dentition.

A summary of the workflow using the Invisalign First appliance is shown (▶ Fig. 3.16).

3.7 Invisalign Treatment with Mandibular Advancement

Early Class II malocclusion treatment has been considered effective in reducing the difficulty of and priority for phase II treatment.[5] The first phase begins in the early mixed dentition between the age of 6 and 10 years old, and the second phase starts in the late mixed or early permanent dentition at approximately age 10 to 12 years old. Some orthodontists maintain that early mixed dentition treatment with phase I orthodontic care can reduce or eliminate the need for full-banded phase II orthodontic treatment at a later age[6] (▶ Fig. 3.17a–d).

Functional appliance therapy with monobloc activators, twin blocks, Frankel, or Herbst appliances has been the most common treatment of choice used to correct skeletal and dental Class II malocclusions. They utilize either varying types of inclined planes or projection rods to posture the lower jaw into a more forward position. With good growth potential, favorable growth patterns, and good patient compliance, good treatment outcomes can be readily achieved. However, fabrication of the appliance may be inconsistent and laboratory dependent.

The discomfort caused by the appliance during active treatment may also put off some patients.

Clear aligners have been renowned to be more esthetic and comfortable than most traditional functional appliances. Recent advancement in research and design has allowed dental movements in deciduous teeth in mixed dentition. The incorporation of attractive magnets in aligners (▶ Fig. 3.18a) worn on the opposing arches and "precision wings" (▶ Fig. 3.18b) incorporated into these clear aligners have attempted to mimic the inclined planes in twin blocks, allowing the forward posturing of the mandible, when activated.

3.7.1 Mandibular Advancement with Precision Wings and Aligners

Conventional twin blocks are effective in correcting the anteroposterior dental relationship, improving patients' skeletal Class II dental profile in young patients displaying favorable growth. Although it is possible to achieve transverse, anteroposterior, and vertical correction with this appliance, individual dental movement including third-order movements cannot be achieved. The bulkiness of the appliance has also somewhat discouraged its widespread use and has reduced wear compliance.

The Invisalign appliance with the mandibular advancement feature (MAF) was developed to overcome some of the problems these traditional twin blocks faced. The precision wings are placed on the buccal aspects of the upper and lower aligners (▶ Fig. 3.19) and mimic the inclined

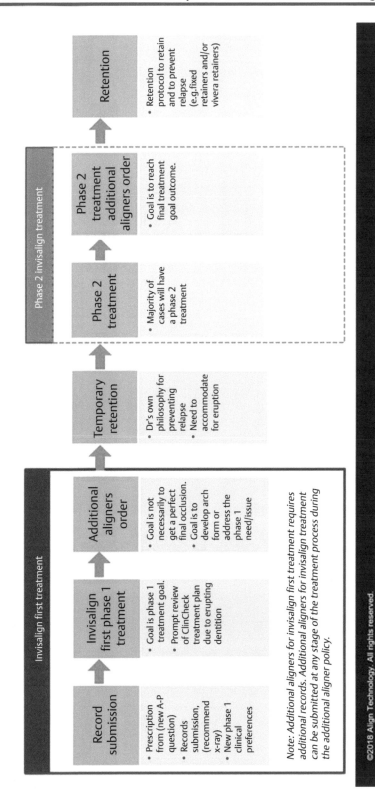

Invisalign first treatment

Record submission
- Prescription from (new A-P question)
- Records submission, (recommend x-ray)
- New phase 1 clinical preferences

Invisalign first phase 1 treatment
- Goal is phase 1 treatment goal.
- Prompt review of ClinCheck treatment plan due to erupting dentition

Additional aligners order
- Goal is not necessarily to get a perfect final occlusion.
- Goal is to develop arch form or address the phase 1 need/issue

Temporary retention
- Dr's own philosophy for preventing relapse
- Need to accommodate for eruption

Phase 2 invisalign treatment

Phase 2 treatment
- Majority of cases will have a phase 2 treatment

Phase 2 treatment additional aligners order
- Goal is to reach final treatment goal outcome.

Retention
- Retention protocol to retain and to prevent relapse (e.g.fixed retainers and/or vivera retainers)

Note: Additional aligners for invisalign first treatment requires additional records. Additional aligners for invisalign treatment can be submitted at any stage of the treatment process during the additional aligner policy.

Fig. 3.16 Overview of workflow using the Invisalign First appliance.

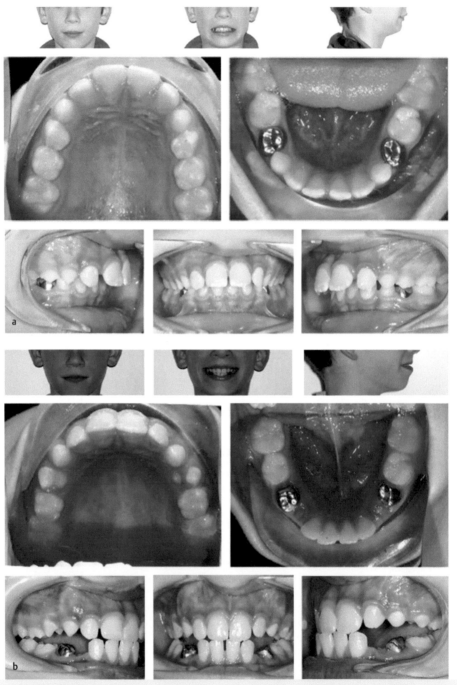

Fig. 3.17 (a) Pretreatment images of a mixed dentition case. (b) After 10 months of functional appliance therapy with twin blocks.

(Continued)

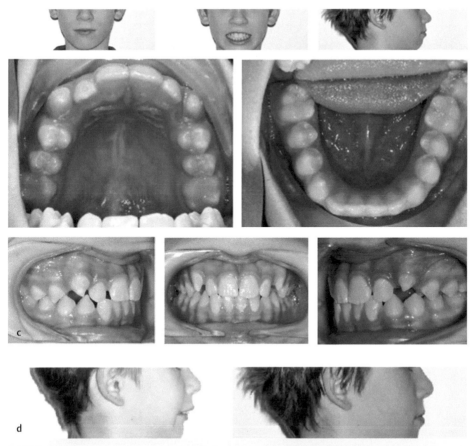

Fig. 3.17 (*Continued*) (**c**) Review images 2 years after functional appliance therapy. Occlusion without further interceptive treatment. (**d**) Comparing before and after images showing profile changes.

planes of the twin block appliance. However, the buccally placed wings (instead of occlusally placed ones in traditional twin blocks) allow for a reduction in the vertical stretching and opening of mouth when the appliance is in place. This improves patient comfort. In activation, the mandible is perpetually postured in a forward position. While the patient changes their aligners weekly, individual dental movements programmed when designing the ClinCheck plans will be expressed simultaneously.

The Invisalign therapy with MAF is indicated for late mixed to early permanent dentition. When indicated for the mixed dentition, the first permanent molars need to be fully erupted. The deciduous molars (Ds and Es)

present need to be firm with approximately at least 1 year from their exfoliation. The permanent canines and molars do not need to be present. It can also be indicated in cases with congenitally missing premolars.

The recommended digital workflow and treatment protocol is shown in ▶Fig. 3.20. It is recommended for the aligners to be worn full time at 20 to 22 hours per day with a weekly change regime. At the commencement of treatment, a compulsory stage of pre-MA (mandibular advancement) is designed. There is a minimal order of at least four active aligners, with no maximum limit of aligners. This stage of treatment is primarily used to level any lower curve of Spee, procline upper incisors in a Class II, division

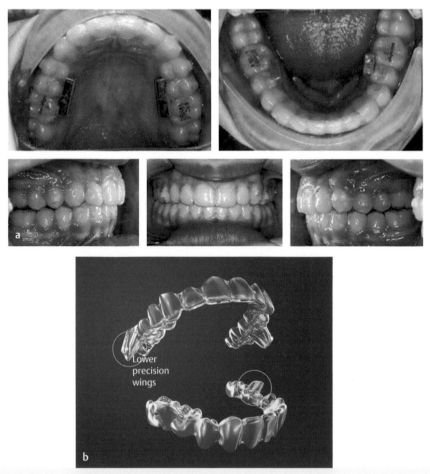

Fig. 3.18 **(a)** Magnets incorporated into clear aligner therapy allowing functional correction. **(b)** "Precision" wings on aligners mimicking the inclined planes in twin blocks.

2 type malocclusion, or any other pre-MA correction that is required. The initiation of the MA is important. The closer the advancement occurs as the patient approaches their growth spurt, the better the treatment outcome. If it is suspected that the patient is about to hit their growth spurt soon, designing a shorter pre-MA stage and commencing MA as soon as possible is recommended. On the other hand, if the peak growth spurt is still a while away, more pre-MA alignment and levelling can be achieved and should be planned.

Mandibular advancement occurs with the progressive activation of the precision wings. This

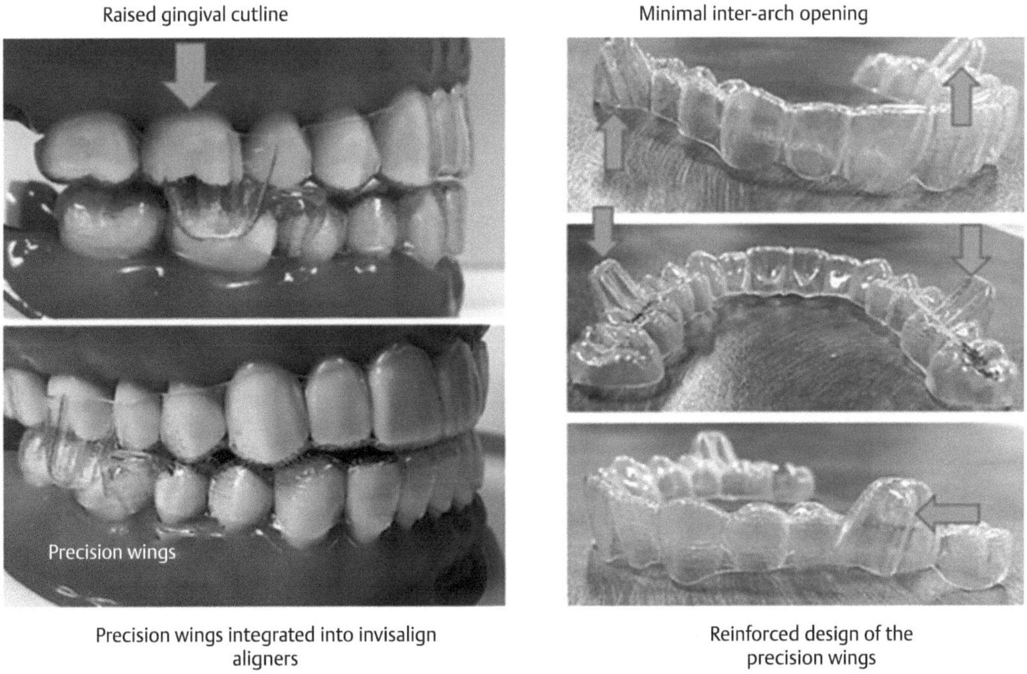

Raised gingival cutline

Minimal inter-arch opening

Precision wings

Precision wings integrated into invisalign aligners

Reinforced design of the precision wings

Fig. 3.19 "Precision" wings integrated into Invisalign aligners. Features include raised gingival cutline, minimal interarch opening, and reinforced precision wings.

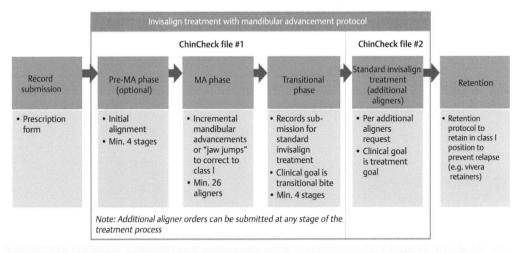

Invisalign treatment with mandibular advancement protocol					
		ChinCheck file #1		ChinCheck file #2	
Record submission	Pre-MA phase (optional)	MA phase	Transitional phase	Standard invisalign treatment (additional aligners)	Retention
• Prescription form	• Initial alignment • Min. 4 stages	• Incremental mandibular advancements or "jaw jumps" to correct to class I • Min. 26 aligners	• Records submission for standard invisalign treatment • Clinical goal is transitional bite • Min. 4 stages	• Per additional aligners request • Clinical goal is treatment goal	• Retention protocol to retain in class I position to prevent relapse (e.g. vivera retainers)

Note: Additional aligner orders can be submitted at any stage of the treatment process

Fig. 3.20 Recommended digital workflow and treatment protocol using Invisalign with mandibular advancement feature.

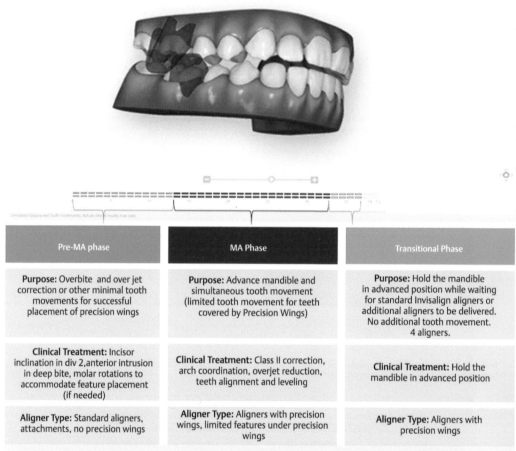

Pre-MA phase	MA Phase	Transitional Phase
Purpose: Overbite and over jet correction or other minimal tooth movements for successful placement of precision wings	**Purpose:** Advance mandible and simultaneous tooth movement (limited tooth movement for teeth covered by Precision Wings)	**Purpose:** Hold the mandible in advanced position while waiting for standard Invisalign aligners or additional aligners to be delivered. No additional tooth movement. 4 aligners.
Clinical Treatment: Incisor inclination in div 2,anterior intrusion in deep bite, molar rotations to accommodate feature placement (if needed)	**Clinical Treatment:** Class II correction, arch coordination, overjet reduction, teeth alignment and leveling	**Clinical Treatment:** Hold the mandible in advanced position
Aligner Type: Standard aligners, attachments, no precision wings	**Aligner Type:** Aligners with precision wings, limited features under precision wings	**Aligner Type:** Aligners with precision wings

Fig. 3.21 A summary of various stages of treatment using Invisalign with mandibular advancement feature.

stepwise advancement occurs at an increment of 2 mm at every eighth aligner unless otherwise requested. There is a minimum of 26 active aligners with no limit to how many active MA aligners that may be requested. However, attachments will not be allowed on any teeth that have precision wings on. Predominantly, these are the upper and lower second premolars, second deciduous molars, and first molars. A summary of the stages in MA treatment is shown in ▶ Fig. 3.21.

There are two subsequent stages after the MA activation stages: (1) transitional bite: no aligners are fabricated; it is to visualize bite in the advanced position (after MA phase); (2) treatment goal: no aligners are fabricated; additional treatment should be requested.

Case Discussion

The patient's age was 12 years 6 months when he commenced orthodontic treatment (▶ Fig. 3.22a–c). He presents a Class II, division 1 malocclusion on a skeletal II base with a permanent dentition and CVS 3. There is an increased overjet, mild degrees of lower dental crowding, and upper dental spacing with proclined upper and lower incisors. There were four pre-MA stages, allowing initial dental retraction and intrusion of the lower incisors. This was followed immediately by 27 active stages of MA with individualized dental movements for further dental retraction, levelling of the lower curve of Spee, and dental arch coordination (▶ Fig. 3.22d).

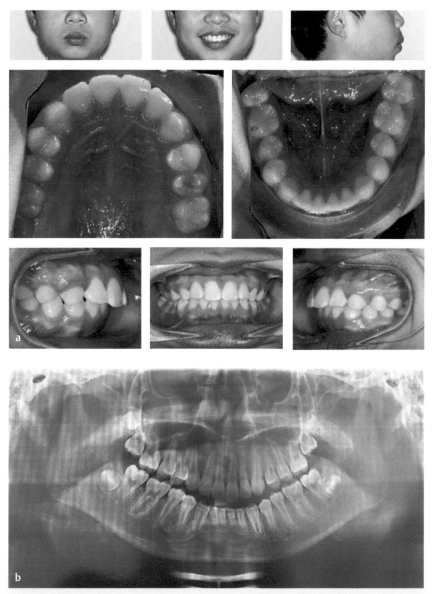

Fig. 3.22 **(a)** Pretreatment images of a young patient at 12 years 6 months, treated using the Invisalign appliance with mandibular advancement feature. **(b)** Pretreatment panoramic radiograph.

(Continued)

Approximately 7 months of active treatment has allowed the overjet and overbite to be normalized as well as improvement of the soft-tissue profile (▶Fig. 3.22e, f). During the additional aligner phase, posterior as well as Class II elastics were utilized to complete the levelling of the curve of Spee, closure of the posterior open bite, and midline correction (▶Fig. 3.22g). The total treatment time was 14 months (▶Fig. 3.22h, i). Fixed upper and lower retainers as well as

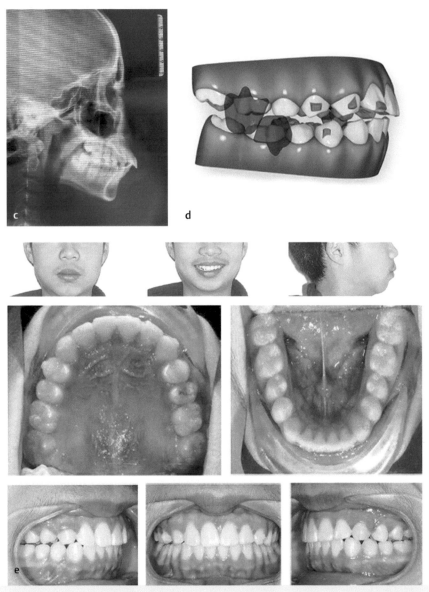

Fig. 3.22 (*Continued*) (**c**) Pretreatment lateral cephalographic radiograph. (**d**) ClinCheck plans with mandibular advancement feature. (**e**) Postmandibular advancement photos.

(*Continued*)

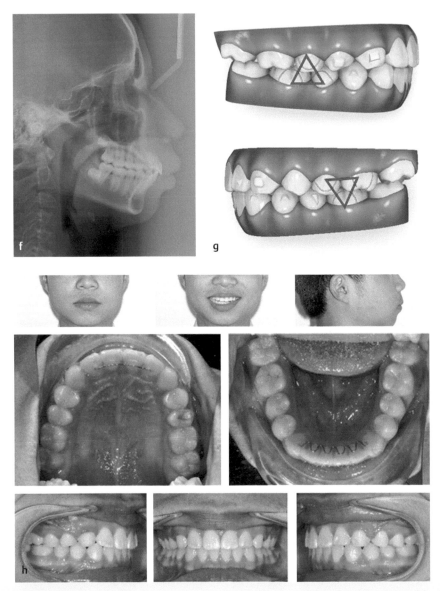

Fig. 3.22 (*Continued*) (**f**) Postmandibular advancement lateral cephalometric radiograph. (**g**) Detailing and finishing mechanics. (**h**) Completion images.

(*Continued*)

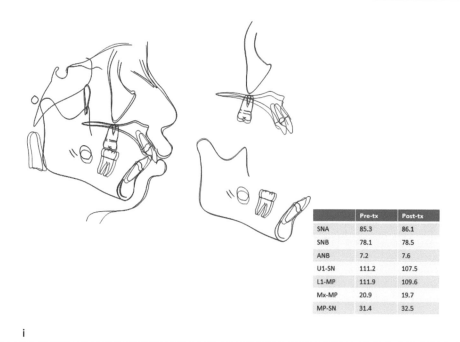

	Pre-tx	Post-tx
SNA	85.3	86.1
SNB	78.1	78.5
ANB	7.2	7.6
U1-SN	111.2	107.5
L1-MP	111.9	109.6
Mx-MP	20.9	19.7
MP-SN	31.4	32.5

i

Fig. 3.22 (*Continued*) **(i)** Overall and regional superimpositions.

Vivera retainers (Align manufactured clear, vacuum-formed retainers) were prescribed thereafter to maintain the orthodontic correction.

This case report demonstrates that mandibular advancement with the Invisalign appliance and their MA features incorporated is successful in achieving a good occlusion, excellent dental interdigitation, and marked facial profile improvements. Traditional twin blocks allow judicious trimming of the bite blocks to encourage vertical dentoalveolar growth/eruption of the lower molars (upward and forward) to allow anteroposterior as well as vertical changes. However, with the Invisalign appliance, the occlusal surfaces of the dentition are covered by the aligners, and this vertical aspect of functional correction cannot be readily achieved. It is thus advisable to level the lower curve of Spee as much as possible during the pre-MA phase, and run posterior elastics to complete this levelling during the post-MA refinement/additional aligner phase. However, if the child is about to hit the peak growth spurt shortly, we may commence the MA phase as soon as possible.

Levelling of the lower curve of Spee will therefore have to be done with posterior elastics during the later, additional aligner phase.

3.7.2 Mandibular Advancement with Magnet-Activated Aligners

The use of magnets in correcting Class II mandibular deficiency problems in growing patients is a known approach and evidence is available in the literature.[7] However, incorporating magnets into sequential aligners for mandibular advancement is novel and yet to be fully tested.

The magnets are designed to be inserted on the palatal/lingual sides of the aligners. Two magnets are placed on the upper aligner, while one is placed on the lower aligner, on either side. A total number of six magnets are incorporated in each set of aligners. The dimensions of the magnets are 7 × 3 × 2 mm with 2 mm of activation (▶ Fig. 3.23).

The advantage of magnetic activation is that when in position, the patient does not need to proactively posture the mandible forward. The attractive forces from the magnets do the job for

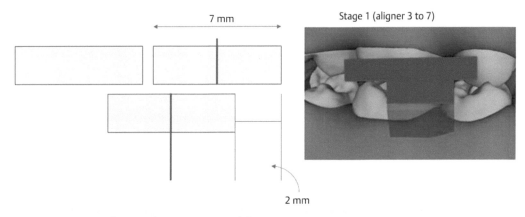

7 mm

Stage 1 (aligner 3 to 7)

2 mm

Fig. 3.23 Magnet configuration for magnet activated aligners.

them. This allows a perpetual and constant forward positioning of the patients' mandible, maximizing the effects of the functional appliance.[8] The aligners are programmed to have the individual dental movements, allowing alignment, levelling, and good interdigitation concurrently.

The magnetic attractive forces also tend to dislodge the appliance from the patient's dentition. This happens especially in younger patients where the clinical crown heights are relatively shorter. Hence, the placement of retention attachments is essential to enforce this anchorage.

Case Discussion

The patient was 12 years and 8 months old when she commenced orthodontic treatment (▶ Fig. 3.24a). She presented a Class II, division 2 malocclusion with a skeletal II growth pattern and normal direction of growth. There is an increased overjet, deep overbite, and mild degrees of upper and lower dental crowding. There are also mild degrees of dental arch constriction, but no posterior crossbites are evident. The ClinCheck plans had the dental arch forms coordinated, overjet and overbite corrected, and teeth aligned. The anteroposterior correction was corrected by the attractive forces of the magnets as described above (▶ Fig. 3.24b, c). The treatment was completed under 24 months. A Class I occlusion with an ideal overjet, overbite with good interdigitation, and arch symmetry was achieved (▶ Fig. 3.24d). The retrusive mandible was normalized. A lower fixed retainer was placed on

the lower canine to canines, with upper and lower nighttime vacuum-formed retainers prescribed as well.

This case report demonstrates that mandibular advancement with magnetic attraction forces is plausible and good dental as well as skeletal and soft-tissue changes can be obtained (▶ Fig. 3.24e, f). Magnets placed on the palatal and lingual surfaces also produces a more "invisible" appliance without any extensions on the buccal surfaces. However, this mode of orthodontic treatment is still in "beta testing mode" and is not available commercially.

3.8 Treatment in Early Mixed Dentition

Early phase I orthodontic treatment occurs when the patient is between 6 and 10 years old, usually right after the upper laterals have fully erupted. Most common phase I corrections include (1) dental arch development, space/crowding (anterior alignment), (2) skeletal—Class II (mandibular advancement), Class III (including functional shift correction), palatal expansion, (3) habit correction (thumb sucking, tongue thrusting), and (4) any other alignment and/or corrections to improve the efficiency of second phase of treatments.

Goals of early treatment can be in the patients' best interests if their problem is one that could become more serious over time, if left untreated—for instance, deep dental overbites contributing

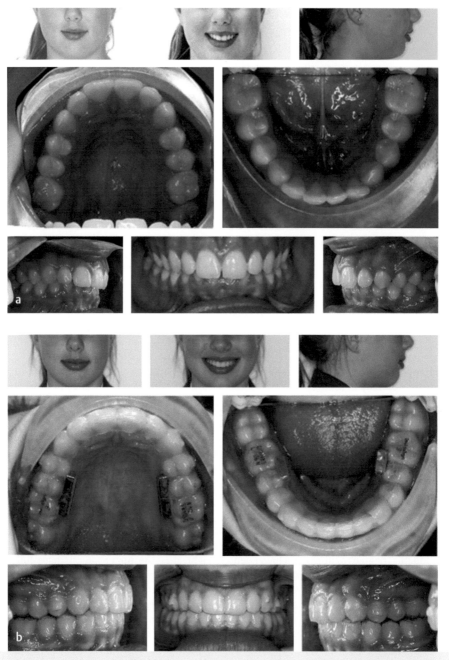

Fig. 3.24 (a) A young, 12-year 8-month-old patient undergoing aligner therapy with magnetic advancement feature. (b) Patient with activated appliance in place.

(Continued)

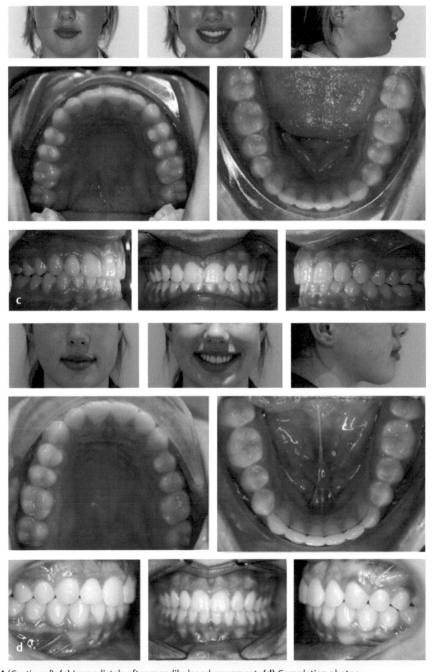

Fig. 3.24 (*Continued*) (c) Immediately after mandibular advancement. (d) Completion photos.

(*Continued*)

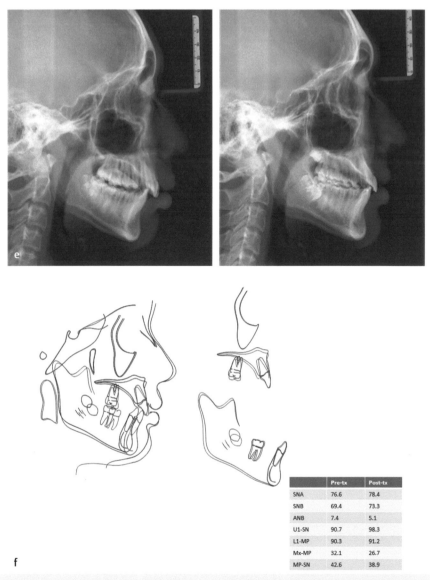

	Pre-tx	Post-tx
SNA	76.6	78.4
SNB	69.4	73.3
ANB	7.4	5.1
U1-SN	90.7	98.3
L1-MP	90.3	91.2
Mx-MP	32.1	26.7
MP-SN	42.6	38.9

Fig. 3.24 (*Continued*) (**e**) A typical pre- and posttreatment cephalometric comparison of a case treated using the Invisalign appliance with magnetic advancement. (**f**) Overall and regional superimpositions.

over a period of 5 years. This allows us to jump in early during the late mixed dentition, commencing orthodontic treatment to first allow for space regaining, arch form development, any early correction of anteroposterior, and transverse, crossbite, and functional shifts.

to increased attrition and wear, or large dental overjets contributing to increased risks of dental trauma. Phase I treatment aims to intercept a developing problem. The diagnosis of the issue(s) and elimination of the cause(s) is paramount. We aim to guide the growth and development of the facial and jaw bones, and also to provide adequate space for erupting permanent teeth. Most patients require a second course of treatment when their permanent teeth have fully erupted.

Case Discussion

This young female patient, age 8 years and 10 months, presented as a Class II, division 1 mal-occlusion with a mild skeletal II base. There is an increased dental overjet, a median diastema, and a constricted upper dental arch with noncoincident dental midlines (▶Fig. 3.25a, b). The deciduous teeth remaining (CEs) are firm and the radiograph shows good root length remaining. The panoramic radiograph also shows that all the permanent teeth are present and appear to be in rather good erupting positions.

Our treatment plans and objectives are to align her dentition, close the median diastema, decrease the overjet, correct the Class II dental relationship, and widen the dental arch forms to allow room for the permanent teeth to erupt uneventfully using the Invisalign First appliance.

The active treatment is estimated to be approximately 12 to 18 months. The ClinCheck plans are shown (▶Fig. 3.25c). There are 21 active aligners planned in this initial stage of treatment. Light Class II elastics were also prescribed. These aligners need to be worn full time (at least 22–20 hours per day) and aligners to be changed weekly. Within this 18-month period, unlimited number of aligners can be ordered with new scans to accommodate for any lack of compliance and/or dental eruption changes. The software default moves the permanent teeth first, followed by the primary dentition to maximize the anchorage requirements. Attachments need to be placed to increase the retention

of the appliance due to the short clinical crown heights. Therefore, the deciduous teeth cannot be mobile or exfoliating during this period of treatment for it to be effective. If they are expected to be exfoliating during this period of treatment, an eruption pontic may be designed to accommodate their dental eruption instead. Once the teeth have erupted through, they may be scanned, captured, and aligned in the next series of aligners during the next additional aligner order stage.

The patient responded very well to treatment, and within approximately 6 months of active treatment, her increased dental overjet has normalized, median diastema closed, and dental arch forms coordinated (▶Fig. 3.25d). The patient can now be placed on temporary retainers as we continue to monitor the growth and eruption of her dentition until she is in permanent dentition. Any further treatment, if necessary, will then be advised and prescribed accordingly.

3.9 Treatment in Late Mixed Dentition

The late mixed dentition is the period of dental eruption where there is the loss of all or almost all deciduous teeth (usually the E's may be the only ones persisting), but the permanent dentition has yet to erupt, or erupt fully (usually the 3's and 5's). This usually occurs between the ages of 10 and 12 years old.

As the deciduous molars are both slightly larger than the succedaneous premolars, maximizing these spaces after the loss of the D's and E's to relieve crowding is useful at this stage of interceptive treatment. If these teeth were lost early and abutment teeth have drifted into the premolar spaces, it would also be essential for space regaining to allow the uneventful eruption of the permanent teeth.

The Invisalign appliance (comprehensive package) now allows for unlimited number of aligners

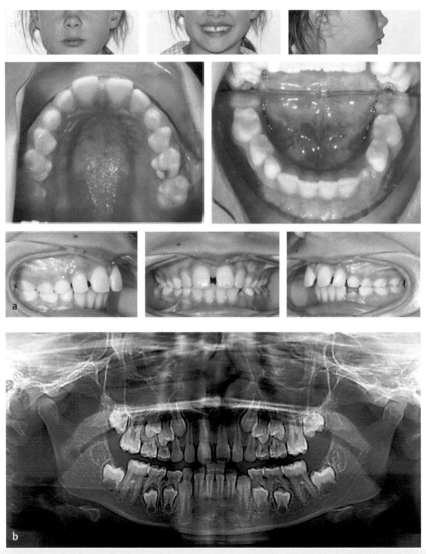

Fig. 3.25 (a) A young preadolescent 8-year 10-month-old patient treated with Invisalign First appliance. (b) Pretreatment panoramic radiograph.

(Continued)

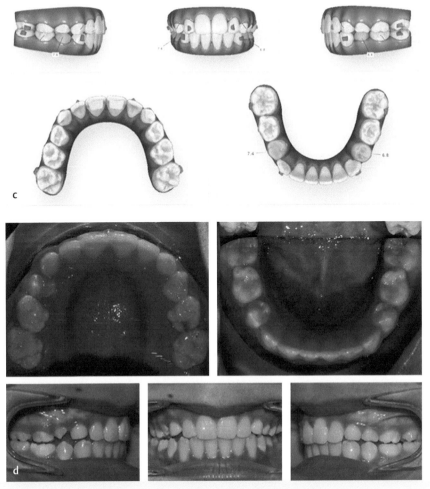

Fig. 3.25 (*Continued*) **(c)** ClinCheck treatment plans. **(d)** After 6 months of active aligner treatment.

Case Discussion

This young male patient was 10 years 1 month old at initial presentation (▶Fig. 3.26a). He presented with the severe loss of space in quadrants 1, 3, and 4. Respectively, the #13, #33, and #43 are blocked out. There is an increased dental overbite, rather constricted upper and lower dental arch forms with noncoincident dental midlines. The upper left and right deciduous second molars are just about to exfoliate.

The panoramic radiograph shows a full complement of teeth (▶Fig. 3.26b). The permanent canines that are blocked out with insufficient eruption space are placed in rather good vertical positions and will erupt through uneventfully, if given the necessary space.

Our treatment plans are to achieve dental alignment, open up the deep overbite, correct the dental midlines, and reestablish space for the eruption of the canines in all four quadrants while persevering space for the eruption of the upper left and right second premolar teeth. The appliance of choice used was the Invisalign Teen appliance. This treatment option allows unlimited number of scans and aligner orders of up to 5 years from the commencement of treatment. The convenience of such a product gives allowance for noncompliance, various changes of growth, and dental eruption, as well as "no treatment" lull periods while awaiting the full eruption of the permanent dentition once the stage I objectives are achieved.

The active treatment consisted of 19 active aligners with a weekly change regime. The ClinCheck

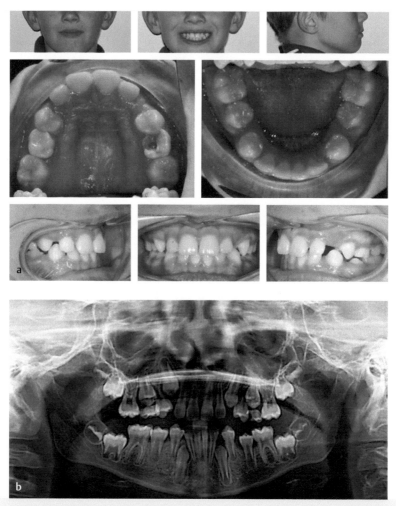

Fig. 3.26 A 10-year 1-month-old patient treatment with Invisalign as a phase I interceptive treatment. **(a)** Pretreatment images. **(b)** Pretreatment panoramic radiograph.

(Continued)

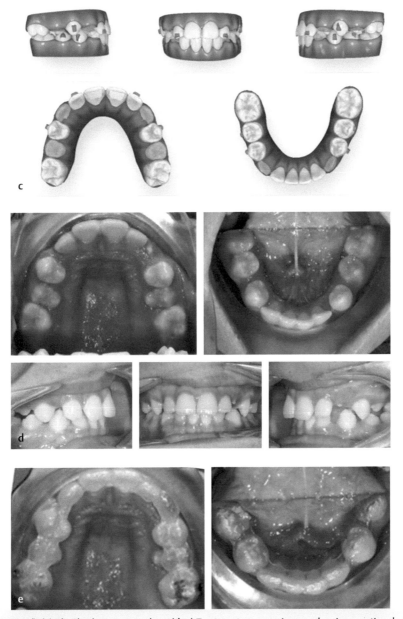

Fig. 3.26 (*Continued*) **(c)** ClinCheck treatment plans. **(d, e)** Treatment progress images showing erupting dentition and eruption compensators.

(*Continued*)

plans shown (▶Fig. 3.26c) demonstrates attachments placed on lateral incisors and premolar teeth. Eruption compensators are placed in areas where unerupted teeth are planned to erupt, namely the upper and lower canines and the upper second premolars.

As treatment progresses, the canines and premolar teeth erupt into the eruption compensators

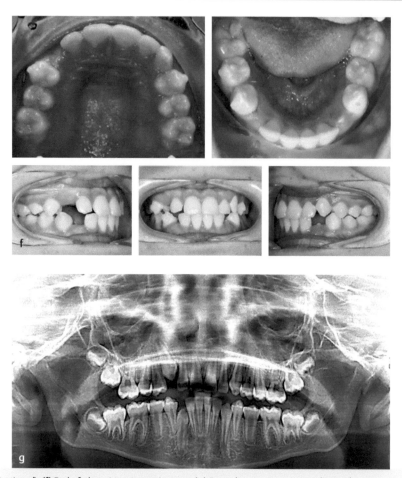

Fig. 3.26 (*Continued*) (**f**) End of phase I treatment images. (**g**) Post phase I panoramic radiograph.

(▶Fig. 3.26d, e). Additional aligners were ordered at the end of 19 weeks. Dental spaces are now created, and preliminary expansion of the arch has been achieved. The upper second premolars and the upper left canine have now erupted.

Once the dental spaces are achieved, we may now wait for the natural eruption of the remaining dentition (▶Fig. 3.26f, g). Temporary retainers will be designed, and once the patient is in his full permanent dentition, further scans and aligners will be ordered to complete the comprehensive treatment. With the dental midlines, alignment and arch forms, ideal overjet, and overbite now achieved, the second stage of active orthodontic treatment becomes much simpler, shorter, and more straightforward.

3.10 Treatment in Permanent Dentition in Young Adolescents

Conventional orthodontic treatment with full fixed appliances in adolescents has been the long stay, mainstream treatment of choice. There remain many advantages fixed appliances have over clear aligner therapy. Operators and parents are concerned that the lack of compliance of aligner wear and the insufficient three-dimensional control will not eventuate in a well-treated case with ideal treatment outcomes. Technology in clear aligner therapy, however, has advanced over the years and it is able to demonstrate outstanding treatment outcomes in full comprehensive orthodontic treatment.

Case Discussion

Case 1

This young female patient presented with two congenitally missing lower incisors. We have been observing her dental eruption since she was 7 years old (▶ Fig. 3.27a, b). The aim is to allow the lower canines to erupt as close to the distal aspects of the lower central incisors to create a better chance of dental substitution without the need for dental implants or other prosthetic replacements in the future. She has a fairly well-balanced facial appearance with a convex profile and a slightly recessive mandible and deep labial mental fold. She presented with a Class II, division 1 malocclusion with a mild skeletal II growth pattern at age 11 and is ready to commence full comprehensive treatment (▶ Fig. 3.27c). Various treatment options were presented to her parents, one of which was the extraction of two upper first premolars. The final treatment of choice was a nonextraction treatment approach, using the Invisalign Teen appliance augmented with Class II elastic traction.

At the commencement of comprehensive treatment, she presented moderate degrees of upper dental crowding, a Class I molar relationship but a full unit Class II canine relationship, with an increased overjet of 13 mm, rather constricted upper and lower dental arch forms, with noncoincidental midlines and a deep dental overbite.

The ClinCheck plans (▶ Fig. 3.27d) show treatment planning with both conventional and optimized attachment designs. Button cutouts are placed on the upper canines and the lower first molars for the prescribed Class II elastics. A sequential staging pattern with upper molar distalization was planned. However, a treatment esthetic start was also designed such that simple upper anterior alignment is also achieved right from the beginning. This allows an esthetic improvement of the patient's smile right from the beginning of treatment instead of the usual sequential staging problem of only seeing an anterior esthetic improvement during the second half of treatment. This is demonstrated by the "arrowhead" staging pattern seen in the figure. With this case, the aligners were worn full time with a 10-day aligner change regime.

At the end of the first group of aligners (47 stages), the overjet and overbite have been fully corrected. Additional aligners were ordered to further correct the dental alignment and coordinate the dental arches as well as the dental midlines (▶ Fig. 3.27e).

The total treatment duration was 24 months. At completion, the overjet and overbite were fully resolved. Dental alignment was well achieved with good arch coordination and dental interdigitation (▶ Fig. 3.27f). As it was a canine substitution case, due to Bolton discrepancy, it was not possible to obtain a fully interdigitated Class I canine relationship.

The before and after lateral cephalometric radiographs (▶ Fig. 3.27g, h) demonstrated good dentoalveolar growth and normalizing of the facial profile. The interincisal angulation and lower lip trap have been corrected. The deep labial mental fold has also been eliminated.

Case 2

Orthodontic treatment requiring extractions and utilizing clear aligner therapy remains a challenge. The lack of full three-dimensional control of dental movements has made many operators have second thoughts at offering this appliance as an alternative to fixed conventional appliances to young patients. However, with the understanding of the inadequacies of the product and slight manipulation of the dental movements during the ClinCheck planning process, good results can still be attainable.

An 11-year-old school girl presented as a Class II, division 1 malocclusion on a skeletal I growth pattern and normal direction of growth (▶ Fig. 3.28a). She has a convex, overall bimaxillary protrusive profile with an incompetent lip. Dentally, there

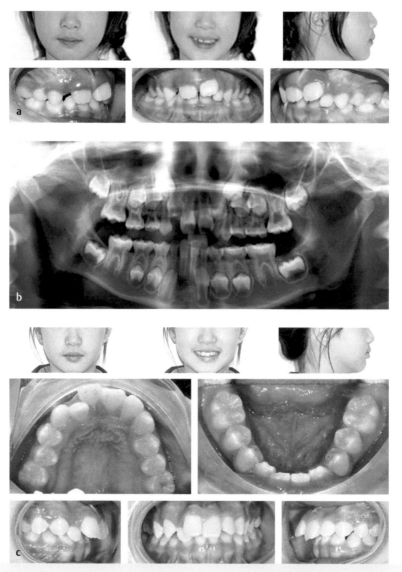

Fig. 3.27 **(a, b)** Pretreatment images and panoramic radiograph at 7 years old. **(c)** Pretreatment images at 11 years old.

(Continued)

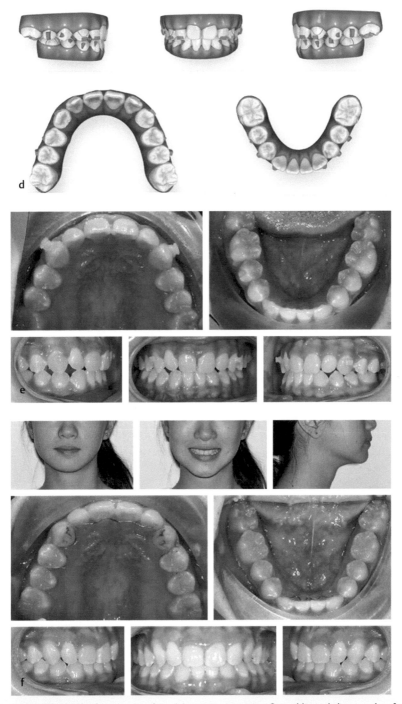

Fig. 3.27 *(Continued)* **(d)** ClinCheck treatment plans. **(e)** Progress images at first additional aligner order after 47 active aligners. **(f)** Posttreatment images.

(Continued)

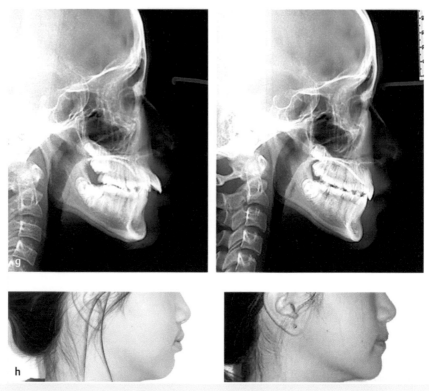

Fig. 3.27 (*Continued*) **(g)** Comparing pre- and posttreatment lateral cephalometric radiographs. **(h)** Comparing pre- and posttreatment profile changes.

was an increased overjet, a constricted upper arch form, and mild upper and lower dental crowding. The canines and molars are in a half-unit Class II relationship.

The treatment plan for this patient was to have the upper first premolars extracted and full comprehensive orthodontic treatment with the Invisalign Teen appliance was prescribed. The ClinCheck plans show the use of various optimized as well as conventional attachments. A simultaneous staging pattern was designed (▶ Fig. 3.28b). "Compensatory" dental movements were also planned to negate the side effects and also to compensate for the lack of three-dimensional control of the appliance, it being a removable one. The

"compensatory" dental movements included (1) increased upper incisor lingual root torque, (2) increased distal root tip of canines, (3) increased mesial root tip of premolar and molars, and (4) increased intrusion of the lower incisors to allow an anterior open bite (▶ Fig. 3.28c). The appliance was worn full time at a two-weekly change interval. Class II elastics was also worn to control the anchorage as treatment progressed.

The completion images show a good harmonious smile with a therapeutic Class II dental occlusion finished (▶ Fig. 3.28d). The canines are in full Class I, while the molars are in full Class II dental relationships. The lip competency has been re-established and overjet and alignment

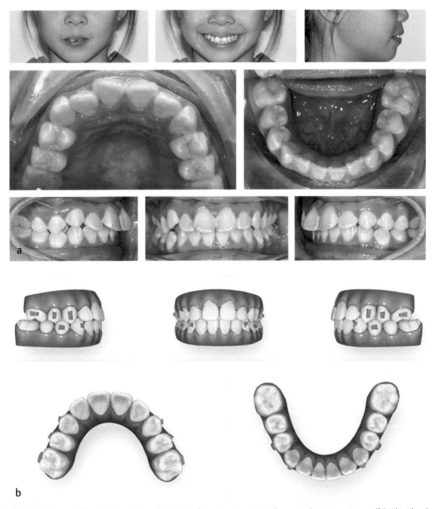

Fig. 3.28 **(a)** An 11-year-old patient undergoing Invisalign treatment with premolar extractions. **(b)** ClinCheck treatment plans.

(Continued)

have been corrected, with arch coordination well achieved. The final radiographs show good axial inclination of the dental roots of all teeth, with the interincisal angle, overjet, and overbite all showing great improvement (▶ Fig. 3.28e, f). The overall treatment duration was 20 months.

3.11 Conclusion

Treatment in younger patients using the Invisalign appliance requires extra patience. We have to first establish if the child will be cooperative with leading questions such as: "do they often lose their

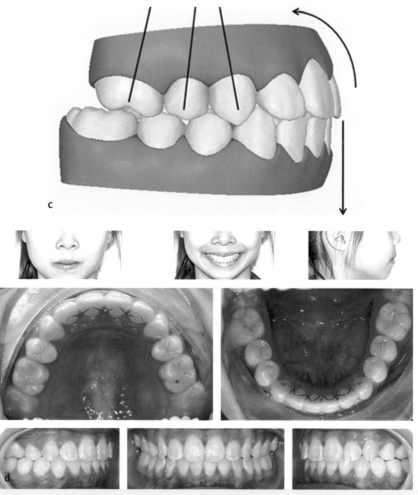

Fig. 3.28 (*Continued*) (**c**) Compensatory movements: (i) increased upper incisor lingual root torque, (ii) increased distal root tip of canines, (iii) increased mesial root tip of premolar and molars, and (iv) increased intrusion of the lower incisors to allow an anterior open bite. (**d**) Posttreatment images.

(Continued)

water bottles or pencil cases in school?" Positive answers would give us a guide as to whether they will be good candidates for Invisalign therapy. Clear and precise instructions should be given to both the child and parent to allow close monitoring of the appliance care and wear away from the dental office. Due to the fast-changing growth of the child, the clinician must be prepared to do multiple scans and reorder additional aligners if the growing/changing dentition varies outside the range of prediction by the ClinCheck plans.

Clear aligner therapy using the Invisalign appliance has seen its expanded portfolio, and has improved its product design over the years. With experience gained with increased exposure within the orthodontic fraternity, clinicians have also increased their confidence and can achieve improved treatment predictability. Orthodontic treatment in younger patients remains quite different from adults due to not only their psychological differences, but also the anatomical and physiological differences.

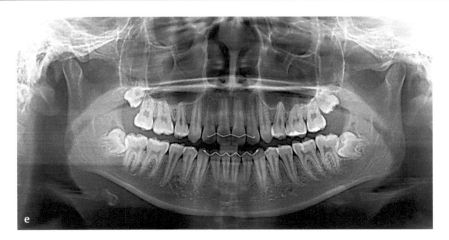

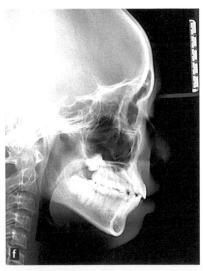

Fig. 3.28 (*Continued*) **(e)** Posttreatment panoramic radiograph. **(f)** Posttreatment lateral cephalometric radiography.

Understanding the biological variations and treating the right patient at the right age all point toward a rewarding experience for both the clinician and patient. No two patients are alike, and therefore no two treatment plans can be exactly identical. However, with close examination and good planning, we can avoid most of the pitfalls that early clear aligner therapy users faced.

References

[1] Patti A, D'Arc GP, Weiss JK. Clinical Success in Early Orthodontic Treatment. Chicago, IL: Quintessence; 2005:3–15
[2] Franchi L, Baccetti T, McNamara JA, Jr. Mandibular growth as related to cervical vertebral maturation and body height. Am J Orthod Dentofacial Orthop. 2000;118(3):335–340
[3] Baccetti T, Franchi L, McNamara JA, Jr. The Cervical Vertebral Maturation (CVM) method for the assessment of optimal treatment timing in dentofacial orthopedics. Semin Orthod. 2005;11:119–129
[4] Dugoni SA, Lee JS, Varela J, Dugoni AA. Early mixed dentition treatment: postretention evaluation of stability and relapse. Angle Orthod. 1995;65(5):311–320
[5] Dolce C, McGorray SP, Brazeau L, King GJ, Wheeler TT. Timing of Class II treatment: skeletal changes comparing 1-phase and 2-phase treatment. Am J Orthod Dentofacial Orthop. 2007;132(4):481–489
[6] Dugoni SA. Comprehensive mixed dentition treatment. Am J Orthod Dentofacial Orthop. 1998;113(1):75–84
[7] Darendeliler MA, Darendeliler A, Mandurino M. Clinical application of magnets in orthodontics and biological implications: a review. Eur J Orthod. 1997;19(4):431–442
[8] Darendeliler MA. Use of magnetic forces in growth modification. Semin Orthod. 2006;12:41–51

4 Teen Treatments with Aligners

Phil Scheurer

Summary

For orthodontic treatments of teens, the same fundamental considerations apply whether the treatment is performed with aligners or with fixed appliances. However, the planning of teen cases with aligners, the definition of treatment strategies, the anchorage situation, and both the possibilities and the restrictions for tooth movements are different between treatments with aligners and treatments with fixed appliances. Therefore, when treating teens with aligners, these different factors and considerations have to be taken into account for a successful treatment. This chapter describes fundamental issues of aligner orthodontics and points out particularities of teen treatments compared to treatments of adults and treatments with fixed appliances.

Keywords: teen treatment, aligner orthodontics, space management, treatment strategies, auxiliaries

4.1 System Check

Aligners can be as effective as brackets and wires for treating patients, both teens and adults, with various kinds of malocclusions. Not all aligner systems on the market show the same range of performance. The following checklist can be a helpful means in determining which aligner system is most appropriate and allows to compare them according to different parameters:

- Material: for comparisons of physical properties, see relevant chapter of this book.
- Tooth movements should be force driven, not shape driven, to be able to treat more complex cases. Specific attachments are required.
- Every aligner should fit the same way. Therefore, a separate model should be produced for each aligner.
- Bodily movements, torque, and sweep (anti-bowing) must be possible to perform by built-in features and altered aligner geometries, which is mandatory for extraction cases and space management.
- Strategies and features for sagittal corrections and vertical corrections must be available.

- The system must be open for auxiliaries such as buttons, hooks, power arms, and elastics. Otherwise, no complex cases can be treated.
- The efficiency of the system must be proven by studies and case galleries.
- No extra fee should be required for midcourse correction (MCC), which is important for teen cases.

What is challenging when treating teens with aligners?
- Growth: we need features and strategies to modify and/or compensate growth.
- Mixed dentition: we might start with deciduous teeth in situ and will have to deal with erupting permanent teeth during the treatment. In almost all cases with erupting teeth, an MCC will be necessary during treatment (▶ Fig. 4.1).
- Compliance: motivation could be less than in adults. Compliance indicators and a progress controlling device are useful.

Why is it favorable to treat teens with aligners?
- Hygiene: with fixed appliances, it is difficult to maintain a high level of oral hygiene. With aligners—even with attachments on the teeth—oral hygiene is as easy to maintain as without appliance.

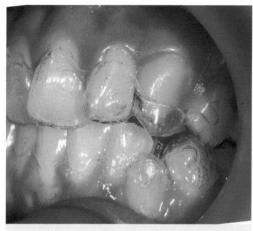

Fig. 4.1 Erupting teeth during aligner therapy.

- Enamel: in many countries, the prevalence of molar incisor hypoplasia is increasing. Patients who have less resistant enamel can benefit from removable appliances and still all types of malocclusions can be treated.
- Allergies: metal-free appliances reduce the risk of allergies and allow performing even complex treatments of patients with such sensitivities.
- Acceptance: not only adults but also teenagers often refuse orthodontic treatments with fixed appliances.
  Aligners are much less visible and much more comfortable.

4.2 Treatment Strategies

4.2.1 Class II Malocclusion Treatment

In most cases, Class II malocclusion therapy consists of both growth modification and dentoalveolar correction. The ideal time for growth modification is mainly in the mixed dentition. The treatment has to start early enough to benefit from the pubertal growth peak. For the treatment of patients with dental and/or skeletal Class II, there are the following options.

Two-Phase Treatment

Phase 1 usually consists of activator (any type), plate-headgear, headgear, any type of distalizing devices (Carriere, Beneslider, Pendulum, distal-jet, etc.), maxillary expansion (forced/rapid), extraction of premolars, etc. Subsequently, this Phase 1 is followed by Phase 2 by means of aligner treatment.

This protocol has the following advantages:
- Parallel to the initial sagittal correction, movements which are less predictable with aligners alone, such as correction of severe deep bites or transversal discrepancies, can be improved simultaneously. The subsequent Phase 2 with aligners will be easier, more predictable, and shorter.
- The estimation of compliance is more precise: a patient who wears headgear respecting the protocol will most likely also wear aligners as required.
- Starting Phase 1 during mixed dentition allows starting the aligner treatment in the permanent dentition and, therefore, the necessity

of an MCC is significantly reduced. Almost all patients starting the aligner treatment during mixed dentition will need an MCC, whereas an MCC after start in the permanent dentition is rare when the planning was correct.

Distalization of Upper Posterior Teeth

With a sophisticated aligner system, the distalization of upper posterior teeth can be performed in a very predictable way. Studies have shown that no significant tipping of teeth will occur when the distal movement of molars is up to 2.5 mm. Clinical experience shows that even movements up to 4.5 mm can routinely be performed successfully. It is recommended to place rectangular vertical attachments on the molars in order to prevent tipping if the distalization exceeds 2.5 mm.

In all cases, use of Class II elastics is mandatory. The standard procedure is to fix buttons on the lower first molars and attach the elastics from these points to hooks located at the upper canines, which are cut directly into the aligners (▶ Fig. 4.2). On both sites, it is possible to place buttons or cuts in order to attach the elastics. The inclination of the incisors will remain very stable for both kinds of attachments of the elastics, cuts and buttons. The decision whether to put cuts or buttons is influenced mainly by the form and the height of the clinical crown of the teeth and by personal preference.

If the skeletal base is only moderate Class II, 12 hours/day of elastic wear can be sufficient for anchorage. Generally, it is recommended to always start with Class II elastics which are worn full-time (24 hours/day). Depending on the progress, the duration can be

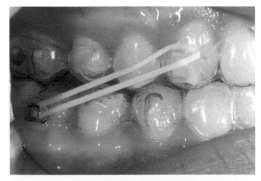

Fig. 4.2 Class II elastics (for anchorage and Class II correction).

reduced during treatment. Careful monitoring is always required for both tipping of teeth and sagittal relation.

The distalization has to be carried out sequentially. A maximum of two pairs of teeth should be distalized simultaneously at the same time. All the other teeth serve as anchorage.

Effect of Class II Elastics Alone

The final result of growth modification alone, in order to correct Class II malocclusions, is highly dependent on the compliance to wear Class II elastics and on growth itself. Both factors are difficult to foresee, and careful steady monitoring is mandatory.

While the inclination of the lower incisors remains very stable, this force system will produce a slight posterior rotation of the maxilla (comparable to a Herren-type activator). Probably, when attaching the elastics on buttons on the teeth, the inclination of the incisors will remain more stable compared to the attachment of the elastics directly on the aligners. However, no scientific data covering this topic are available yet.

Combination of Distalization in the Maxilla and Effect of Class II Elastics

For most cases with Class II malocclusion, the strategy of combining both distalization and skeletal effect of Class II elastics seems to be the most suitable.

The predictability of growth is limited. Therefore, clinically we can see more or less of growth modification by the effect of Class II elastics than expected or than the treatment plan requires.

The amount of distalization of the upper posterior teeth could be too much if the effect of the elastics is higher than planned or if more sagittal growth occurs than included in the treatment plan. Should this be the case, it is necessary to undertake an MCC.

It is recommended to correct Class II malocclusion 2/3 by distalization in the maxilla and 1/3 by effect of Class II elastics. If the treatment plan is designed accordingly, the clinician has more flexibility during the treatment phase.

Extraction of Premolars

In cases with severe crowding, the extraction of upper first and lower second premolars can be useful in order to obtain a Class I molar and canine relationship. This treatment will require attachments and auxiliaries to prevent undesired molar tipping, particularly in the mandible (see Section 4.3 and Section 4.6.1).

Mandibular Advancement Feature

Align Technology has released this newly designed treatment option for Class II treatments with aligners for teens. The aligners are constructed comparable to a Twin Block appliance.

The precision wings (▶ Fig. 4.3) keep the mandible in a slightly protruded position.

Advantages:
- The appliance is worn for 22 to 24 hours (only removed for eating and cleaning), which makes it more effective than comparable appliances worn at nighttime.
- The anterior teeth can be fully aligned at the same time.
- Reduced treatment time.

First clinical studies show:
- A good effect on the sagittal relation.
- No posterior rotation of the maxilla.
- No unwanted proclination of the lower incisors.
- Very good control of the incisors in both jaws in all dimensions.

4.2.2 Class III Malocclusion Treatment

The treatment of Class III patients almost always consists of a two-phase therapy: the first phase consists of growth modification in preadolescent age and the second phase will follow afterward in the permanent dentition (camouflage or surgery).

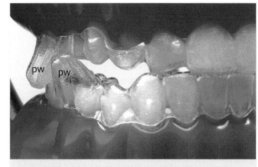

Fig. 4.3 Precision wings of the mandibular advancement feature (Invisalign).

The most commonly used appliances for the first phase treatment are still functional appliances such as Fränkel III, Delaire face mask, Tandem Traction Bow appliance, or Chin Cup treatment.

For both the first and the second phase of treatment, aligners offer very interesting opportunities.

First Phase Treatment of Class III

According to the present skeletal pattern, either maxillary deficiency or mandibular protrusion or a combination of both, different appliances have been designed. Clinically and cephalometrically, it is difficult, however, to separate the effects of an appliance, for example, the Delaire face mask, to the jaws. We will always find effects in both dental arches/jaws.

Clinically, the focus should be on growth modification (skeletal effect) and avoiding camouflage or compensation. It is important not to protrude the upper incisors when trying to obtain or keep a positive overjet.

Aligner treatment in this phase consists of a pair of passive aligners provided with buttons for the application of Class III elastics. In the lower jaw, it is recommended to bond buttons or hooks directly on to the first primary molars. This prevents the lower aligner from disconnecting. In the upper jaw, alternatively, a palatal plate can be used. This device has the advantage that the position of the upper incisors can simultaneously be improved (mainly derotation of lateral incisors) and some expansion can be done when needed. Poncini clasps are strong enough to keep the plate in place with the elastics hooked directly on them. To improve compliance, the labial arch can be left out.

Aligner therapy in the first phase of Class III treatment is advantageous due to the following reasons:

- The appliance can be worn full time, showing faster and higher effect.
- Lower forces are needed (4 ounces instead of 12 ounces recommended for the Delaire mask).
- Compliance is much higher as the appliance is less bulky and much less visible than all other Class III appliances.
- The costs are much lower, even when the aligners have to be replaced when worn out.

Second Phase of Class III Treatment

In the permanent dentition, we naturally only have limited possibilities left for growth modification. When starting the second phase of Class III treatment, the first question to answer is whether the available therapeutic possibilities are sufficient to correct the present malocclusion with orthodontics alone or if orthognathic surgery is needed as well. In the latter case, treatment start would be delayed until growth is almost over.

Distalization of Lower Posterior Teeth

Class III treatment with aligners is an interesting option also in the permanent dentition, regardless of whether there is still growth occurring or not. The main reason for this is that with aligners it is very easy to distalize posterior teeth in the mandible. Just as in the upper dental arch, the distalization has to be performed sequentially and Class III elastics are mandatory for anchorage—and/ or for its skeletal effect. If distalization exceeds 2.5 mm, rectangular attachments on the molars are highly recommended.

Extraction of Premolars

In cases with severe crowding, the extraction of upper second and lower first premolars can be useful in order to obtain a Class I molar and canine relationship. This treatment will require attachments and auxiliaries to prevent undesired molar tipping (see Section 4.3 and Section 4.6.1).

Extraction of a Lower Incisor

If there is not much growth left and, therefore, only limited possibilities remain to influence the growth pattern, the extraction of a lower incisor is a treatment option. The respecting considerations leading the planning, such as Bolton analysis, space analysis, and inclination of the upper and lower incisors, are the same as when treating the patient with any other technique. Treatments with aligners are highly predictable when choosing and working with an appropriate aligner system that allows control of the axis during translation as well as control of torque. Usually, such kinds of treatment last about 6 months.

4.3 Space Management

Space management basically describes how to deal with the discrepancy between the space available and the space needed. The first step is always to establish an analysis of the situation in the dental arches. Orthodontic textbooks describe a variety of systems and techniques in order to get a resulting score when there is a lack or an excess of space. Handling this result is a key factor in the planning. Thus, when treating teens with aligners, the following factors should be taken into account when establishing the treatment plan.

4.3.1 Spacing (Excess of Space)

The considerations whether or not to close spaces, regarding Bolton analysis, dental arch width, and occlusion, are the same as for the planning with any other appliance. When treating with aligners, however, space closure might be more difficult when mesial movement of molars is needed (▶Fig. 4.4). If lip posture and profile are proportionate, it is preferable to move teeth distally in order to close spaces. Highly developed features for planning are helpful and should be used to find the optimal proportions of sagittal movements of the teeth and designing anchorage, attachments, and auxiliaries in order to get realistic and predictable results.

4.3.2 Lack of Space

Basically, there are two options: creating more space or removing dental substance (extraction or interproximal enamel reduction).

Nonextraction Solution

By expanding the dental arches transversally and sagittally, it is possible in many cases to create enough space for aligning the teeth.

In the upper dental arch, a variety of appliances exists for distalizing posterior teeth and expanding the dental arch in order to get space. Aligners are also an interesting option to create space, knowing that both distalizing and transversal expansion can be performed in a very predictable way. Transversal expansion requires the placement of attachments on the molars (rectangular horizontal) for buccal root torque. For distalization exceeding 2.5 mm, it is recommended to place attachments on the posterior teeth to avoid tipping.

In the lower dental arch, solving crowding problems—which is a very frequent procedure—usually consists of the proclination of the anterior teeth ("blow-up"). This may likewise require proclination of the upper incisors even when according to the treatment plan this would not be necessary. Another problem related to the proclination of the front teeth is the higher risk of gingival recessions on these teeth. The risk is probably lower in teens than in adults, but there is only little information regarding this aspect in the literature. Also, there is still very scarce information about long-term stability, both of the alignment and of the level of the gingival margin, after considerable proclination of lower front teeth. Therefore, these movements should be avoided in order to limit the risk of recessions. When working with fixed

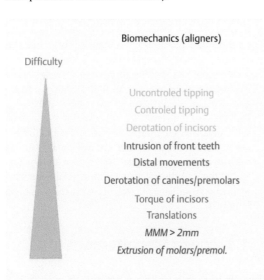

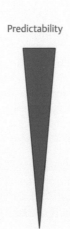

Biomechanics (aligners)

Difficulty

Predictability

Uncontroled tipping
Controled tipping
Derotation of incisors
Intrusion of front teeth
Distal movements
Derotation of canines/premolars
Torque of incisors
Translations
MMM > 2mm
Extrusion of molars/premol.

Fig. 4.4 Biomechanics, predictability of aligners. MMM, mesial movement of molars.

appliances, the alternative to proclination and expansion is extraction. Extraction in the lower dental arch usually implies extraction in the upper arch as well, even without space problems.

With aligners, however, it is possible to distalize posterior teeth in the lower dental arch in a very predictable way. Hence, aligner orthodontics is an interesting treatment strategy in cases with lower incisor crowding. It allows keeping the teeth within the biological envelope and thus reducing the risk of recessions. Furthermore, it is possible to treat more cases without extractions while still not overexpanding the arch. Nonextraction therapy can be desirable in the lower dental arch in order to avoid extraction in the upper dental arch as well.

Correspondingly to the procedure in the maxilla, the posterior teeth must be moved by sequential distalization. Equally, attachments are required when the amount of distalization exceeds 2.5 mm and elastics should be applied for anchorage.

Extraction Solution

Treating patients with aligners when teeth have to be extracted can be challenging. The removal of teeth always leaves a large gap within the dental arch. Even if overall there is a distinct amount of missing space, the problem of closing the spaces created by the extractions in a reasonable and predictable way still occurs. The first step in the planning process is how and how much, and in what mesiodistal direction the adjacent teeth should be moved into the extraction gap. When treating patients with aligners, a sophisticated software program is mandatory to define the amount of movement, the anchorage, the attachments, and the auxiliaries.

Extraction and subsequent space closure often implies the need to perform less predictable movements, in particular mesial movements of molars (▶ Fig. 4.4). In order to avoid this, it might be reasonable to distalize posterior teeth in both dental arches, thereby averting extractions.

While extraction of premolars leaves significant spaces to close, and thus less predictable movements may take place, the extraction of a lower incisor can be an interesting treatment strategy if both the occlusion and the Bolton analysis permit this solution. However, very often the extraction of premolars cannot be avoided and requires satisfying solutions.

If the decision to extract can be taken early, i.e., in the early mixed dentition, it is favorable to perform the extraction as early as reasonably possible and to then wait until the permanent dentition stage before starting the aligner treatment. In the meantime, vertical or transversal problems can be solved (Phase 1 treatment). The extraction gaps will be significantly reduced by natural tooth migration and thus Phase 2 will be easier to manage.

In cases where space closure is to be performed from mesial to distal, i.e., high anchorage cases, Invisalign offers an elaborated solution with optimized attachments placed on the posterior teeth for building up anchorage, optimized attachments for bodily distalization of the canines, and integrated features in the aligners to prevent extrusion and lingual tipping of the incisors during their retraction. Other aligner systems require auxiliaries.

In cases where reciprocal space closure or mesial movement of posterior teeth of more than 2 mm is planned, attachments and auxiliaries such as lever arms and temporary anchorage devices (TADs) are mandatory in order to get the desired perfect results (see below).

As summary for extraction cases, we can say that in order to keep predictability high when treating with aligners:
- Extract early.
- Consider nonextraction therapy if possible and reasonable, distalize posterior teeth.
- Consider extraction of a lower incisor.
- Use auxiliaries.

4.4 Vertical Problems

When treating teens, we always have the advantage that it is possible to influence both tooth position and skeletal pattern, and we can design the treatment plan accordingly. On the other hand, we always have the risk that unexpected growth may interfere with our plans in an undesired manner. Careful monitoring during the treatment is always imperative. When treating teens with aligners, we only have limited possibilities to intervene once the whole set of aligners is ordered. It might be necessary to change the set of aligners during the course of treatment.

4.4.1 Open Bite

Initially, the basic analysis has to reveal if the lack of vertical contact between the teeth is due to

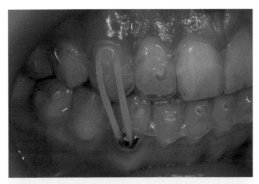

Fig. 4.5 Vertical elastics (for anchorage and supporting extrusion).

dental or skeletal reasons. In addition, the role of the tongue is always a key factor during the planning of the treatment strategy.

In general, when treating open bites with aligners, the following options are given:
- Extruding anterior teeth in the upper and/or in the lower dental arch.
- Intruding posterior teeth in the upper and/or in the lower dental arch.
- A combination of both.

Both movements, intrusion of posterior teeth and extrusion of anterior teeth, can be performed with aligners.

Intrusion of posterior teeth is assisted by the fact that the aligners lie occlusally on the teeth and effect some intrusive force by their sheer presence. Therefore, sequential intrusion of posterior teeth works well with aligners.

Extrusion of anterior teeth requires the placement of attachments due to the anatomy of the teeth (horizontal, gingivally beveled). When extruding frontal teeth simultaneously to the intrusion of posterior teeth, there is optimal effect as each movement anchors the opposing movement. Thus, if the exposure of the anterior teeth is favorable to the lips, simultaneous extrusion of the incisors and intrusion of the posterior teeth is the most efficient way to close an anterior open bite. Additionally, vertical intermaxillary elastics can be useful for additional anchorage and enhancing the effect of the aligners (▶ Fig. 4.5).

4.4.2 Deep Bite

The basic analysis first has to reveal the origin of the problem, whether the deep bite is due to the skeletal pattern or to overeruption of teeth or a combination of both.

In general, when treating deep bites with aligners, the following options are given:
- Intrusion of anterior teeth in the upper and/or in the lower dental arch.
- Extrusion of lateral teeth in the upper and/or in the lower arch.
- A combination of both.

In order to take a decision which of these possibilities should be chosen, several factors should be considered:
- The exposure of the upper anterior teeth. (How much intrusion of the upper incisors is esthetically judicious?)
- The inclination of the incisors (relative vs. absolute intrusion).
- The overjet.
- The age of the patient (to hold the incisors vertically during natural extrusion of the posterior teeth).
- The depth of the curve of Spee.
- The amount of movement needed.

Intrusion of anterior teeth can be performed with aligners in a predictable way up to the amount of 3 mm. It is recommended to place attachments for anchorage on the premolars to enhance the effect of the aligners. If it is planned to carry out this amount of intrusion in both dental arches, up to 6 mm of interincisal overlapping can be corrected easily with aligners.

What is helpful when correcting open bites, namely the intrusive force of aligners when biting on them, is a problem in cases of deep bites—especially, if a deep bite should be corrected not only by the intrusion of anterior teeth, but also simultaneously by extrusion of posterior teeth. Occlusal forces annihilate the possible effect of extrusion by the aligners. Thus, the posterior teeth have to be prevented from getting into contact. The placement of bite ramps is a key element for posterior extrusion; during the time when the aligners are worn, the posterior teeth are out of vertical contact (▶ Fig. 4.6).

Bite ramps are more effective in teens as growth and natural extrusion of the teeth may express more than in adults and thus make it easier to correct deep bites. Additionally to the bite ramps, attachments are useful to improve the extrusive effect of the aligners. In many cases, Class II elastics should be applied in order to compensate the

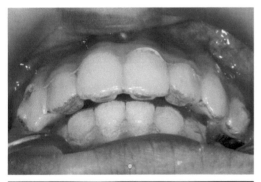

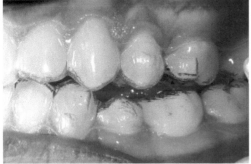

Fig. 4.6 Bite ramps for disocclusion of the posterior teeth.

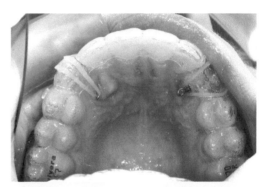

Fig. 4.7 Treatment of impacted canines.

effect of posterior rotation of the mandible caused by the bite ramps.

Bite ramps are an essential tool when treating deep bites with aligners, especially for the treatment of teens. Aligner systems without this feature are by far less effective. Intrusion of front teeth can be performed in a good way with aligners, but in many cases this approach is too limited for the problem.

For teens with severe skeletal and dental deep bites, a two-phase treatment is advantageous.

4.5 Dislocated Impacted Canines

The treatment strategy and the protocol for deimpacting and aligning dislocated canines are personal preferences of each orthodontist. Orthodontic bibliography describes many different ways and solutions for this problem, and the considerable number of case reports illustrates the variety of suitable clinical procedures.

When working with aligner orthodontics, similarly, different protocols are convenient in order to align dislocated canines. Basically, there are three approaches to this clinical problem:

- Two-phase treatment: after surgical placement of a button with a chain on the impacted canine, a lever arm delivers the extrusive force. Anchorage is built up by a fixed appliance such as Nance appliance, sectional appliance with braces, and miniscrews. Once the canine has reached its position, in the second phase, all the remaining tasks are solved with aligners.
- Three-phase treatment: in the first phase, a first set of aligners solves the local problems, such as creating enough space in the arch for the displaced canine, in order to allow proceeding to surgery and the procedure described in the previous approach. During the second phase, with the extrusion of the canine by means of a lever arm, retention aligners have to be worn. Finally, a second set of aligners finishes the case.
- Treatment with aligners alone: surgical exposure of the canine by removing the covering gingiva and placement of a hook on the canine. The patient attaches elastics from this hook onto the aligners. The orthodontist instructs and monitors the force and the direction of these elastics (▶ Fig. 4.7). During the time the canine reaches its position, orthodontic treatment can proceed as usual, as regular change of the aligners is still possible. Once the canine can be guided not only by the elastics, but also by the aligners, it will be integrated into a new set of aligners.

4.6 Interdisciplinary Treatments

With a highly developed aligner system, it is possible to produce all the necessary tooth movements

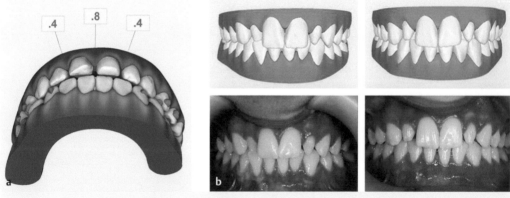

Fig. 4.8 (a, b) Precise planning prior to prosthodontics.

which are required to get functionally and esthetically perfect results. These elaborated systems usually also provide excellent planning tools. In cases with deformed or missing teeth, these tools allow to define and visualize the final position of all teeth. When the planning is correct and the movements are predictable, the result can be foreseen precisely (▶Fig. 4.8a, b). In this way, the cooperation between the orthodontist and the prosthodontist is technically easy and the patient can significantly be benefitted from it.

4.6.1 Auxiliaries

Treating complex cases with aligners first requires a high-performing aligner system:
- Material delivering a flat load–deflection curve.
- A distinct force system producing defined moments, so that the movements are force driven and not shape driven.
- Specific ("optimized") attachments.
- Built-in biomechanics such as compensatory intrusion and torque when retracting incisors.

Secondly, auxiliaries are needed. With aligners alone, it is not possible to achieve all required movements in complex orthodontic cases. Auxiliaries allow enhancing the predictability of less predictable movements (▶Fig. 4.4). The same holds true for fixed appliances. With braces and wires alone, not all cases or problems can be solved—the use of auxiliaries is essential. Elastics, TADs, lever arms, buttons, and springs are the most common auxiliaries used in both techniques. In order to allow the attachment of auxiliaries such as buttons

or lever arms, the borders of the aligners should not overlap the gingival margin. There are systems where it is possible to order a cutout of a specific tooth, which allows an easy application of these auxiliaries.

4.6.2 Elastics

Intermaxillary elastics are applied for sagittal corrections and for anchorage (see above). These are by far the most common and the most frequent reasons to use elastics. Elastics can also be used for localized problems such as elongation (extrusion) of single teeth or derotation of teeth (▶Fig. 4.9a, b) and thus can be compared with the use of power chains for local movements of teeth when working with fixed appliances.

4.6.3 TADs

In the upper dental arch, the insertion of a palatal implant or miniscrews is useful as anchorage (▶Fig. 4.10a) when teeth have to be moved over longer distances, distally or mesially (for molars, the critical amount of mesial movement is as low as 2 mm; ▶Fig. 4.4).

In the lower dental arch, the insertion of a miniplates or miniscrews is recommended for the same reasons.

When using an aligner system with the borders of the aligners not overlapping the gingival margins, the presence of TADs does not interfere with the aligners and tooth movements can be combined for both, movements requiring TADs and other movements. A Beneslider, for example,

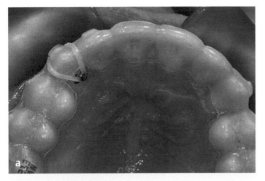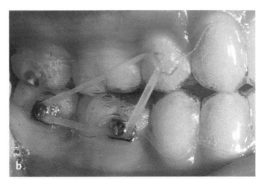

Fig. 4.9 (a, b) Auxiliaries: elastics.

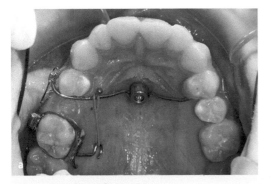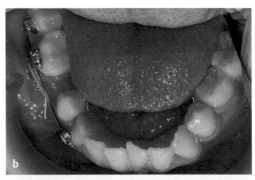

Fig. 4.10 (a, b) Auxiliaries: TADs.

can be used in combination with standard aligner therapy. TADs can also be used together with other auxiliaries such as a sectional arch with braces in order to close a space prior to aligner therapy (▶ Fig. 4.10b).

4.6.4 Power Arms/Lever Arms

Uprighting movements of molars are difficult to achieve with aligners. The application of an appropriate attachment (horizontal, gingivally beveled) is mandatory, but is only effective in a minor range of movements (up to 5 degrees). Mesially tipped molars or molars to be moved mesially need a power arm producing an uprighting moment (▶ Fig. 4.11). The power arm should be long enough to reach the level of the center of rotation of the tooth. Depending on the uprighting moment needed, it is possible to bend it more mesially to get more effect. The force is applied by elastics. In a Class II malocclusion situation, the elastics can be attached on the upper canine (either on a precision cut or on a button), whereas in a Class I malocclusion situation

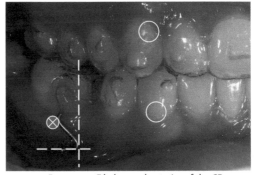

Powerarm: F below and anterior of the CR => uprighting moment

Fig. 4.11 Biomechanics of power arms.

they are to be attached on a button on the lower canine (▶ Fig. 4.12a, b). With this technique, mesial movements of molars up to 4 mm can be accomplished in both jaws without significant tipping. In the lower dental arch, the undesired moment of rotation (mesial in) is compensated by the aligner

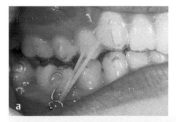
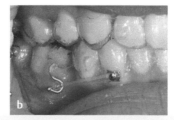
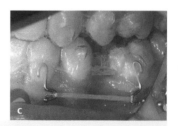

Fig. 4.12 (a–c) Mesial movement of lower molars with auxiliaries.

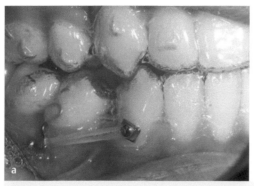
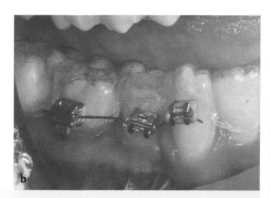

Fig. 4.13 (a, b) Uprighting of premolars with auxiliaries.

and can be neglected. In the upper dental arch, due to the anatomy of the roots, additional compensation is needed.

4.6.5 Braces, Sectionals

Undesired tipping may still occur. This happens most frequently when closing spaces after extraction of premolars. Uprighting of tipped premolars or molars can be achieved by means of a lever arm or by a sectional fixed appliance (▶Fig. 4.13). The insertion of braces can be considered an element in the solution to a localized unforeseen problem; it is unusual to plan the insertion of braces from the beginning on.

4.7 Retention

Long-term and efficient retention is mandatory at the end of every orthodontic treatment. This is particularly true for teens. Even though the final planned result is achieved, growth may still change the occlusion. The retention protocol must keep not only the alignment stable, but also the sagittal, vertical, and transversal dimension of the occlusion. Furthermore, it might be challenging to keep motivation and compliance high when "everything already looks good."

The most logical appliance for retention is aligners. The patients are used to having them and the same appliance that brought the teeth into the final position is designed to keep them there. If needed, sagittal elastics still can be applied in a simple manner. When occlusal contact was established by intrusion of posterior teeth, aligners might prevent a vertical relapse better than a retainer which does not cover the occlusal surfaces of the teeth. A Hawley retainer in the upper dental arch is preferable, on the other hand, when a severe deep bite or a severe transversal problem was corrected. Many practitioners set fixed retainers canine-to-canine by default. These can be combined with aligners or any other retention device.

5 Routine Mechanics and Aligners (Extraction/ Nonextraction)

Eugene K. Chan and M. Ali Darendeliler

Summary

Clear aligner therapy has become a common treatment modality within the orthodontic practice. Cases ranging from simple Class I malocclusion to complex Class II and Class III malocclusions, with or without extractions, may be attempted. Although computer-aided appliance design and digital virtual treatment planning have helped us in many ways to improve our skills in treating patients with this relatively new technique, it is still not foolproof. This chapter highlights the essence of routine orthodontic treatment in various types of malocclusions, offering concise explanations on staging patterns, the use of elastics and their various configurations, attachment designs, and other important considerations.

Keywords: orthodontics, Invisalign, complex cases, extractions

5.1 Introduction

Modalities of orthodontic treatment have changed much over the last 10 to 15 years. With the advent of digital technology, fast internet speeds, and various digital mobile platforms, modern orthodontic treatment planning and execution have never been so much at our fingertips. However, with the convenience of advanced technology, the biology of dental movement still has not changed and the complex nature of orthodontic treatment should not be trivialized.

Aligner treatment has broadened our scope of choice of orthodontic appliances. Especially esthetically conscious adult and/or adolescent patients who may never have considered orthodontic treatment with conventional therapies now have a viable option. It is important for the clinician to understand the intricacies of digital treatment planning and their innate shortfall to allow a seamless incorporation of such techniques into their daily orthodontic practices.

5.2 Initial Appointments and Informed Consent

ClinCheck virtual treatment plans do not translate absolutely into clinical outcomes. Dental movements cannot be completely mimicked by digital manipulation, at least not yet. The biology of orthodontic movement is complex, involving a cascade of exchange of biochemicals, hormone precursors, and enzymes.[1] The components of the periodontium supporting this movement have different physical properties, and the dynamic nature of this system, namely, the constant changing of stress/strain patterns within the periodontal ligament, has made its *in vitro* duplication difficult, if not impossible.

Hence, it is essential for new clinicians to present a more realistic treatment goal to the patient during the initial consultation appointments. Without fully considering the patient's dental biology, studying the physical anatomy of the dentition, and understanding the intricacies of aligner mechanotherapy, it would be unwise to assume that the virtual treatment outcomes can be readily achieved.

Routinely, it is important to note patients' chief concerns and relate to them if that was achievable. Generous treatment time frames, absolute compliance with appliance wear (including elastics for anchorage), the need to place attachments, and/or other auxiliaries need to be intimately discussed. Skeletal versus dental discrepancies contributing to the malocclusion need to be carefully considered. Additional aligners, multiple staging patterns with updated impressions, or intraoral scans will be required. Retention appliances and regimes need to be discussed during these initial appointments as well.

5.3 Nonextraction Plans (Class I, II, and III Malocclusions)

Nonextraction treatment plans do not always mean a shorter treatment duration or an easier orthodontic journey. There are different considerations in Class I, II, and III dental malocclusions.

5.3.1 Class I Malocclusion Considerations

The essences in obtaining space in a Class I malocclusion characterized by dental crowding are (1) dental arch expansion, (2) anterior dental proclination, and (3) interproximal reduction (IPR).

Dental Arch Expansion

Scrutinizing the dentoalveolus to ensure all expansion done is kept within the thickness of the bone is important. Existing buccal recession and/or bone loss is a contraindication. Successful cases are those where the buccal segments are lingually inclined (▶Fig. 5.1). Cases with bilateral posterior crossbites with no functional shift need not always be corrected (▶Fig. 5.2a, b).

The soft- and hard-tissue resistance to dental arch expansion has to be considered. Although for every 1 mm of dental arch expansion the dental arch perimeter increases by approximately 0.7 mm,[2] the tissue resistance prevents us from obtaining this. Therefore, during the ClinCheck planning process, it is important to have a certain degree of overexpansion planned—usually, approximately 50% more dental expansion, or about 2 mm more on either side. However, due to the lack of rigidity of the aligners at the terminal molars, overexpansion has to be greater there as compared to the midarch (premolar) regions.

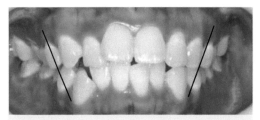

Fig. 5.1 Case showing lingually rolled in buccal segments ideal for dental arch expansion.

During upper dental arch expansion, the center of rotation of the maxilla is positioned superior to the palatal vault. The inevitable buccal tipping of the posterior dentition usually results in the palatal cusps of these teeth being extruded, increasing the vertical dimension. In a case that has a vertical or hyperdivergent skeletal pattern, or with an anterior open bite tendency, this would worsen the anterior open bite and makes its correction extremely difficult. Therefore, during the ClinCheck treatment planning process, overcorrection movements including increased buccal root torque and intrusion of the posterior dentition need to be considered (▶Fig. 5.3a–c).

Anterior Dental Proclination

Anterior labial recession, low gingival attachments, and bone loss are contraindications of anterior dental proclination. Otherwise, this is a very efficient way to gain space in a crowded arch. Retroclined incisors are effectively proclined using the aligner appliance. For every 1 mm of incisor proclination, there is approximately 2 mm of dental arch perimeter obtained. This translation from the digital planning clinically is usually absolute due to less tissue resistance of the dentoalveolus in the anterior region (▶Fig. 5.4a–c).

In a case where lower anterior crowding is accompanied by a deep dental overbite, the proclination of the lower incisors while relieving the lower dental crowding will inevitably help in opening the deep overbite. The proclination of the lower incisors effectively allows an intrusion moment

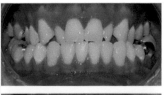
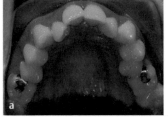
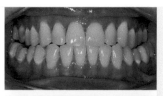
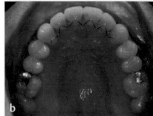

Fig. 5.2 (a) Before and **(b)** after images of bilateral posterior crossbite left uncorrected.

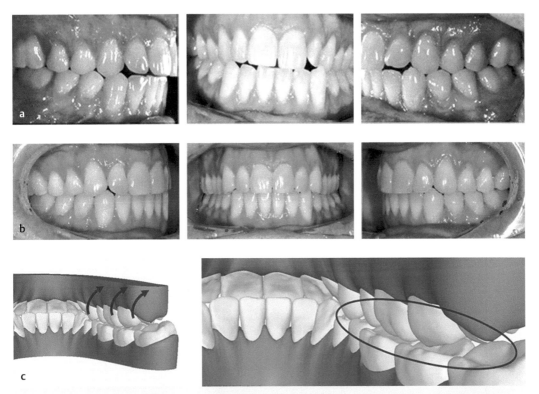

Fig. 5.3 Images of **(a)** before and **(b)** after treatment with bilateral posterior arch expansion, in a case with an anterior open bite. **(c)** ClinCheck planning with increased buccal root torque of the upper posterior teeth and no occlusal contacts between the upper palatal cusps and the lower central fossae.

as well. This relative intrusion (proclination and intrusion), as opposed to absolute intrusion, is more readily achieved clinically (▶ Fig. 5.5a–c).

Interproximal Reduction (IPR)

Upon submitting the prescription form, if we select all three ways to create space in a nonextraction crowded condition, IPR will be the default, last consideration. If space was not sufficient after dental arch expansion and anterior dental proclination, IPR will be indicated (▶ Fig. 5.6a–c). This is a nonreversible clinical procedure and has to be indicated with care. Traditional orthodontic therapies using fixed appliances seldom require IPR, usually only in cases where Bolton discrepancy is eminent.

IPR is contraindicated in cases in which this procedure was done in previous orthodontic treatment, in cases with thin and slender

dental anatomy, or in cases where there is poor oral hygiene or other enamel defects such as dental imperfecta.

5.3.2 Class II Malocclusion Considerations

There are many various plans to correct nonextraction Class II malocclusions. How the anteroposterior correction is performed or staged is the crux of treatment planning in these cases. The decision largely lies on the age of the patient and the severity of the correction required.

Staging Patterns

The staging pattern in Class II malocclusion correction could be (1) sequential staging pattern, (2) simultaneous staging (elastic simulation), or (3) simultaneous staging (*en masse* movement).

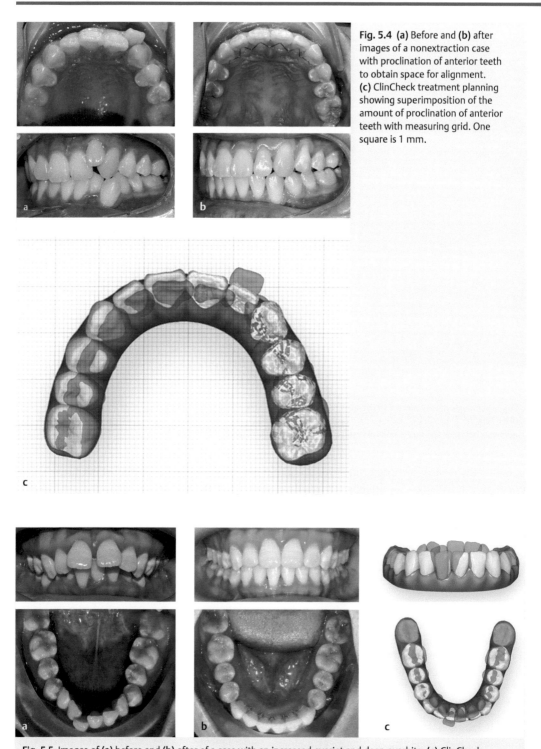

Fig. 5.4 (a) Before and **(b)** after images of a nonextraction case with proclination of anterior teeth to obtain space for alignment. **(c)** ClinCheck treatment planning showing superimposition of the amount of proclination of anterior teeth with measuring grid. One square is 1 mm.

Fig. 5.5 Images of **(a)** before and **(b)** after of a case with an increased overjet and deep overbite. **(c)** ClinCheck treatment plans showing the degree of intrusion obtained with the proclination of the lower incisors.

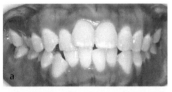
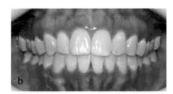
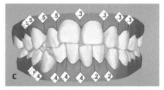

Fig. 5.6 (a) Before and (b) after images of a nonextraction case with IPR creating sufficient space for dental alignment. (c) ClinCheck treatment plans showing the range of IPR required for alignment.

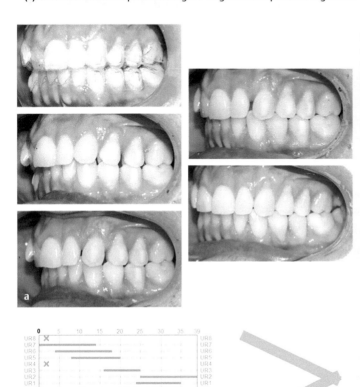

Fig. 5.7 (a) Treatment progress of a Class II malocclusion, upper molar distalization case demonstrating the sequential movement of the posterior teeth backward supported with Class II elastics clinically. (b) ClinCheck plans showing the staging pattern with a "V"-shaped pattern.

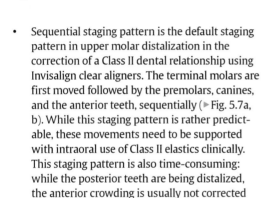

- Sequential staging pattern is the default staging pattern in upper molar distalization in the correction of a Class II dental relationship using Invisalign clear aligners. The terminal molars are first moved followed by the premolars, canines, and the anterior teeth, sequentially (▶ Fig. 5.7a, b). While this staging pattern is rather predictable, these movements need to be supported with intraoral use of Class II elastics clinically. This staging pattern is also time-consuming: while the posterior teeth are being distalized, the anterior crowding is usually not corrected

till the later stages of treatment. This may contradict our patients' chief concern which usually is the anterior crowding. To overcome this slight roadblock, request for an "esthetic start" while planning the ClinCheck treatment. This will allow the commencement of simple alignment of the anterior teeth while the terminal molars and premolars are distalizing (▶ Fig. 5.8).

- The anchorage control in Class II dental correction in adolescence is usually less demanding as there remains vertical dentoalveolar growth which helps with the anteroposterior correction. It is useful to use peak growth charts as guidelines (▶ Fig. 5.9a, b) and also ask leading questions during the consultation appointment. For instance, how rapidly the child has grown recently? Whether clothes and/or shoe sizes have changed? Age of sexual maturation in older siblings. Comparison of the child's height–weight with parents/older siblings. Planning active orthodontic treatment to coincide with the child's growth spurt often makes the treatment more effective.[3,4]

The compliant wear of aligners and Class II elastics can usually correct routine half-unit molar Class II relationship, and sometimes a full-unit molar correction is possible if conditions are ideal (▶ Fig. 5.10a, b). Ideal conditions include good clinical crown heights, good biological response, and compliant wear of aligners and elastics. Features of the Invisalign product for suitable younger patients (Invisalign Teen or Invisalign First) includes compliance indicators, free replacement aligners, and compensatory eruption tabs, which help to overcome some roadblocks in teen treatment. Recent release of the mandibular advancement feature with precision wings (▶ Fig. 5.11) also attempts orthopedic correction in these growing patients.

Elastic simulation staging is effective in adolescent Class II correction and is the staging pattern of choice. Augmented with compliant elastic wear, routine half-unit correction is easily achieved (▶ Fig. 5.12a–c).

• *En masse* Class II malocclusion correction requires more anchorage and it can be augmented by having temporary anchorage devices (TADs) placed in concurrent with elastics wear (▶ Fig. 5.13a, b).

Elastic Wear and Configuration

Elastic wear with traditional fixed orthodontic treatment is common. It can be configured in many different ways to achieve our desired orthodontic movements (▶ Fig. 5.14a–c). Similarly, with aligner therapy, elastics help to coordinate dental arch forms as well as anteroposterior correction (▶ Fig. 5.15a, b).

Precision cuts (precision hooks and button cutouts) designed during the ClinCheck planning process will assist in prescribing the elastics during treatment (▶ Fig. 5.16a, b). These precision cuts may be placed immediately at the start of the treatment in cases where elastics are required early or at any stage later during the active treatment. Bear in mind that with any precision cuts, there will be

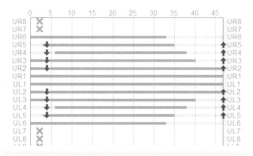

Fig. 5.8 Staging pattern of a Class II malocclusion, molar distalization case showing modified sequential staging with an "esthetic start."

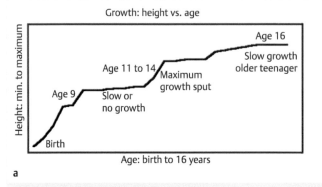

a

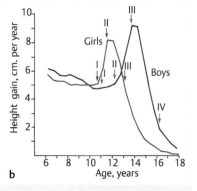

b

Fig. 5.9 (a, b) Peak-height growth in adolescence.

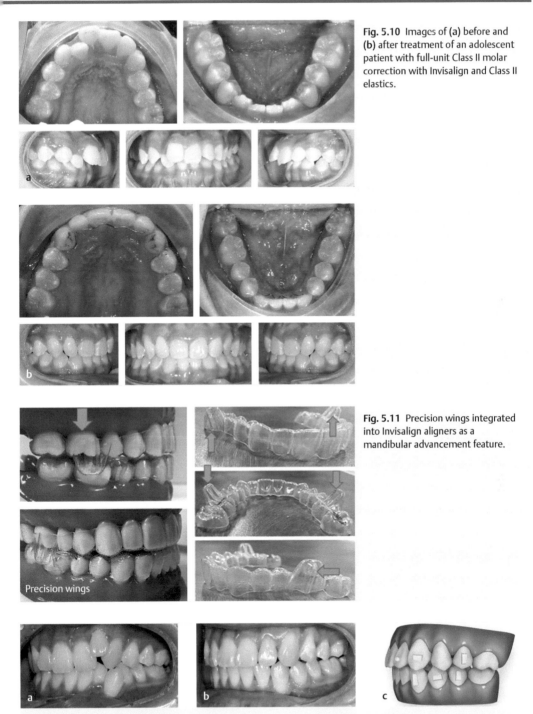

Fig. 5.10 Images of **(a)** before and **(b)** after treatment of an adolescent patient with full-unit Class II molar correction with Invisalign and Class II elastics.

Fig. 5.11 Precision wings integrated into Invisalign aligners as a mandibular advancement feature.

Precision wings

Fig. 5.12 Images of **(a)** before and **(b)** after of a half-unit Class II correction in an adolescent case. **(c)** ClinCheck plans showing an "elastic simulation" in the staging profile.

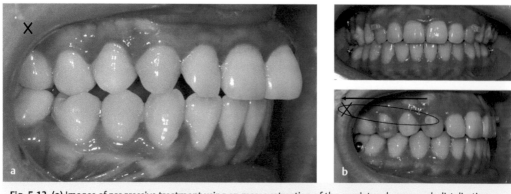

Fig. 5.13 (a) Images of progressive treatment using en masse retraction of the overjet and upper arch distalization with the placement of a TAD on the upper posterior segment. Position "x" is the position of the TAD, and elastics are worn to an esthetic button bonded on the canines. **(b)** An attachment is placed on the canine tooth to negate any side effects of the elastic traction.

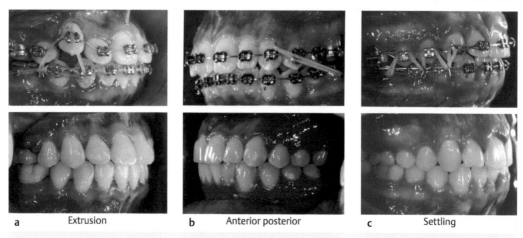

a   Extrusion   b   Anterior posterior   c   Settling

Fig. 5.14 (a) Before and **(b, c)** after images of cases treated with conventional fixed appliances utilizing elastics for extrusion, anteroposterior correction, and settling.

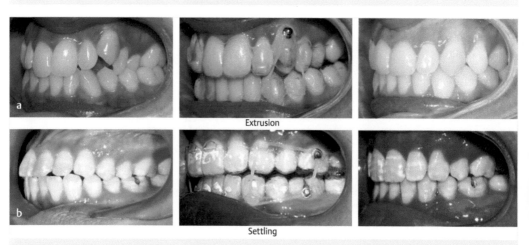

Extrusion

Settling

Fig. 5.15 (a) Before and **(b)** after images of cases treated with Invisalign appliances utilizing elastics for extrusion and settling.

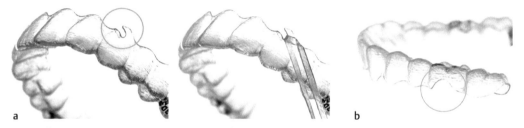

Fig. 5.16 Precision cuts on aligners with **(a)** precision hooks and **(b)** button cutout.

reduced plastic contact between the aligner and the dentition, thereby potentially reducing the control of dental movements. Therefore, in cases where clinical crown heights are short, these precision hooks should be placed only when elastic traction is required.

Due to the damping effect of the aligner system, elastic strength used in aligner therapy is usually slightly stronger than traditional fixed orthodontic appliances for the similar intended effect. When elastics are worn to a precision hook, they tend to displace the aligner away from the dentition, thereby reducing the absolute control of the dental movements. Therefore, if stronger elastics are used, it should be worn to a button bonded to the tooth and a button cutout prescribed instead. An attachment (either buccally or lingually placed) may also be necessary to increase the retention of the aligners.

In cases with shorter clinical crown heights, the aligner retention in these cases will be diminished. Hence, elastics are usually worn from a button rather than a precision hook. In cases where the maxillary canines require complex movements such as vertical as well as rotational corrections, it is advisable to have the elastics worn from the maxillary first premolars to the mandibular second molars instead (▶ Fig. 5.17). In order to improve esthetics and also for the comfort of the patient, we may also consider placing the buttons for elastics on the palatal surfaces of the maxillary canines, provided they do not contribute to occlusal interference (▶ Fig. 5.18a, b).

5.3.3 Class III Malocclusion Considerations

Nonextraction Class III dental malocclusions are often tricky to address in conventional orthodontics. It is essential to diagnose the case correctly

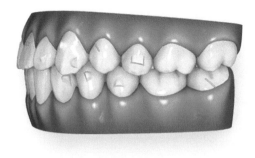

Fig. 5.17 Precision cuts (precision hooks) indicated in blue demonstrating Class II elastics worn from the upper first premolars to the lower second molars.

prior to the prescription of the exact treatment plans.

Functional Shifts

Cases with an anterior premature contact and functional shift may be much easier to tackle. Using conventional methods such a "Dawson bimanual technique,"[5] try to locate the patients' premature contact and track its functional shift. If the patient can move from a reverse overjet to an edge-to-edge bite, the chances of successful treatment will be much higher (▶ Fig. 5.19a, b). It is essential to look out for sufficient periodontal support of the upper and lower anterior teeth. Ensure sufficient thickness of the dentoalveolus to allow compensatory movements such as the proclination of the upper anterior teeth and the retroclination of the lower-anterior teeth.

Class III Elastics

Even though such dental movements in correcting these pseudo-Class III dental malocclusions

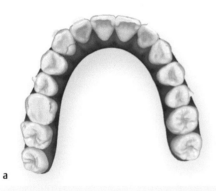
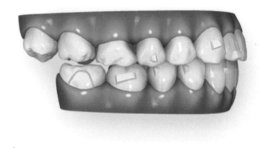

Fig. 5.18 Precision cut (button cutouts) indicated in blue demonstrating Class II elastics **(a)** worn from the lingual surface of the upper right canine to the lower right second molar **(b)**.

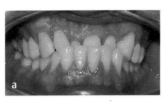
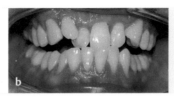

Fig. 5.19 Isolating the anterior functional shift **(a)** by manipulating the lower jaw downward and backward **(b)**.

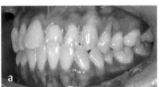
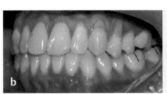

Fig. 5.20 Images of **(a)** before and **(b)** after treatment of an adult Class III case with functional shift supported with Class III elastics.

can be predictable, it is also essential that Class III elastics are applied to support the anteroposterior correction as planned in the ClinCheck treatment plans. The general principles of using Class III elastics in such cases are similar to those of Class IIs, as described above—particularly in the strength of the elastics and the choice between engaging the elastics from elastic hooks of the aligners and a button bonded on the tooth (▶Fig. 5.20a, b).

IPR

The use of Class III elastics with lower dental IPR also allows for more capacity to retract the lower dentition backward in order to facilitate more anteroposterior correction. All the pros and cons of IPR correction as described previously will also apply in these instances (▶Fig. 5.21a–c).

Increasing the Dental Arch Length of the Upper Dentition

Patients with congenitally missing teeth or upper anterior Bolton discrepancy may often end up having an "edge-to-edge" bite or even a reverse dental overjet. The upper anterior segments are usually more retrusive and retroclined, with the upper dental midline often deviated to the side with the missing dentition. The ability to plan Class III elastics, and/or lower anterior IPR, and to open up the dental space to replace the missing tooth with a dental prosthesis (dental implant, cantilever bridge, full veneer bridge, bonded bridge, or even a single tooth denture—depending on case suitability) can restore the functionality as well as esthetics of the case. The deviated dental midlines, reverse overbite, and the poor interincisor angulation will be corrected simultaneously (▶Fig. 5.22a–d).

TADs and Lower Molar Distalization

Molar distalization for anteroposterior correction in Class III malocclusions is less successful as compared to Class IIs. However, this can still be attempted in cases where the lower wisdom teeth are extracted and TADs are placed. Elastics can be worn from the TADs directly to the precision hook from the aligner at the premolar region to allow for anchorage control during lower dental retraction (▶Fig. 5.23a–e).

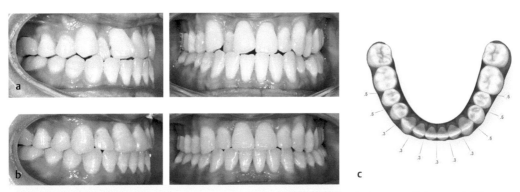

Fig. 5.21 Images of **(a)** before and **(b)** after treatment of an adult Class III malocclusion case with lower arch IPR supported with Class III elastics clinically. **(c)** ClinCheck plans showing the range of IPR indicated.

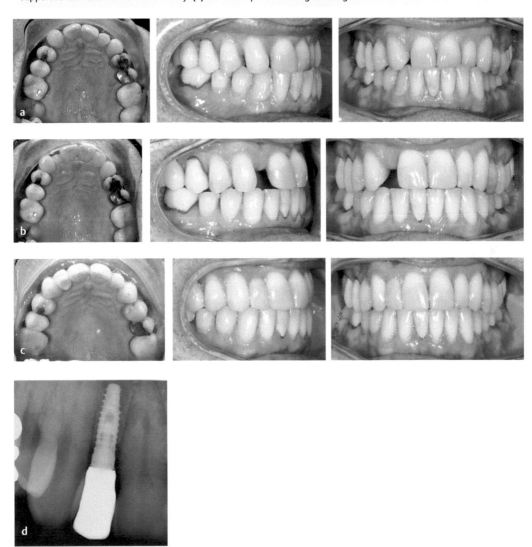

Fig. 5.22 Images of **(a)** before and **(b)** after treatment of an adult Class III malocclusion case with upper anterior Bolton discrepancy and a missing upper right lateral incisor. **(c, d)** Images of case after the placement of the implant and final restoration.

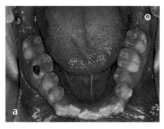
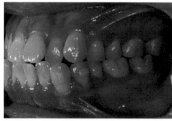

Fig. 5.23 Images of **(a)** before treatment and **(b)** panoramic radiograph after placement of TADs. **(c)** Application of elastics to TAD with the aligners. **(d)** Images of after treatment with **(e)** panoramic radiograph. (The images are provided courtesy of Dr. Tsai SJ.)

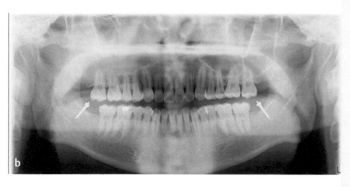

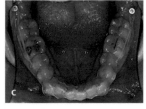
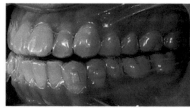

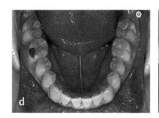
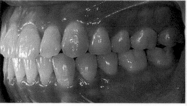

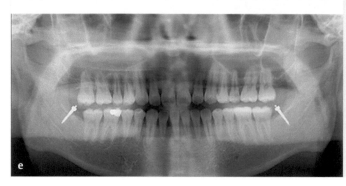

5.4 Extraction Plans (Extraction Plans, Anchorage Control, Compensatory Movements)

Extraction treatment therapy using the aligner system is challenging, and it is the least predictable of all treatment modalities within the aligner treatment plans. Invisalign uses surface area contact points to "grip" the surfaces of the dentition, the shape memory, while the aligner plastic is distorted upon insertion of the active aligners, thus allowing the subsequent release of energy, putting an orthodontic force on the teeth. There is no direct bond between the appliance and the dentition, and being a removable appliance, the three-dimensional control of dental movement is difficult to achieve. Absolute compliance with aligner wear is required to ensure optimal light consistent orthodontic forces to be applied within the system. Anything less than ideal will be a compromise and the treatment goals will not be achieved.

5.4.1 Considerations in Extraction Plans

The complexity of the plan lies in the nature of the case. These are some factors that we cannot control as a clinician. For instance, metabolism, cellular turnover, and the density of the bone and dentoalveolus differ in age, gender, and racial diversity and are factors affecting bone physiology.[6] The dimension and anatomical form of the dentition, both crowns and roots, also affect the way teeth move through bone. Case selection is hence important and it begins at the consultation appointment. Absolute compliance needs to be adhered to and explained clearly to the potential patient at this stage.

The appropriate attachment selection, sound sequencing, and staging of dental movement are essential parts of the ClinCheck treatment planning process. The need for auxiliary use such as elastics, TADs, and/or sectional fixed appliances may also arise.

5.4.2 ClinCheck and Treatment Planning

A ClinCheck treatment plan allows us to plan and visualize both treatment progress and treatment outcome. It is, however, strongly guided by software defaults and limitations. Trained aligner technicians may be unaware of patients' individual dental biology, biomechanics that is involved, and other clinical limitations and/or variations. The final position of the dentition in the approved ClinCheck plans does not necessary translate fully to the actual orthodontic treatment. Common trouble situations are often reported: (1) difficulty in obtaining the correct amount of dental expansion, (2) inability to achieve sufficient anterior torque in premolar extraction cases, (3) inability to fully correct deep overbite dental malocclusions, and (4) inability to resolve severe dental crowding (including premolar rotations) without multiple refinements or additional aligners.

Recovery techniques are therefore concocted to overcome these situations. Sectional or full arch fixed appliances, fixed bonded power arms incorporated with power chains, and/or pull coils, button, and elastics, etc., are often the "get out of trouble" consequence. Clinicians have to spend more time and overheads to prepare and plan for such situations. Patients who are not prewarned of such situations are often not impressed with the prolonged treatment duration, extra costs involved, and the placement of a more visible appliance in order to complete the case to perfection.

We strive to achieve predictable, repeatable, outstanding results without the need for such predicaments. We can come close to avoiding such situations by going back to the basics: understanding the true biology of tooth movement and relating it back to aligner treatment and biomechanics.

5.4.3 Planning and Execution

With an expansive market within the field of dentistry, Invisalign has made orthodontics easily available for the masses. As the product evolves into the cosmetic dental environment, the science behind dental movement is slowly eroded.

"Is Invisalign Orthodontics?"

Using preset defaults within the ClinCheck software and allowing technicians to dictate clinical treatment may allow the new clinician to get away with treating simple Class I malocclusion cases. However, when faced with more complex situations, the age-old debate comes about: "How much orthodontics should you know before using the Invisalign appliance, especially when tackling extraction cases?"

The decision on which tooth and/or teeth to extract, or even to extract or not, lies heavily on a few factors. It is often pertinent to choose the tooth and/or teeth that help with your anchorage control. It is also useful to note the prognosis and longevity of the tooth within the oral cavity. Look out for dental decay, large fillings, teeth that have anatomical defects (e.g., *dens invaginatus*), history of previous trauma, reduced periodontal support, and even signs of increased attrition and wear.

Other important considerations include: (1) the final position of the upper incisor in relation to the upper lip position, (2) the degree of dental crowding, (3) the amount of retraction required, (4) midline correction and/or preservation, and (5) the amount of overjet and overbite present.

The Invisalign system prefers a maximum anchorage setup. Protraction and mesialization of the posterior segments forward is unpredictable and therefore should be discouraged, unless it is augmented by auxiliaries such as TADs and sectional fixed appliances mechanics (▶ Fig. 5.24a–c).

A classic case would be a routine bimaxillary protrusive, dental crowding case that requires four premolar extractions. The space that remains after the extraction would be utilized for either dental retraction or relieving dental crowding, or both. It is essential to have treatment plans lined up with the diagnosis. Cephalometric tracings, soft-tissue analyses, and patients' chief concerns should all be addressed accordingly.

Four first premolar extractions are usually necessary in cases with severe dental crowding associated with lip incompetency. Where space acquired by dental arch expansion and/or IPR is either not feasible or insufficient, extractions will be indicated. In cases in which there is a need to protect the profile from being overly retracted and in which IPR is contraindicated or insufficient for retraction, four second premolar extractions may be considered.

5.4.4 Shape-Driven Orthodontics

The bread and butter of orthodontic treatment is the application of forces and force systems to alter tooth positions or to produce physiologic bony changes. The application of scientific biomechanics improves the quality of treatment and treatment efficiency.

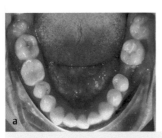
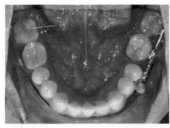
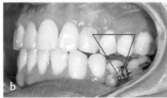
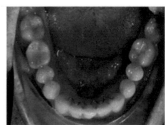
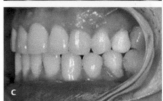

Fig. 5.24 Images of **(a)** before and **(c)** after treatment with aligners to mesialize the lower left second and third molars to close the lower left first molar space using a TAD as anchorage. **(b)** Running triangular elastics to sectional braces used in concurrent with aligner therapy.

Historically, orthodontic appliances were developed, described, and taught as shape-driven. In the era of shape-driven appliances, we were taught how to bend or twist a wire or how to properly position a bracket. That is all geometry and driven by shape.

The best approach is to first determine our orthodontic goal, what we want to achieve, and then determine the force system that is required to produce that result. Subsequent to that we can design our appliances. It is important to have a shape, but it is more important that the shape produces the desired force system. Often, that resultant shape will look nothing like the ideal finish.

5.4.5 Compensatory Movements

Understanding the side effects and the inadequacies of the aligner system is extremely important in treating of complex cases such as cases requiring extractions. As Invisalign is also a removable appliance; the degree of "play" between the appliance and the dentition affects the true tracking of the appliance.

During dental space closure using any aligner system, the anterior teeth are extruded and retroclined, contributing to an increase in dental overbite and deepening of the curve of Spee, often leading to an anterior interference and posterior open bite. The axial control of the dental translation during space closure is also difficult to manage (▶ Fig. 5.25).

Hence, compensatory movements in the ClinCheck plans are required when handling these extraction cases. Common compensatory movements include the following:

- Increased upper anterior lingual root torque, and further intrusion of the lower incisors. As a result, an anterior open bite is often seen in the final ClinCheck plans. These two compensatory movements will prevent the "dumping" of the anterior teeth as the dental spaces are closing. G5 precision bite ramps could also be included on the upper anterior teeth to assist the control in the vertical dimension as retraction occurs.
- Teeth mesial to the extraction sites need increased distal root tip movements, while teeth distal to the sites require increased mesial root tip movements. Essentially, we are trying to counteract the crown "dumping" of the abutment teeth as the extraction spaces are closed. Due to the damping effect of the aligner system, the farther the teeth are away from the extraction space, the less of these increased tipping movement is required (▶ Fig. 5.26).[7]

However, there is no formula to calculate the amount of compensation required in such extraction cases. Every individual case is different. The degree of compensation relies on various factors. These include factors affecting bone density, basal metabolic rates, and dental anatomy of the patient. The age, gender, ethnic group, crown height versus root dimensions, and other factors such as pregnancy, and if the patient is on any medication which may affect any cellular turnover and other metabolic changes are considered. The anchorage control in the maxilla and mandible often differs. The left may also differ from the right side within the same arch of the same patient as well. The use of asymmetrical

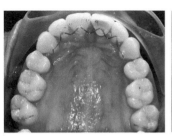
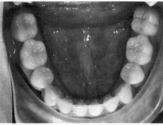
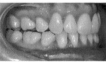
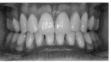
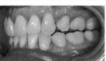

Fig. 5.25 A four first premolar extraction case treated with aligner therapy showing the inadequacies of the appliance. Bite deepening (deepening of curve of Spee) causing anterior interference and posterior open bite, and the losing control of axial inclination of the posterior teeth (often known as "dumping").

mechanics (e.g., stronger elastics on one side compared to the other) or asymmetrical extraction patterns will be necessary in cases where an innate asymmetry exists.

When we consider ClinCheck plans for the extraction of first premolars versus second premolars, the degree of compensation required for the second premolars case has to be greater on the dentition distal to the extraction sites. This is due to the increased anchorage demands in resistance to protraction of the posterior molars forward. Hence, it has to be adjusted accordingly.

5.4.6 Attachment Designs

Attachments are made up of composite resin material and are adhered to the surface of teeth in order to increase the surface area contact between the aligners and the dentition. This allows a better three-dimensional control of the dental movements desired. Attachments are generally indicated for (1) intrusion, (2) retention, (3) rotation, (4) tooth uprighting, and (5) significant space closure.

Attachments can be classified as either passive or active. Passive attachments are indicated for indirect anchorage (e.g., on posterior teeth for anterior intrusion) (▶ Fig. 5.27) or for aligner retentiveness (e.g., to resist displacement when elastics are worn directly to the aligners via precision hooks) (▶ Fig. 5.28). Active attachments are placed on the teeth that actually move during treatment (e.g., the rotation of cylindrical teeth, root control in tipping and/or translation, and dental extrusion).

Conventional attachments included elliptical, rectangular, and beveled-type attachments. With recent improvement in digital designs, optimized attachments are computer-aided designs that are customized for each tooth, requiring different type of dental movements. They are largely based on three parameters: (1) the mesial–distal width of the tooth, (2) the long axis of the tooth (arbitrary), and (3) the buccal contour of the tooth. Optimized attachments are designed for dental movements such as: incisor, premolar, and molar extrusion; incisor, canine, and premolar tip correction; lateral incisor multiplane control; and canine and premolar rotations.

Although computer-aided designs have helped greatly with the selection of the type of attachments required for the desired dental movements, it is still essential to check clinically for any biological variations prior approval of the ClinCheck plans. Considerations include the crown and root dimensions, worn incisor edges, root dilacerations, bifurcations, and the degree of dental crowding/spacing present. The time of placement of attachments has to be considered as well.

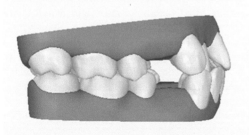

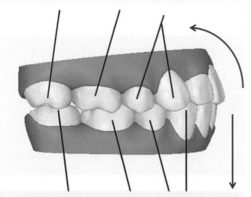

Fig. 5.26 Compensatory movements indicated for a four first premolar extraction case during the ClinCheck planning process.

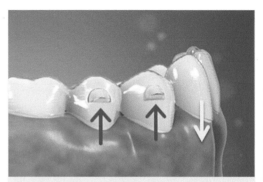

Fig. 5.27 Image showing optimized attachments supporting the intrusion of the lower incisors when leveling the curve of Spee.

5.4.7 Class I Malocclusion Considerations

Four Premolars Extraction

A typical Class I malocclusion four premolar extraction case is either with severe upper and lower dental crowding or cases with a bimaxillary protrusive dentofacial profile. The case demonstrated is an adult male patient of Asian background. He presented with a bimaxillary protrusive

Class I dental malocclusion on a skeletal Class I base and normal skeletal pattern. He had a protrusive dental profile, incompetent lips, an anterior crossbite with minimal overjet, and overbite (▶ Fig. 5.29a–c).

The treatment plan was to have four first premolars extracted. The Invisalign ClinCheck treatment plan was set up with both optimized and conventional attachments with simultaneous staging. A vertical rectangular attachment was placed on the lingual surface of the upper right lateral incisor for esthetic reasons (▶ Fig. 5.29d).

The compensatory movements in this case included an increased upper incisor lingual root torque of 4 degrees, further intrusion of the lower incisors of 0.6 mm, and increased mesial and distal root tip of the abutment teeth distal and mesial to the extraction sites, respectively, of between 4 and 8 degrees (▶ Fig. 5.26).

Class II elastics were used initially to allow anchorage control and also to maintain a Class I canine relationship. During the refinement stages, posterior box elastics were used in conjunction with the upper anterior precision bite ramps (G5 feature) in order to control the vertical settling of the occlusion (▶ Fig. 5.29e).

The total treatment duration was 26 months with 83 aligners (30 + 17 + 12 + 24) and 3 lots of

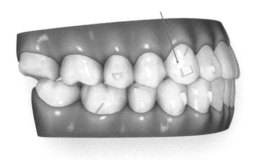

Fig. 5.28 Image showing a conventional attachment on the canine placed to prevent displacement of the aligners during elastic traction.

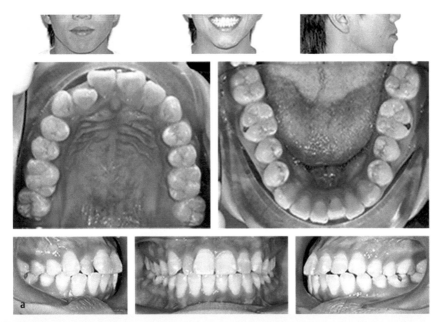

Fig. 5.29 (a) Pretreatment images of an adult Class I malocclusion treated with four first premolars extractions.

(Continued)

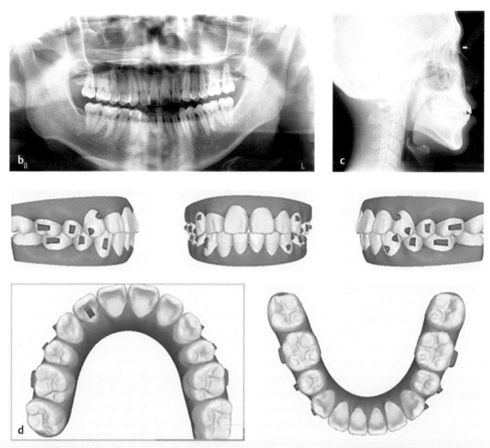

Fig. 5.29 (*Continued*) (**b**) Pretreatment panoramic radiograph, (**c**) pretreatment lateral cephalogram, and (**d**) ClinCheck plans.

(*Continued*)

refinements/additional aligners (▶Fig. 5.29f–i). The refinement/additional aligners were changed weekly.

5.4.8 Class II Malocclusion Considerations

Extraction of Two Upper First Premolars

One of the treatment plans in treating Class II malocclusion cases is the extraction of two upper premolars and completing the case in a therapeutic Class II occlusion. The case demonstrated is an adolescent Asian female with a Class II, division 1 dental malocclusion with a skeletal Class 1 pattern and a vertical to normal growth pattern (▶Fig. 5.30a–c). Her chief concerns were that her upper front teeth stuck out and she wanted to have them retracted with an improvement in her dentofacial profile. She also presented with severe upper and moderate lower dental crowding, a deep lower curve of Spee, and incompetent lips. Her dental midlines were noncoincident.

The upper first premolar teeth were extracted and Invisalign Teen was prescribed. The ClinCheck plans with conventional attachment designs and staging patterns are shown (▶Fig. 5.30d).

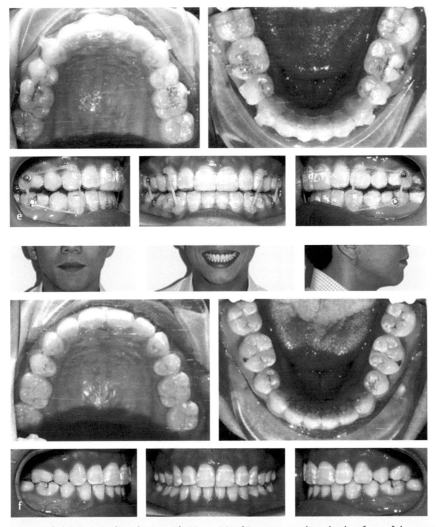

Fig. 5.29 (*Continued*) **(e)** Posterior box elastics with G5 precision bite ramps on the palatal surfaces of the upper incisors. **(f)** Posttreatment images of the case.

(*Continued*)

Class II dental elastics were also used to control the anchorage during space closure. Precision buccal cutouts were designed and buttons were placed to enable controlled retraction and space closure.

The compensatory movements planned in this case were: increased lower incisor intrusion by 0.8 mm, increased distal root tip of the upper canines 6 degrees, and increased mesial root tip of the upper second premolars and first molars by 8 and 6 degrees, respectively.

The case was treated well in 24 months with a total of 51 (37 + 14) aligners with 1 lot of refinement/additional aligners (▶Fig. 5.30e–h).

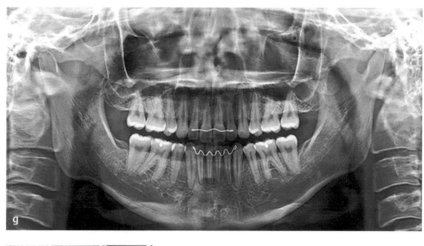

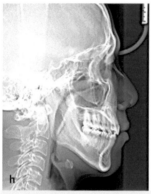

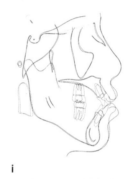

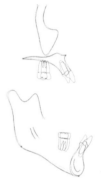

Fig. 5.29 (*Continued*) **(g)** Posttreatment panoramic radiograph. **(h)** Posttreatment lateral cephalogram. **(i)** Overall and regional superimpositions.

5.4.9 Class III Malocclusion Considerations

Extraction of Two Lower Premolars

Lower two premolar extractions in vertical Class III skeletal and dental malocclusion cases is a good camouflage treatment modality for patients who are within the realms of nonsurgical treatment envelope.

This case demonstrated is an adult female patient of Asian descent. Her chief concerns were her crowded dentition. She presented as a Class III dental malocclusion on a skeletal Class III base with a vertical growth pattern. She had bilateral posterior and anterior crossbites, moderately severe upper and lower dental crowding, and minimal overbite and overjet with deviated dental midlines (▶ Fig. 5.31a–c).

A camouflage treatment plan was designed with the extraction of the lower left first and lower right second premolars. The ClinCheck plans show a mixture of optimized and conventional attachment designs, IPR, and simultaneous staging (▶ Fig. 5.31d).

Compensatory movements were planned with increased mesial root tip of the immediate dentition distal to the extraction spaces and increased distal root tip of the immediate dentition mesial to the extraction spaces (▶ Fig. 5.31e). Class III elastics were used to control the anchorage. The plan was to complete the occlusion with a Class I canine and Class III molar dental relationship.

The treatment duration was 22 months with 47 (32 + 15) active aligners with 1 refinement (▶ Fig. 5.31f–i).

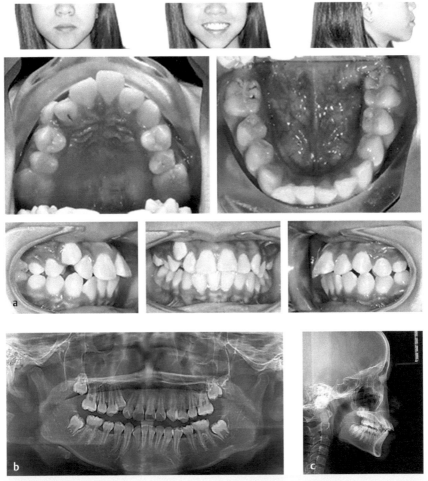

Fig. 5.30 (a) Pretreatment images of a growing child with Class II malocclusion treated with two upper premolars extractions. (b) Pretreatment panoramic radiograph and (c) pretreatment lateral cephalogram.

(Continued)

5.5 Conclusion

Contrary to popular belief, there is no "cookbook formula" to the successful outcome of orthodontic treatment. Biological variation, patient compliance, and the clinicians' expertise all play equally big roles. Hence, the title "routine mechanics for aligner therapy" may be a misnomer after all. Although digital technology, biomaterials, appliance designs, and computing interfaces are improving and ever-changing, the biology of dental movements does not. Therefore, it is essential to fully understand what truly affects the treatment outcome—be it a dilacerated root, the growth potential of the patient, or even certain preexisting parafunctional habits or conditions.

This brief chapter showcases and demonstrates nonextraction and extraction considerations in various scenarios with Class I, Class II, and Class III dental malocclusions. The full extent of treatment with aligner cannot be completely contained within a book. Clinical experience increases over time and it is still important to learn from our mistakes, understand where we have gone wrong, and how to do it right the next time.

Digital-aided orthodontics is here to stay, and aligner therapy remains one of the mainstream orthodontic treatment options within this space.

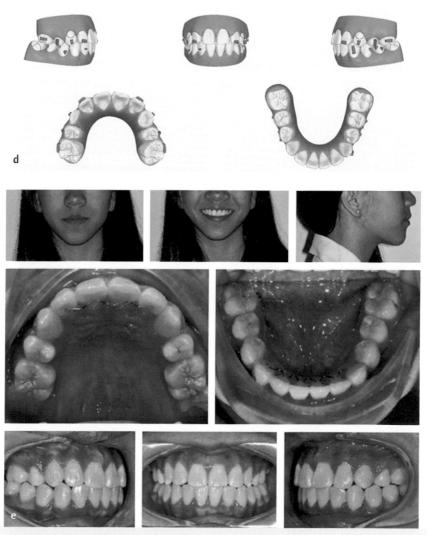

Fig. 5.30 (*Continued*) **(d)** ClinCheck plans. **(e)** Posttreatment images of the case.

(*Continued*)

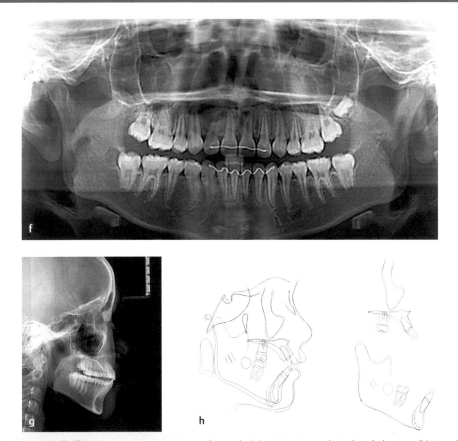

Fig. 5.30 (*Continued*) **(f)** Posttreatment panoramic radiograph. **(g)** Posttreatment lateral cephalogram. **(h)** Overall and regional superimpositions.

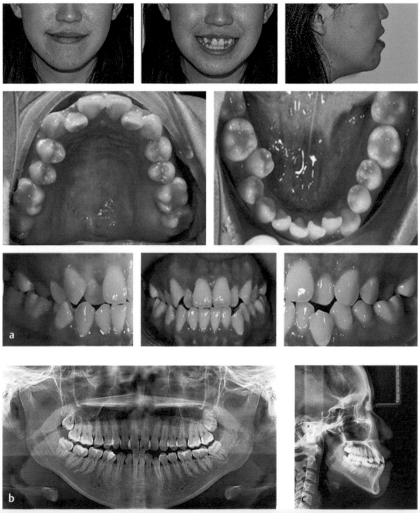

Fig. 5.31 (a) Pretreatment images of an adult Class III malocclusion treated with two lower premolars extractions. (b) Pretreatment panoramic radiograph and (c) pretreatment lateral cephalogram.

(*Continued*)

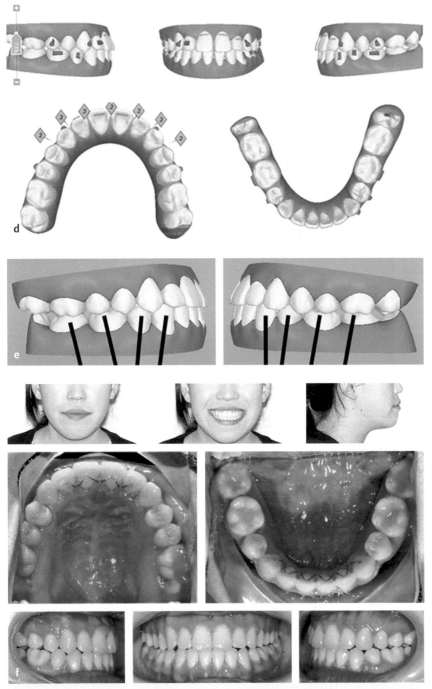

Fig. 5.31 (*Continued*) (**d**) ClinCheck plans. (**e**) Compensatory movements. (**f**) Posttreatment images of the case.

(*Continued*)

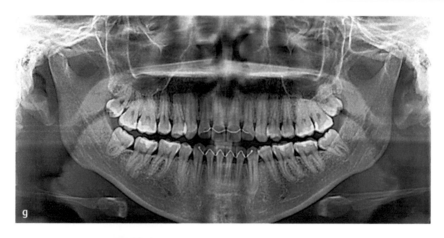

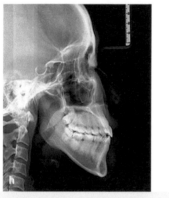
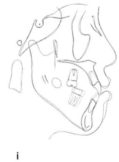
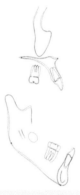

Fig. 5.31 (*Continued*) **(g)** Posttreatment panoramic radiograph. **(h)** Posttreatment lateral cephalogram. **(i)** Overall and regional superimpositions.

References

[1] Meikle MC. The tissue, cellular, and molecular regulation of orthodontic tooth movement: 100 years after Carl Sandstedt. Eur J Orthod. 2006;28(3):221–240

[2] Adkins MD, Nanda RS, Currier GF. Arch perimeter changes on rapid palatal expansion. Am J Orthod Dentofacial Orthop. 1990;97(3):194–199

[3] Baccetti T, Franchi L, Toth LR, McNamara JA, Jr. Treatment timing for Twin-block therapy. Am J Orthod Dentofacial Orthop. 2000;118(2):159–170

[4] Baccetti T, Lorenzo F, McNamara JA, Jr. The Cervical Vertebral Maturation (CVM) method for the assessment of optimal treatment timing in dentofacial orthopedics. Semin Orthod. 2005;11:119–129

[5] Dawson PE. New definition for relating occlusion to varying conditions of the temporomandibular joint. J Prosthet Dent. 1995;74(6):619–627

[6] Roberts WE, Turley PK, Brezniak N, Fielder PJ. Implants: Bone physiology and metabolism. CDA J. 1987;15(10):54–61

[7] Chan EK, Darendeliler MA. The Invisalign appliance today: A thinking person's orthodontic appliance. Semin Orthod. 2017;23:12–64

6 Precautions with Aligner Treatment

Tony Weir, Haylea Louise Blundell, Raj Gaddam, and Amesha Maree

Summary

The acceptance and ratings regarding clear aligners, in particular, are high for both adolescents and adults. Young adults with aligners are considered more attractive and rated higher for intellectual ability and attractiveness than those with the visible buccal fixed appliances. Moreover, current research has given insights on the effects of aligner treatment on parameters known only to the patient, such as quality of life, pain experience, and satisfaction with treatment. As orthodontic treatment with fixed appliances has been associated with impacts on these domains known only to the patient, it is logical to assume that malocclusion correction with clear aligners might be different in terms of patients' experience. Although initial data might indicate positive outcomes on health-related quality of life assessments, pain perception, and satisfaction with treatment, further research is warranted to enhance our insight on clear aligner treatment from the patient's perspective.

Keywords: orthodontic aligners, orthodontic treatment, malocclusion, health-related quality of life, oral health-related quality of life

6.1 Special Care with Aligner Therapy

Much of the current knowledge about Invisalign remains anecdotal. Evidence on clinical outcomes with aligner treatments is sparse and generally of low quality. The available published data are mostly anecdotal case reports, clinician commentaries, in vitro material studies, clinician surveys, and retrospective comparative cohort studies. While there is no doubt that clinically excellent outcomes can be achieved with clear aligners, the routine predictability, parameters, and clinical efficacy and efficiency of aligner treatment are still in doubt. The limitations of aligner therapy have been discussed in the literature[1,2,3,4,5,6,7,8] where the efficacy of such treatment remains controversial. While some clinicians believe aligners can only successfully treat mild to moderate malocclusions,[2,9,10] others have demonstrated their use in the treatment of more severe malocclusions.[11,12,13] Align Technology maintains

an online International Case Gallery which supposedly contains examples of excellent outcomes, yet analysis of this hand-picked cases reveals less than ideal finishes and finishes obtained only after up to five sets of additional aligner orders. Clearly, then, there are challenges in obtaining excellent clinical outcomes routinely with aligners.

The primary author is an accredited provider with four clear aligner products and has previously published a review article comparing and incorporating data from 29 clear aligner products.[14] Due to the introduction of Invisalign as the first and currently the most widely employed clear aligner in the world, most evidence regarding clear aligner efficacy, and hence most of the discussion in this chapter, will be focused on Invisalign appliances. However, it is believed that many of the features displayed by Invisalign aligners with regard to treatment efficacy could be applied to other aligner products, although it seems that currently Invisalign is the most sophisticated and comprehensive appliance available.[14] Most clear aligner products do not have features analogous to Align's ClinCheck program, but most have a predetermined endpoint to the sequence of treatment aligners.

The principal author's role as Clinical Consultant to Invisalign Australia/New Zealand and to Invisalign South Asia has resulted in assessment of in excess of 12,000 cases from other doctors, in addition to approximately 1,000 cases treated by the author. Many of the cases from the above sources are reviewed precisely because they achieve less than ideal outcomes after the initial phase or phases of aligner treatment. This results in a unique and voluminous perspective on problems with aligner treatment outcomes across a large number of doctors in multiple countries with ethnically diverse populations. In turn, this enables assessment and categorization of the routine problems that doctors experience with aligner treatments. This chapter will therefore be more directly pertinent to treatments with Invisalign aligners, although the features identified and some of the studies quoted are applicable to other aligner products.

The reasons why teeth may not be aligned to the same degree as the ClinCheck plan depiction after an initial course of aligner treatment include:

patient cooperation; failure of the ClinCheck plan to translate to reality due to problems with the default protocols applied by Align Technology; failure of aligners to clinically express 100% of movements shown in ClinCheck; and therefore doctor's inexperience regarding what to prescribe in the ClinCheck treatment plan. It is also important to realize that aligner systems are limited in four dimensions in a way that does not apply to fixed appliances. Each of these points will be discussed in this chapter.

It is outside the scope of this chapter to discuss patient cooperation, other than to make the point that aligner treatments in general involve the ultimate compliance appliance, as opposed to the plethora of noncompliance strategies available with fixed appliance therapy.

Regarding the remaining three reasons for failure to completely achieve the originally depicted treatment outcome, it is first necessary to understand some basic features. The failure of full expression of prescribed movements requires the recognition of exactly what ClinCheck is and what aligners are. Conceptually, the teeth and any attachments that may be applied to the teeth are equivalent to brackets in fixed appliance treatment—that is the means by which a force is applied to the teeth. The force itself comes from the aligners, and hence the entire series of aligners equates to the world's most superelastic full-size arch wire, tied into all brackets at the start of treatment and not changed in any way

through treatment, until additional aligners are ordered. Therefore, the ClinCheck plan is equivalent to the arch wire design to achieve an ideal clinical outcome, not the ideal clinical outcome in itself—i.e., a ClinCheck plan should not be the final finished outcome. With fixed appliances, we place overexpanded arch wires to correct transverse discrepancies, and reverse-curved of Spee arch wires to open bites, not because we want the final occlusion to match the shape of the arch wire, but because we recognize the need to place overcorrections within our fixed appliance systems to overcome the shortfalls in expression inherent in those systems.

Align Technology lays claim to having treated 6.8 million patients as of Q1 2019,[15] and describes the Invisalign appliance as a "bespoke" individually tailored appliance, constructed using the accumulated experience derived from the data from all the treatments to date. However, Align Technology makes more than 250,000 aligners per day, which equates to approximately 5,000 cases per day. Thus, all attachment and malocclusion protocols applied by Align Technology are, to some unavoidable extent, based on averages—a "one size fits all" approach. Since the mean is a lonely place statistically, reliance by the doctor on standard protocols for tooth movements and attachments is not likely to result in consistently excellent clinical outcomes (▶ Fig. 6.1). The use of overcorrection and the limitations of the aligner as an arch wire, plus the current limited

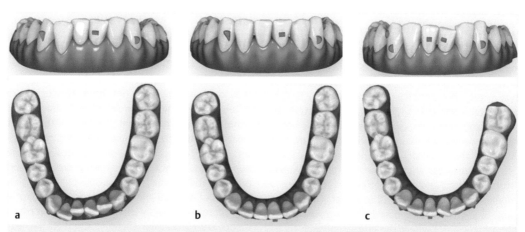

a   b   c

Fig. 6.1 (a) Initial alignment. Note Align default protocol places an optimized extrusion attachment on 31. Failure to upright 31 is the more critical movement as uprighting will determine the arch length required for 31 to fit into the aligner. (b) Planned final alignment according to the accepted ClinCheck plan. (c) Actual alignment achieved as depicted at the beginning of an additional aligner order. Note failure to upright, rotate, or extrude 31 due to arch length issues. Note also the same default attachment is again placed!

suite of attachments available for selection, can negatively impact the treatment outcome.

The clinical outcomes with aligner treatments that are routinely less than desirable include rotations (of incisors as well as more rounded teeth), transverse expansion, correction of deep overbites, and movement of roots through bone (root uprighting and torque)[6,10,13,16–35] (see also Appendices A, B, C, D, E, F). Overcorrections as a part of the ClinCheck plan are therefore an essential approach to overcome the routine shortfalls experienced in these areas if lengthy additional aligner orders are to be avoided.

The single most important biomechanical concept that is necessary to know about aligners is that, to a much more significant extent than fixed appliances, aligners limit tooth movement in four dimensions, namely length, breadth, height (vertical), and in timing of movements. Dental arches are three-dimensional objects, as are aligners. The dental arches must fit entirely within the three-dimensional constraints of the aligner, and if they do not, we get intruding and nontracking teeth. With fixed appliances, unless the arch wire is absolutely cinched back and is totally full-sized in the bracket slot, teeth can tip and move around the arch (▶ Fig. 6.2). Therefore, failure to provide the space required by the three-dimensional constraints of the aligner, by failing to either appropriately upright a tooth (▶ Fig. 6.3) or do planned interproximal reduction (IPR) accurately (▶ Fig. 6.4), results in a tooth becoming too

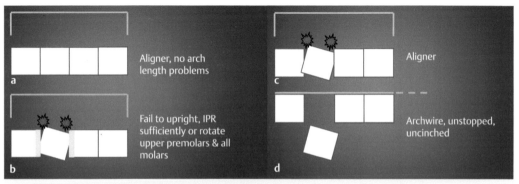

Fig. 6.2 The importance of the three-dimensional limitations imposed by aligners. **(a)** The objects ("teeth") fit uniformly into the "aligner." **(b)** A nonaligned tooth may require space to be made via uprighting or rotation or interproximal reduction or expansion. **(c)** If the required space is not made, the tooth cannot fit within the confines of the aligner. **(d)** With an arch wire, unless absolutely full-sized and completely cinched back, the teeth can move along the arch wire and align with fewer serious consequences.

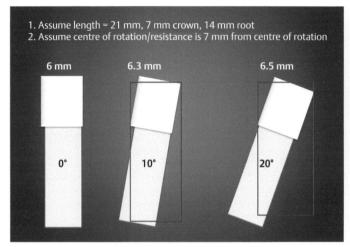

Fig. 6.3 The effect of mesiodistal tip of a theoretical lower incisor on arch length occupied.

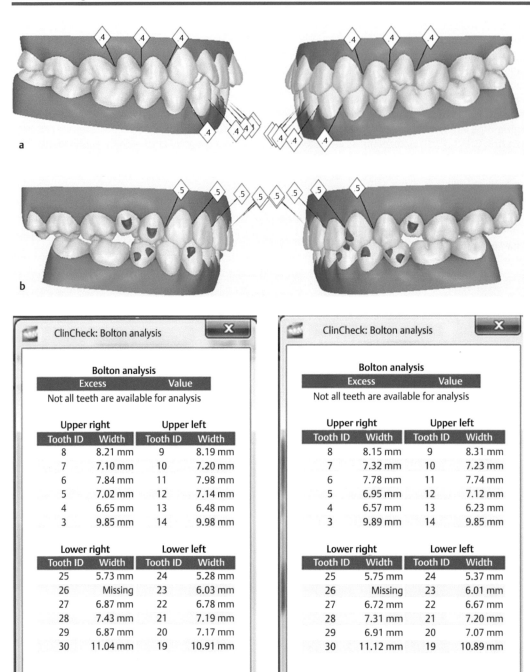

Fig. 6.4 (a) Initial alignment. Note IPR planned for upper arch. **(b)** Alignment achieved after initial course of treatment. **(c)** Tooth size measurements at treatment start. **(d)** Tooth size measurements at additional aligners. Note the 1.2 mm of IPR on each side of the upper arch was essentially NOT performed to any meaningful degree. This results in 15, 25 not having room to align and thus intruding (the watermelon seed effect).

big to fit in the aligner and stops tracking. With fixed appliances, the teeth can adjust around the arch wire. A similar situation exists when expansion is used to align teeth and fails to fully express according to the aligner dimensions. Essentially, this means that exquisite levels of detail are required in designing a ClinCheck plan and in carrying out treatment with aligners—details that are less important with fixed appliance treatments which are inherently less constrained in the four dimensions outlined above.

The dimension of time is important because with fixed appliances teeth are free to move, with arch wires that have a reasonable range of action, at the rate biology permits. With aligners, teeth are constrained to move at the rate that aligners permit depending on the prescribed rate of change. This may mean a patient is better suited to less or more than two-weekly aligner change, and there is certainly no published evidence for shorter than two-weekly intervals of aligner change with Invisalign.[1,31] Some patients may even benefit from longer than two-weekly change depending on biologic, anatomic, and movement complexity factors. With fixed appliances, the desired movement happens at the rate it happens. With aligners, either the movement happens at the rate of aligner change or it stops tracking. Thus, aligners are less forgiving in all four dimensions as far as alignment is concerned.

Uprighting an anterior tooth increases the space available for subsequent derotation.[36] In relation to a maxillary central incisor, uprighting can influence dental arch length. Careful visual inspection of the need for uprighting should be performed. Hussels and Nanda in 1987 formulated a simple mathematical equation for maxillary central incisor angulation and inclination as described earlier in the review.[37]

In addition, Align Technology default protocols mean that often teeth that require significant uprighting get no attachment or an attachment unsuited to uprighting the tooth.

Since tooth uprighting is required for adequate space availability prior to rotational movement, incisor uprighting must also be factored in. It has been determined by basic mathematical analysis that each 5-degree shortfall in root uprighting of a lower incisor reduces the space available for rotation or other alignment of the incisor by 0.2 to 0.3 mm. Incomplete incisor uprighting may therefore affect the ability of aligners to complete rotational movements (▶ Fig. 6.3).

Shortfalls in movements with aligners when comparing intended outcomes to actual clinical outcomes have been noted in the literature. Tables highlighting the published literature are presented in the Appendices. It would appear that aligner treatment allows certain tooth movements such as crown tip for alignment to be conducted with efficiency and accuracy (Appendices A and B), but it struggles to achieve desirable root movements (Appendices B, C, and D), extrusion (Appendix E), intrusion (Appendix F), and rotations (Appendix G). The best synthesis of these tables is that movements requiring root movement through bone such as root uprighting and torque generally express at 60 to 80% of the amount predicted by the ClinCheck. Similarly, data for rotations and transverse expansion indicate shortfalls of similar magnitude and thus clinical significance. Potentially, the most problematic shortfall for all aligner treatments, however, is in the treatment of deep bites.

As previously mooted, little published evidence is available for non-Invisalign aligner treatments. Lombardo and co-workers in 2017 determined that the average accuracy of movements achieved with F22 aligners was 73.6%. The accuracy of tooth movement in ascending order was 66.8% for rotation, 72.9% for labiolingual tipping movements, and 82.5% for mesiodistal tipping.[38] Weir in 2017 was unable to find any published evidence at all for the vast majority of the 29 clear aligner products reviewed, and hence it is likely that these products perform no better than Invisalign and likely much worse.[14] Clearly, further study in this area is needed to substantiate the claims made by the providers of clear aligners for the efficacy of their appliances.

6.2 Conclusion

Knowledge of shortfalls in movement expression with aligners would allow doctors to incorporate the appropriate overcorrections into their ClinCheck treatment plans to hopefully avoid at least some of the problems associated with under-expressed movements. Similarly, knowledge of problems with ClinCheck default protocols should result in improved protocols or else the treating doctor must carefully adjust the protocols for each patient based on both research and experience. Finally, recognition of the significant four-dimensional constraints that aligners place upon tooth movement and their effects on those subsequent movements should result in improved clinical outcomes.

Aligner treatment remains a relatively new option in the orthodontic armamentarium, and the quality of the appliances constructed and the research knowledge base related to treatment outcomes are still far from ideal. Doctors with significant experience, often gained as a result of personal trial and error, can produce routine good outcomes with aligners. Reliance on the manufacturers for appliance construction and tooth movement planning will not result in such routine desirable outcomes. Aligner treatment is not easy, is prone to poor outcomes, and, without an extremely high level of competence on the part of the treating doctor, remains significantly weaker in terms of clinical outcomes.

References

[1] Zheng M, Liu R, Ni Z, Yu Z. Efficiency, effectiveness and treatment stability of clear aligners: A systematic review and meta-analysis. Orthod Craniofac Res. 2017;20(3):127–133

[2] Boyd RL, Vlaskalic V. Three-dimensional diagnosis and orthodontic treatment of complex malocclusions with the invisalign appliance. Semin Orthod. 2001;7:274–293

[3] Boyd RL, Miller RJ, Vlaskalic V. The invisalign system in adult orthodontics: Mild crowding and space closure cases. J Clin Orthod. 2000;34:203–212

[4] Rossini G, Parrini S, Castroflorio T, Deregibus A, Debernardi CL. Efficacy of clear aligners in controlling orthodontic tooth movement: a systematic review. Angle Orthod. 2015;85(5):881–889

[5] Rossini G, Parrini S, Deregibus A, Castroflorio T. Controlling orthodontic tooth movement with clear aligners: An updated systematic review regarding efficacy and efficiency. J Aligner Orthod. 2017;1:7–20

[6] Kravitz ND, Kusnoto B, BeGole E, Obrez A, Agran B. How well does Invisalign work? A prospective clinical study evaluating the efficacy of tooth movement with Invisalign. Am J Orthod Dentofacial Orthop. 2009;135(1):27–35

[7] Galan-Lopez L, Barcia-Gonzalez J, Plasencia E. A systematic review of the accuracy and efficiency of dental movements with Invisalign®. Korean J Orthod. 2019;49(3):140–149

[8] Papadimitriou A, Mousoulea S, Gkantidis N, Kloukos D. Clinical effectiveness of Invisalign® orthodontic treatment: a systematic review. Prog Orthod. 2018;19(1):37

[9] Gu J, Tang JS, Skulski B, et al. Evaluation of Invisalign treatment effectiveness and efficiency compared with conventional fixed appliances using the Peer Assessment Rating index. Am J Orthod Dentofacial Orthop. 2017;151(2):259–266

[10] Djeu G, Shelton C, Maganzini A. Outcome assessment of Invisalign and traditional orthodontic treatment compared with the American Board of Orthodontics objective grading system. Am J Orthod Dentofacial Orthop. 2005;128(3):292–298, discussion 298

[11] Wheeler TT. Orthodontic clear aligner treatment. Semin Orthod. 2017;23:83–89

[12] Vlaskalic V, Boyd RL. Clinical evolution of the Invisalign appliance. J Calif Dent Assoc. 2002;30(10):769–776

[13] Li W, Wang S, Zhang Y. The effectiveness of the Invisalign appliance in extraction cases using the the ABO model grading system: a multicenter randomized controlled trial. Int J Clin Exp Med. 2015;8(5):8276–8282

[14] Weir T. Clear aligners in orthodontic treatment. Aust Dent J. 2017;62(Suppl 1):58–62

[15] Q1 2019 Align Corporate fact sheet. Available at: https://www.aligntech.com/documents/Align%20Technology%20Corp%20Fact%20Sheet%202019%20Q1.pdf. Align Technology, 2019

[16] Pavoni C, Lione R, Laganà G, Cozza P. Self-ligating versus Invisalign: analysis of dento-alveolar effects. Ann Stomatol (Roma). 2011;2(1–2):23–27

[17] Krieger E, Seiferth J, Marinello I, et al. Invisalign® treatment in the anterior region: were the predicted tooth movements achieved? J Orofac Orthop. 2012;73(5):365–376

[18] Grünheid T, Gaalaas S, Hamdan H, Larson BE. Effect of clear aligner therapy on the buccolingual inclination of mandibular canines and the intercanine distance. Angle Orthod. 2016;86(1):10–16

[19] Solano-Mendoza B, Sonnemberg B, Solano-Reina E, Iglesias-Linares A. How effective is the Invisalign® system in expansion movement with Ex30' aligners? Clin Oral Investig. 2017;21(5):1475–1484

[20] Grünheid T, Loh C, Larson BE. How accurate is Invisalign in nonextraction cases? Are predicted tooth positions achieved? Angle Orthod. 2017;87(6):809–815

[21] Houle JP, Piedade L, Todescan R, Jr, Pinheiro FH. The predictability of transverse changes with Invisalign. Angle Orthod. 2017;87(1):19–24

[22] Clements KM, Bollen AM, Huang G, King G, Hujoel P, Ma T. Activation time and material stiffness of sequential removable orthodontic appliances. Part 2: Dental improvements. Am J Orthod Dentofacial Orthop. 2003;124(5):502–508

[23] Kassas W, Al-Jewair T, Preston CB, Tabbaa S. Assessment of Invisalign treatment outcomes using the ABO Model Grading System. J World Fed Orthod. 2013;2:e61–e64

[24] Buschang PH, Ross M, Shaw SG, Crosby D, Campbell PM. Predicted and actual end-of-treatment occlusion produced with aligner therapy. Angle Orthod. 2015;85(5):723–727

[25] Simon M, Keilig L, Schwarze J, Jung BA, Bourauel C. Forces and moments generated by removable thermoplastic aligners: incisor torque, premolar derotation, and molar distalization. Am J Orthod Dentofacial Orthop. 2014;145(6):728–736

[26] Tai C. How Accurate Is Invisalign? Are Predicted Tooth Positions Achieved? [Dissertation]. Minneapolis, MN: University of Minnesota;2017

[27] Castroflorio T, Garino F, Lazzaro A, Debernardi C. Upper-incisor root control with Invisalign appliances. J Clin Orthod. 2013;47(6):346–351, quiz 387

[28] Zhang XJ, He L, Guo HM, Tian J, Bai YX, Li S. Integrated three-dimensional digital assessment of accuracy of anterior tooth movement using clear aligners. Korean J Orthod. 2015;45(6):275–281

[29] Ravera S, Castroflorio T, Garino F, Daher S, Cugliari G, Deregibus A. Maxillary molar distalization with aligners in adult patients: a multicenter retrospective study. Prog Orthod. 2016;17:12

[30] Garino F, Castroflorio T, Daher S, et al. Effectiveness of composite attachments in controlling upper-molar movement with aligners. J Clin Orthod. 2016;50(6):341–347

[31] Hennessy J, Garvey T, Al-Awadhi EA. A randomized clinical trial comparing mandibular incisor proclination produced by fixed labial appliances and clear aligners. Angle Orthod. 2016;86(5):706–712

[32] Duncan LO, Piedade L, Lekic M, Cunha RS, Wiltshire WA. Changes in mandibular incisor position and arch form resulting from Invisalign correction of the crowded dentition treated nonextraction. Angle Orthod. 2016;86(4):577–583

[33] Zhou N, Guo J. Efficiency of upper arch expansion with the Invisalign system. Angle Orthod. 2019:(e-pub ahead of print)

[34] Charalampakis O, Iliadi A, Ueno H, Oliver DR, Kim KB. Accuracy of clear aligners: A retrospective study of patients who needed refinement. Am J Orthod Dentofacial Orthop. 2018;154(1):47–54

[35] Katchooi M, Cohanim B, Tai S, Bayirli B, Spiekerman C, Huang G. Effect of supplemental vibration on orthodontic treatment with aligners: A randomized trial. Am J Orthod Dentofacial Orthop. 2018;153(3):336–346

[36] Siatkowski RE. Incisor uprighting: mechanism for late secondary crowding in the anterior segments of the dental arches. Am J Orthod. 1974;66(4):398–410

[37] Hussels W, Nanda RS. Effect of maxillary incisor angulation and inclination on arch length. Am J Orthod Dentofacial Orthop. 1987;91(3):233–239

[38] Lombardo L, Arreghini A, Ramina F, Huanca Ghislanzoni LT, Siciliani G. Predictability of orthodontic movement with orthodontic aligners: a retrospective study. Prog Orthod. 2017;18(1):35

[39] Khosravi R, Cohanim B, Hujoel P, et al. Management of overbite with the Invisalign appliance. Am J Orthod Dentofacial Orthop. 2017;151(4):691–699.e2

[40] Kravitz ND, Kusnoto B, Agran B, Viana G. Influence of attachments and interproximal reduction on the accuracy of canine rotation with Invisalign. A prospective clinical study. Angle Orthod. 2008;78(4):682–687

Appendices (Aligner Efficiency in Individual Tooth Movements)

Adapted from Rossini et al[5]

Appendix A: Alignment

Study	Accuracy of predicted movement, improvement achieved with treatment, and comments
Clements et al[22]	Overall weighted PAR reduction by 31% Weighted PAR reduction with 2-week wear with hard material: 43.74%
Djeu et al[10]	No statistical difference in OGS-ABO scores
Kassas et al[23]	Statistically and clinically significant improvement in ABO model grading scores (pretreatment 15.16 ± 5.00 vs. posttreatment 6.00 ± 3.78)
Buschang et al[24]	4.0 point deductions in ABO-OGS scores for aligners in comparison to 1.0 deduction with fixed appliances. Fixed appliances usually deliver a superior level of finishing and detailing to that achieved with aligners
Li et al[13]	ABO-OGS points lost in posttreatment: mean: −9.91; SD: 3.56 Significant improvement in alignment

Appendix B: Labiolingual Inclination: Tipping

Study	Accuracy of predicted movement, improvement achieved with treatment, and comments
Kravitz et al[6]	Mesiodistal tip average of 40.5%, mandibular canines worst at 26.9% Retracting teeth is almost twice as accurate as labial expansion Invisalign is efficient in closing anterior spaces, especially in the mandibular arch, when compared to correction of crowding by labial proclination
Kassas et al[23]	Space closure of up to 6 mm by tipping teeth into extraction spaces Invisalign is efficient in tipping movement
Hennessy et al[31]	Mandibular incisor proclination: Statistically insignificant difference between fixed appliances and aligners Marginally higher protrusion of lower incisors with fixed appliances is due to canine tip in the brackets and to the force application in the Invisalign group being close to the long axis of teeth Results show Invisalign capability in relieving mandibular incisor crowding by protrusion is no larger, but indeed smaller than fixed appliances
Duncan et al[32]	Mandibular incisor proclination in different categories of crowding: <6 mm (mild, moderate): no significant lower incisor proclination >6 mm (severe): mandibular incisor proclination is seen by almost 4 degrees

Appendix C: Labiolingual Inclination: Torque

Study	Accuracy of predicted movement, improvement achieved with treatment, and comments
Djeu et al[10]	ABO-OGS scores: Invisalign lost 4.19 points, while fixed appliances lost 2.81
Kravitz et al[6]	Labial crown tip worse than palatal crown tip (37.6 vs. 53.1%), especially with maxillary incisors Overcorrection can be planned for proclining maxillary central incisors but can be avoided while retroclining flared maxillary lateral incisors among Class II, division 2 patients
Kassas et al[2,3]	Statistically and clinically significant improvement in ABO model grading scores (pretreatment 7.00 ± 3.14 vs. posttreatment 6.26 ± 3.58)
Castroflorio et al[27]	Mean torque values for upper incisors at T0 were 20.95 degrees on the virtual setups and 21.12 degrees on scanned casts; at T1, torque values were 10.55 and 10.53 degrees, respectively. Mean change in torque for the virtual setups between T1 and T0 represented the torque prescription, 10.4 degrees Preliminary study of Power Ridges demonstrates that when torque correction of about 10 degrees is required, torque loss is negligible

(Continued)

Study	Accuracy of predicted movement, improvement achieved with treatment, and comments
Simon et al[25]	Incisor torque accuracy (%) Torque loss approximately 50% Study of old aligner material (Ex30) not current SmartTrack LD30
Buschang et al[24]	4.0 point deductions in ABO-OGS scores in comparison to 3.0 deduction with fixed appliances.
Li et al[13]	ABO-OGS points lost in posttreatment: Buccolingual inclination: Invisalign: mean: –3.55 degrees, SD: 1.36 degrees Fixed appliances: mean: –5.85, SD: 2.68 Root angulation: Invisalign: mean: –4.79 degrees, SD: 1.45 degrees Fixed appliances: mean: –4.68 degrees, SD: 2.32 degrees Root control with Invisalign is statistically significantly inferior to fixed appliances
Zhang et al[28]	Achieved vs. predicted mean difference in tooth position Crown: Maxilla: mean: 0.376 mm, SD: 0.041 mm Mandible: mean: 0.398 mm, SD: 0.037 mm Root: Maxilla: mean: 2.062 mm, SD: 0.128 mm Mandible: mean: 1.941 mm, SD: 0.154 mm ClinCheck overestimates root positions that could be delivered by the appliance
Ravera et al[29]	Maxillary central incisor edge was retracted by 2.23 mm ($p < 0.01$) with insignificant vertical change ($p = 0.43$) Maxillary incisors did not significantly change in terms of angular relationship with palatal plane (pretreatment: mean 109.60 degrees with SD 6.70 degrees, posttreatment mean 106.70 degrees with SD 6.66 degrees, $p < 0.05$)
Garino et al[30]	Root movement (1.86 mm) was pronounced in comparison to crown movement (0.13 mm at tips and 0.83 mm at crown centre) when posterior teeth have square attachments on first molars and premolars Crown movement (2.48 mm at tips and 1.58 mm at crown centre) was more pronounced than root movement (1.31 mm) when square attachments are placed on canines, premolars, and molars More proclination of maxillary incisors than torque (root movement) in the Invisalign group with attachments on canines, premolars, and molars than the group with attachments only on premolars and first molars
Grünheid et al[20]	Maxillary central incisors: mean: 1.75 degrees, SD: 2.86 degrees (0.86, 2.65) of difference between predicted and actual outcome Clinically significant difference was noticed with maxillary second molars, with a torque difference of >2 degrees Maxillary central incisors tipped rather than moved bodily. Maxillary lateral incisor position was accurate despite smaller size of the teeth
Tai[26]	Statistically significant difference between predicted and achieved outcome Maxillary teeth: Canines: 1.75 ± 2.86 degrees Second premolar: –1.18 ± 3.27 degrees First molar: –1.45 ± 3.37 degrees Second molar: –2.13 ± 4.19 degrees Mandibular teeth: Canine: –1.60 ± 2.04 degrees First molar: –0.85 ± 2.41 degrees Second molar: –1.09 ± 2.13 degrees
Zhou and Guo[33]	Bodily expansion efficiency of the maxillary first molar was 36.35 ± 29.32%, and the ratio of the expansion movement between the root and crown was approximately 2:5. The maxillary first molar buccally tipped 2.07 ± 3.27 degrees after expansion

Appendix D: Transverse Plane

Study	Accuracy of predicted movement, improvement achieved with treatment, and comments
Kravitz et al[6]	Lingual constriction: 47.1%, with best results in mandibular canine (59.3%) and mandibular lateral incisor (54.8%)
Pavoni et al[16]	Average expansion obtained: Invisalign: Canine cusp width 0.50 mm, canine gingival width 0.05 mm First premolar cusp width 0.05 mm, First premolar gingival width 0.15 mm Second premolar cusp width 0.45 mm, second premolar cusp width 0.30 mm, Molar cusp width 0.5 mm, molar cusp width 0.05 mm Fixed appliances (self-ligating): Canine cusp width 3.15 mm, canine gingival width 0.8 mm First premolar cusp width 3.4 mm, first premolar cusp width 2.45 mm Second premolar cusp width 2.5 mm, second premolar cusp width 2.15 mm, Molar cusp width 0.9 mm, molar gingival width 0.3 mm
Kreiger et al[6]	Intercanine distance: Less by −0.13 ± 0.59 mm (maxillary) and −0.13 ± 0.59 mm (mandibular) Dental midline deviation: Less by −0.24 ± 0.46 mm Statistically and clinically insignificant
Grünheid et al[18]	Increase in intercanine width (mean: 0.7 mm, SD: 1.5 mm from Invisalign in comparison to fixed appliances (mean: −0.1 mm, SD: 2.4 mm) Difference too small to be clinically relevant
Solano-Mendoza et al[19]	Achieved expansion in comparison to predicted ClinCheck values was less: Mandibular arch: maximum of −1.817 mm (molar cusp tips) to minimum of −0.678 mm (cuspid tips). Maxillary arch: maximum of −1.32 mm (molar cusp tips) and a minimum of −0.35 mm (canine gingival margin). Average expansion achieved: cuspid canine width 1.38 mm, canine gingival width 0.54 mm, first premolar gingival width 1.39 mm, second premolar gingival width 1.25 mm, and molar gingival width 0.56 mm Invisalign overestimates the expansion in molar area compared to cuspid area in ClinCheck models
Grünheid et al[20]	Maxillary posterior teeth more lingually positioned with greater than predicted buccal crown torque Maxillary molars tipped rather than moved bodily
Houle et al[21]	Transverse changes in maxillary arch: 72.8% overall, 82.9% accurate at cusp tips, and 62.7% near the gingival margins. At the first molar gingival margin, accuracy was least (52.9%) Transverse changes in mandibular arch: Overall accuracy 87.7%, with 98.9% at cusp tips and 76.4% near the gingival margin. Mandibular canines have the largest prediction error: 62% accuracy Authors recommend overcorrecting maxillary arch posterior expansion
Charalampakis et al[34]	Interpremolar expansion was accurate for both arches, as was mandibular canine expansion. Maxillary canine expansion was not
Zhou and Guo[33]	Significant differences between the expected and actual expansion amounts Average expansion efficiencies of the upper canine crown, first premolar crown, second premolar crown, and first molar crown were 79.75 ± 15.23%, 76.1 ± 18.32%, 73.27 ± 19.91%, and 68.31 ± 24.41%, respectively. The average efficiency of bodily expansion movement for the maxillary first molar was 36.35 ±29.32%

Appendix E: Vertical Plane: Intrusion

Study	Accuracy of predicted movement, improvement achieved with treatment, and comments
Kravitz et al[6]	Maxillary central incisors 44.7% and mandibular central incisors 46.6% Despite improvements in overbite, deep bite correction seems to be difficult
Krieger et al[17]	Achieved overbite correction is less than predicted correction in ClinCheck models by −0.71 ± 0.87 mm Vertical tooth movements are more difficult to achieve with the Invisalign technique than transverse or sagittal tooth movements
Khosravi et al[39]	Median overbite opening of 1.5 mm by proclination of mandibular incisors and maxillary incisor intrusion Mandibular plane angle remained unchanged with minimal vertical changes in molars The severe deep bite cases in this study were not able to be corrected with Invisalign restricting the benefits to mild to moderate cases only
Tai[26]	Differences between the predicted and actual outcome is less than 0.5 mm Good vertical predictability, but the discrepancy in maxillary central incisors, being more occlusal, could be relevant, which could need some overcorrections

Appendix F: Vertical Plane: Extrusion

Study	Accuracy of predicted movement, improvement achieved with treatment, and comments
Kravitz et al[6]	Extrusion accuracy 29.6%, with lowest being maxillary canines (18.3%) and mandibular central incisors (24.5%)
Khosravi et al[39]	Open bite patients had an average bite deepening of 1.5 mm by maxillary and mandibular incisor extrusion (change in U1 - palatal plane = 0.9 mm, change in L1 - mandibular plane = 0.8 mm) as noted in posttreatment cephalometric analysis Mandibular plane angle experienced insignificant changes. There were similar findings with the molars in vertical height

Appendix G: Rotations

Study	Accuracy of predicted movement, improvement achieved with treatment, and comments
Kravitz et al[40]	Mean accuracy of canine rotation: Overall Invisalign: 35.8% (SD: 26.3%) IPR only group: 43.1% Attachment only group: 33.3% No attachments, no IPR group: 30.8% Difference between individual groups is not statistically significant
Kravitz et al[6]	Rotation accuracy of maxillary canines (32.2%) and mandibular canines (29.1%), maxillary central incisors (54.2%). Approximately one-third of predicted rotation achieved in maxillary and mandibular canines. Rotational accuracy for canines was significantly lower than that of all other teeth, with the exception of the maxillary lateral incisors. Accuracy for maxillary canines was significantly reduced at rotational movements greater than 15 degrees
Krieger et al[17]	Predicted outcomes were achieved even in severe pretreatment crowding cases (≥10 mm of contact point deviation under Little's Irregularity Index).
Simon et al[25]	Mean accuracy of premolar derotation with attachments: <15 degrees: 43.3% (SD: 0.24) >15 degrees: 23.6% (SD: 0.15) Mean accuracy of premolar derotation without attachments: <15 degress:42.4% (SD: 0.24) >15 degrees: 37.5% (SD: 0.15) Study conducted using old aligner material (Exceed30), in comparison to the later version (Smart-Track LD30)
Solano-Mendoza et al[19]	No statistically difference between the predicted and the final outcome values seen
Grünheid et al[20]	Mean 1.71 mm, SD: 2.91 mm of reduced final outcome in comparison to predicted rotations in mandibular first premolars Rotation of rounded teeth may be incomplete
Tai[26]	Statistically significant difference between predicted and actual outcome is only seen in mandibular arch Lower incisors: −0.99 ± 2.28 mm Canines: 0.88 ± 3.14 mm First premolars: −1.71 ± 2.91 mm Second premolars: 0.88 ± 3.86 mm Rounded teeth are difficult to get complete rotational correction
Charalampakis et al[34]	All achieved rotations were significantly smaller than predicted ones. Canines had the greatest discrepancies—3.05 degrees (maxillary) and 2.45 degrees (mandibular). The maxillary premolars had the lowest discrepancy of only 0.9 degrees

7 Clear Plastic Appliances as Retainers

Simon J. Littlewood

Summary

Clear plastic appliances have been used as retainers for over 50 years. They are esthetic, and are easy and economical to manufacture. There are three main types of plastic that can be used: polyethylene, polypropylene, and polyurethane. The commonest design involves full occlusal coverage of the dentition, and there is good evidence to suggest that they only need to be worn at night. There is a lack of high-quality evidence to compare them to other types of retainers. The best current evidence would seem to suggest that, at least in the short term, compared to Hawley retainers clear plastic retainers are equally effective at retaining the maxillary dentition and possibly slightly better at retaining the mandibular dentition. Patients may prefer wearing them to Hawley retainers as they are less embarrassing to wear, and they may be more cost-effective. Compared with bonded retainers, they are equally effective at retaining the upper arch, but may be very slightly less effective at retaining the lower arch. However, patients find them easier to look after than bonded retainers and maintenance is simpler. Interestingly, persuading patients to wear clear plastic plastics in the long-term has been shown to be a problem. Occlusal settling is slower with clear plastic retainers due to full occlusal coverage, but will happen if worn at night only. Current evidence would seem to suggest they are relatively safe, provided the patients keep them clean and avoid drinking cariogenic drinks while wearing them. The longevity of clear plastic retainers is unknown, and patients must know how to identify problems with them and who to contact when they need replacements.

Keywords: orthodontic retainers, polyethylene, polyp-ropylene, polyurethane, vacuum-formed, thermoplastic, compliance, longevity

7.1 Introduction

Clear plastic appliances have been used as removable retainers for many years. In fact, the use of clear plastic as retainers predates the recent growth in popularity of clear plastic aligners. The aim of this chapter is to provide an overview of the use of clear plastic appliances as retainers, describing a contemporary overview of the different materials that are used, a guide to their clinical management, and the current evidence to support their use.

7.2 Historical Background to Clear Plastic Retainers

For many years, variations of the Hawley retainer, a removable retainer fabricated from acrylic and stainless steel wires, were the most popular retainers in orthodontics. However, in the late 1950s, Nahoum[1] developed a "vacuum-formed dental contour appliance" that could be used to retain teeth, with Ponitz[2] describing it as invisible retainer in the orthodontic literature in 1971. Initially, the popularity of these vacuum-formed retainers was limited by reliability problems, with the plastic often failing or cracking. However, by the early 1990s, specific plastics were developed that were better suited to the properties required from a retainer.[3] These new plastics showed less distortion and were less prone to cracking.

The newer retainers, known commercially as "Essix" retainers, proved to be more reliable and mechanically sound, and helped to increase the popularity of clear plastic as retainers. Since this time, there has been a gradual increase in the use of clear plastic retainers, with manufacturers trying to improve the qualities of improved esthetics, increased mechanical strength and resistance to stress relaxation, and increased wear resistance, while at the same time ensuring the clear plastic retainers were biocompatible, and easy and economical to make. This chapter will describe different types of plastics that are used to manufacture retainers.

7.3 Worldwide Use of Clear Plastic Retainers

The use of orthodontic retainers differs markedly throughout the world, as shown from surveys of orthodontic clinicians' retention practice.[3,10,11,12] Clear plastic retainers are the most popular retainers in both arches in the United Kingdom,[8] Malaysia,[4] and Ireland,[11] and are the first-choice retainers in the upper arch in Australia and New Zealand.[12] They are also often used in a form of "dual retention," along with a bonded retainer.[10] It is unclear why clear plastic retainers are used differently around the world. This may relate to differences in patient expectation, health care systems, malocclusions, or clinician choice.[13]

7.4 Types of Materials and Methods of Production

There are essentially three types of plastics commonly used to make clear plastic retainers:
- Polyethylene (polyethylene terephthalate-glycol).
- Polypropylene.
- Polyurethane.

7.5 Polyethylene and Polypropylene Retainers

Polyethylene and polypropylene are both known as thermoplastics. Thermoplastics are plastics that can be reheated and changed back into their original state. Usually, they are initially manufactured as small pellets, which can then be heated and formed into the desired shape.

In contrast, polyurethane is a thermoset plastic. This means it is generally formed using heat, but once cooled and set, it cannot be returned to its original state.

The properties of polyethylene and polypropylene retainers differ:
- Polyethylene is clearer and therefore slightly more esthetic (▶ Fig. 7.1).
- Polyethylene is stiffer. This means any significant undercuts need to blocked out on the cast with a thermally stable material, before the retainer is formed. In contrast, polypropylene is typically slightly more flexible, making it more comfortable when engaging and removing from multiple undercuts.

- Polyethylene is more resistant to wear. This has been shown in laboratory wear tests,[14,15] suggesting that polyethylene retainers may be more resistant to wear in the long term than polypropylene retainers. It should be noted that clear plastic retainers are not as resistant to wear as traditional Hawley retainers, made of polymethyl methacrylate,[16] although the latter is more brittle and prone to fracture.
- It is possible to bond acrylic to polyethylene retainers, which may be useful when adding adjuncts to clear plastic retainers.

7.6 Polyurethane Retainers

Polyurethane is a thermoset plastic. Current commercial examples include Vivera retainers produced by Align Technology and Zendura retainers by Bay Materials LLC. Polyurethane retainers were developed to try and improve on the material properties offered by polyethylene and polypropylene retainers—for example, better crack resistance, better stain resistance, increased clarity, and better stress retention. Align Technology claims that Vivera retainers are 30% stronger and twice as durable as other competitor retainers on the market, but this has yet to be investigated with independent testing.

Further independent research is needed to investigate how well polyurethane retainers perform against the more established polyethylene and polypropylene retainers.

7.7 Multilayer Clear Plastic Retainers

In an effort to incorporate a range of different properties in the same retainer, a multilayer vacuum-formed retainer formed from different types of plastics has been developed.[17] A similar multilayer approach has been used to develop an active

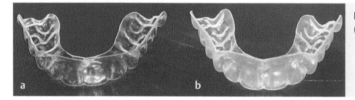

Fig. 7.1 (a) Polyethylene right and (b) polypropylene right.

retainer that also has the ability to offer mild tooth movements.[18]

These multilayer retainers are more complex, and are more time-consuming and expensive to manufacture. The clinical implications of these multilayer retainers are yet to be fully investigated.

7.8 Thickness of Retainers

The ideal thickness of retainers is not known. The plastic needs to be thick enough to resist fracture and wear, but still thin enough to be comfortable and well tolerated. The ideal thickness may differ for different types of plastic. Initial pilot clinical studies suggest a thickness of 1 mm is preferable to 0.75 mm.[19] As a result, most clear plastic retainers are slightly thicker than aligners that are used to correct malocclusions.[19]

7.9 Production of Retainers

Polyethylene and polypropylene retainers are typically formed from a sheet of plastic which is then shaped around a model of the patient's dentition. The sheet can be shaped either by applying pressure to the sheet (pressure-formed retainers) or by using a vacuum (▶ Fig. 7.2) to suck down the heated sheet over the model (vacuum-formed retainers).

The vacuum-forming process involves heating a sheet of plastic to the correct temperature and then "sucking" it down over a cast of the patient's teeth. The advantage of this process is that it is possible to get rapid access to the plastic immediately after formation. This may be important in controlling the temperature during the cooling phase. Some plastics need active cooling with an external refrigerant spray, to prevent the plastic cooling away from the cast. This process will help to improve the quality of the fit of the retainer. It is also possible to use an instrument to actively mold the plastic into areas of undercut to improve the fit of the retainer while it is still warm.

Pressure machines force heat-softened plastic over the cast in a sealed pressure chamber. More pressure can be applied, so there is a greater potential for detailing and adaptation of the plastic to the teeth and gingival margins. However, these machines are often more expensive.

The conventional approach for both vacuum-formed and pressure-formed retainers begins with the patient having an impression of their teeth, usually using alginate, and from this impression a plaster model is cast up. The retainer is then produced on this plaster model. A digital alternative to this approach involves taking an intraoral scan or scanning the impression, thus allowing the production of digital "virtual" models. These virtual models can be used to produce study models using a 3D printer. The retainer can then be thermoformed on these 3D printed models. The method of production of the 3D models may be important. For those printed using an additive process, for example, Vivera retainers, the surface of the models shows slight ridges, caused by the models being produced in layers during 3D printing. This may lead to slight ridges on the retainers, which may have implications for retention of bacteria.[20,21] The clinical implications of this are yet to be tested and will be discussed further in a later section of this

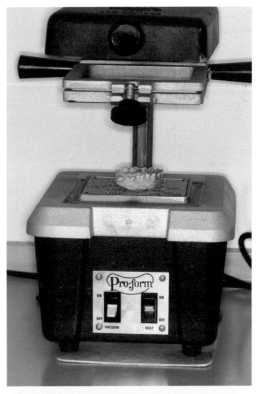

Fig. 7.2 Vacuum (suck-down) machine.

chapter. Models that are 3D printed using continuous liquid interface production may lead to a smoother finish.

7.10 Design of Clear Plastic Retainers

When Sheridan et al[3] popularized the vacuum-formed retainers in the early 1990s, they described two types of design:

- Full coverage (▶Fig. 7.3).
- Cover of only the anterior teeth, to allow posterior settling (▶Fig. 7.4).

There are concerns that using canine-to-canine clear plastic retainers may result in differential eruption of teeth, leading to a step in the occlusion. As a result, most operators use full coverage clear plastic retainers, including partial coverage of the most distal teeth (▶Fig. 7.3), even if the most distal teeth have not been aligned as part of the orthodontic treatment. This will prevent the overeruption of the most distal teeth. If teeth erupt after orthodontic treatment has been completed, consideration should be given to making new retainers to cover these most distally erupted teeth.

Clear plastic retainers are retained by the plastic engaging areas of undercut, in particular the area between the contact point and the papilla. It is therefore important that the plastic is finished beyond this point (▶Fig. 7.3), unlike bleaching trays, which are often trimmed along gingival margins. The plastic is typically finished 1 to 2 mm above the gingival margins. If the retainer is difficult to remove, some operators trim the plastic to expose the gingival third of the canine

crowns labially, to allow finger nails to disengage the appliance. Alternatively, transparent buttons can be attached to the buccal surface of first molars on the study models, so that when the thermoplastic retainer is created, the button is incorporated within the plastic, making the retainer easier to remove.[22]

Minor modifications can be made to the design of clear plastic retainers. One common example is the incorporation of a stainless steel wire insert to increase the transverse rigidity of the retainer (▶Fig. 7.5). This is particularly useful in cases where considerable expansion has taken place, and where a traditional clear plastic retainer may not be rigid enough to maintain this transverse correction.

7.11 How Often to Wear Clear Plastic Retainers?

For many years, there was disagreement about how many hours per day patients should wear removable retainers. A Cochrane review of retention

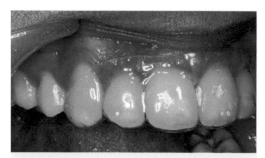

Fig. 7.4 Upper canine-to-canine clear plastic retainer.

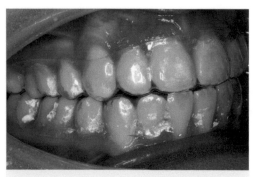

Fig. 7.3 Full coverage upper and lower clear plastic retainers.

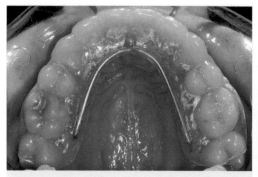

Fig. 7.5 Upper clear plastic retainer reinforced with a stainless steel wire.

concluded that there was no evidence that wearing thermoplastic retainers part-time led to any more relapse than full-time wear.[23] Based on the results of high-quality randomized clinical trials, it has been shown that patients only need to wear their clear plastic retainers at night.[24,25] This is important for two reasons. Firstly, it helps preserve the longevity of the retainers as they will not be worn so many hours per day, and secondly it means a lower burden of compliance for the patient.

While there is good evidence to support the number of hours of wear needed per day, it is less clear how long into the future the clear plastic retainers need to be worn. There is, however, a growing acceptance of the unpredictability of long-term relapse, largely as a result of life-long low-level growth and soft-tissue changes. For the majority of patients, orthodontic treatment should perhaps not be viewed as a life-long "cure" for the malocclusion. Instead, the appliance phase of treatment is the first phase that corrects the malocclusion, and then the retention phase (an integral part of the whole treatment plan) is used to control the result. As a result, a number of orthodontists now advise patients to wear their retainers "for as long as they want straight teeth."[26] This protocol of use has major implications for the patient, supervising dentist, and orthodontist, in terms of longevity of the retainer and the patient's compliance.

7.12 Indications for Use

There is a lack of high-quality evidence on what is the best type of retainer.[23] There has been a growing popularity of clear plastic retainers over the last 20 years, with some operators using them for retaining the majority of cases. However, there are cases where alternative retainers may be preferable and these will be briefly discussed in this section.

As clear plastic retainers are removable, they will never be worn completely full-time. There are a number of corrected malocclusions that are thought to be so unstable that full-time (fixed) retainers are usually preferred.[27] Examples of these high-risk relapse cases, where removable clear plastic retainers alone would therefore be unsuitable, include:

- Closure of markedly spaced dentition (including a median diastema).
- After correction of severely rotated teeth.

- Where there has been substantial movement of the lower labial segment, either in terms of change of intercanine width, or with either excessive proclination or retroclination of the lower labial segment.
- Where the final periodontal support for the teeth is substantially reduced due to previous periodontal disease.
- When an overjet has been reduced, but the upper incisors are not controlled by the lower lip at the end of treatment due to lip incompetence.

In these cases, a bonded retainer may be used instead of the clear plastic retainer, or in addition to the clear plastic retainer, sometimes referred to as dual retention (▶ Fig. 7.6).

Clear plastic retainers are retained by the plastic engaging areas of undercut, in particular the area between the contact point and the papilla. If the patient's oral hygiene has not been good during treatment, this area of undercut may be obscured by hyperplastic gingivae, meaning that the clear plastic retainers may be poorly retained. In these cases, it may be sensible to choose another type of retainer, at least until the hyperplastic gingivae resolve.

Traditional clear plastic retainers have full occlusal coverage (▶ Fig. 7.3), which means that settling of the occlusion after removal of the appliances is delayed.[28] Attempts to improve settling of the teeth with clear plastic retainers are discussed in detail in a later section, but if rapid settling of the occlusion is desired at the end of treatment, the use of bonded retainers, positioners, or Hawley or Begg retainers may be better alternatives to clear plastic retainers.

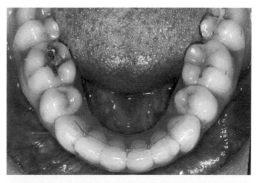

Fig. 7.6 Dual retention: clear plastic retainer in addition to bonded retainer.

7.13 Clear Plastic Retainers: An Evidence-Based Approach

An evidence-based approach[29] means considering the following:
- Best research evidence.
- Clinical expertise.
- Patient's values, expectations, and circumstances.

This section will focus on the best research evidence to support the use of clear plastic retainers, but it is important to remember that an evidence-based approach is also affected by factors related to the clinician's expertise and the patient's expectations. In fact, in the absence of sufficient high-quality research evidence, the approach to retention may be strongly influenced by a clinician's expertise and experience with different retainers, and patient's values, expectations, and circumstances.[13]

Retention is arguably the most important topic in orthodontics. However, there is still a shortage of high-quality evidence to support our choice of approaches to retention, including our use of clear plastic retainers.[23] In this section, we will consider the high-quality evidence from randomized controlled clinical trials that compare clear plastic retainers with other retainers in terms of stability, patient satisfaction, survival of the retainers, oral health, cost-effectiveness, and occlusal settling.

7.14 Clear Plastic Retainers versus Hawley Retainers

The largest randomized controlled clinical trial comparing patients wearing clear plastic retainers and Hawley retainers was published in 2007.[30,31] In this trial, 397 patients were randomly allocated to either upper and lower Hawley retainers or upper and lower clear plastic retainers. The study was undertaken in a single orthodontic practice, and all the patients were treated by one orthodontist. The patients were followed up for 6 months, and the key outcomes were stability, retainer survival, patient satisfaction, and cost-effectiveness.

In terms of stability, there was no statistically significant difference in intercanine or intermolar widths in both arches. However, they did find a statistically significant difference in Little's Irregularity Index in the upper arch, with 0.25 mm more relapse in the Hawley retainer group. In the lower arch, there was 0.56 mm more relapse in the Hawley group. The clinical significance of these differences is unclear, as the values are very small. The authors suggested that the difference may be clinically significant in the lower arch, if the irregularity was restricted to one tooth contact.

Clear plastic retainers survived better over the 6 months of the trial, with 32 Hawley retainers needing repairs, compared to 12 clear plastic retainers, giving a risk ratio of 2.96 (95% confidence interval [CI], 1.58–5.55; $p = 0.000072$).[23]

Patient satisfaction is a particularly important outcome in relation to removable retainers, as this may affect the patient's compliance with wearing the retainers. In this study, the patients preferred the clear plastic retainers, saying they were more likely to be able to wear them than Hawley retainers and they were less likely to feel embarrassed wearing clear plastic retainers.

Finally, in terms of cost-effectiveness, the clear plastic retainers were found to be more cost-effective for the patient, the orthodontic practice providing the appliance, and the national health service system under which the treatment was provided.

A further randomized controlled trial compared the ability of upper Hawley retainers with upper clear plastic retainers to retain teeth that have been derotated.[32] There were 218 patients that were followed up for 1 year. The authors found that clear plastic retainers maintained corrected rotations better than Hawley retainers (risk ratio, 4.88; 95% CI, 1.13–21.07; $p = 0.034$).[23,32] These results should be viewed with some caution as there is a risk of bias due to a large dropout rate and selected reporting of outcomes.

A further randomized controlled trial from China compared the survival time of clear plastic retainers and Hawley retainers over 1 year.[33] Unlike the Rowlands study discussed above,[30] they found a great failure rate with the clear plastic retainers. However, in this study the patients were asked to wear the clear plastic retainers full-time (instead of night only), which may have affected the longevity of the retainers.

7.15 Clear Plastic Retainers versus Begg Retainers

One randomized controlled trial from India randomly allocated 224 patients to either upper and lower clear plastic retainers or upper and lower Begg retainers.[34] It was found that clear plastic retainers appeared to retain the teeth better over 6 months. There was slightly more irregularity in the lower arch with Hawley retainers, and a reduction in the quality of the final result, measured using the Peer Assessment Rating (PAR) index. The findings of this study, however, are difficult to fully interpret, as the patients also had bonded retainers fitted in the lower arch in both groups.

7.16 Clear Plastic Retainers versus Bonded (Fixed) Retainers

A study from the United Kingdom has compared upper and lower clear plastic retainers with upper and lower bonded (fixed) retainers in a randomized controlled trial.[35,36] Sixty patients were followed up for 1 year in retention. After 1 year, both retainers were successful at maintaining a reasonable level of stability. There was slightly more relapse in Little's Irregularity Index in the lower arch with the clear plastic retainer (1.69 mm) compared to the bonded retainer (0.77 mm). There was no difference in survival rates in the upper arch, but greater failure rate of the mandibular bonded retainers than the mandibular clear plastic retainer. The authors suggest that this increased failure rate of the lower bonded retainers may have been due to the relative inexperience of the operators. In terms of patient satisfaction, the patients found the clear plastic retainer interfered with speech more, required more compliance, and were less comfortable than the bonded retainers, but reported that the clear plastic retainers were easier to keep clean. After 1 year, the patients with bonded retainers showed greater accumulation of plaque and calculus and slightly more gingival inflammation, but no clinically significant, adverse periodontal health problems.

A further randomized controlled trial from the United Kingdom comparing lower clear plastic retainers with lower bonded retainers over 18 months found both clear plastic retainers and bonded retainers were very effective at reducing relapse.[37] There was a statistically different increase in relapse with the clear plastic retainers, but the amount was so small as to be clinically insignificant. Interestingly, 4 years later, 67% of the patients were no longer wearing their vacuum-formed retainers, and as a result, there was 1.64 mm more irregularity in the vacuum-formed retainer group compared with the bonded retainers group (p = 0.02; 95% CI, 0.30–2.98 mm).[38]

A randomized controlled trial based in a hospital setting in Ireland compared patients wearing a mandibular clear plastic retainer with patients wearing a mandibular bonded retainer.[39,40] It was found slightly better stability with the lower bonded retainer,[39] and patients reported that in this study they felt the lower bonded retainers was easier to wear and easier to keep clean.[40]

7.17 Clear Plastic Retainers: Full Coverage versus Modified Clear Plastic Retainers

As discussed previously, one of the concerns about clear plastic retainers is that they may prevent settling due to their full occlusal coverage. Settling may be considered as favorable relapse that happens after removal of the appliances to improve the occlusal contacts. Previous research had suggested that clear plastic retainers may slow this settling process,[28] so a team in Turkey investigated clear plastic retainers that had been modified by removing the occlusal and half of the lingual and buccal surfaces over the premolars and molars to encourage faster settling.[41] The modified clear plastic retainers also had a stainless steel wire lingually to reinforce them. Patients were randomly allocated to conventional full-coverage clear plastic retainers or to the modified design. Both groups wore the retainers full-time for 6 months; then, both groups wore them at nights only for the following 6 months. They measured the change in occlusal contacts to assess the degree of settling. Interestingly, there was no difference between the groups, and settling only occurred during the nights-only phase of wear, suggesting that part-time wear of clear plastic retainers is more important than the design in terms of encourage settling of the occlusion.

7.18 Safety and Clear Plastic Retainers

As with all health interventions, the first priority is to do no harm. Clear plastic retainers may have the potential to compromise health by changing the level and nature of cariogenic and periodontal microorganisms intraorally. It is also important that the plastic is biocompatible, with no adverse tissue effects caused by the plastic material or risk of an allergic response.

Any appliance in the mouth has the potential to change the oral microflora, which may in turn lead to diseases such as caries or periodontal disease. Studies have shown that the level of *Streptococcus mutans* increases in the mouth after fixed appliances are removed and retainers are fitted.[42,43] It has been suggested that the smoothness of the clear plastic surface may affect the retention of bacteria. Retainers created by incremental layers during a 3D printing process, such as Vivera retainers, may have a corrugated surface with ledges and recesses that can harbor bacteria.[20,21] It is unclear whether there are any clinical implications to this.

There are certainly isolated case reports of extensive damage caused to the dentition as a result of patients drinking cariogenic drinks with clear plastic retainers in place.[44] Clear patient instructions to avoid eating, and particularly drinking, with the clear plastic appliances in place is vital.

One of the concerns of long-term wear of clear plastic appliances is the leaching out of components of the material that may by cytotoxic or estrogenic.[44-46] Studies on clear plastic aligners would seem to suggest that the risks are so low that there is no safety issues, but longer term studies on clear plastic retainer wear may be indicated.

Allergies to methyl methacrylate and nickel in orthodontics are well documented, but more research may be indicated to investigate allergies to clear plastics, particularly in retainers which will be worn long term.

7.19 Longevity of Clear Plastic Retainers

As our understanding of relapse has improved, there has been a realization that long-term post-treatment changes are unpredictable. This has meant that there has been a move to advising patients to wear their retainers long term—"for as long as you want straight teeth." This has major implications for the type of materials used for retainers and how often the retainers need to be replaced.

High-quality, long-term research is notoriously difficult to undertake in orthodontics, so it is difficult to provide accurate data about how long clear plastic retainers will last. Perhaps it is more important to educate patients to recognize problems with their retainers (cracks, poor-fitting, etc.) and explain how and where to seek advice for replacements. Long-term maintenance of retainers will have inherent costs, including any costs for retainers that need replacing or repairing. It is the orthodontist's responsibility to ensure the patient is made aware of any long-term costs before the patient commits to treatment.[26]

Another approach is to set up a regular review and replacement of retainers after debonding, rather than waiting for problems to arise. This can be arranged by the orthodontist, or commercial companies can offer this service—for example, Align Technology offers a subscription service for regular replacement of Vivera retainers.

Patients should be educated about how best to clean their clear plastic retainers. Toothpaste is often regarded as too abrasive, so brushing with a toothbrush and water is usually advised, along with regular use of specially designed retainer cleaning product recommended by the manufacturer for the particular type of retainer plastic that is used. It is important to avoid other cleaning products that may damage the plastic and shorten the retainer's lifespan.[47]

7.20 Compliance with Clear Plastic Retainers

Patient compliance is arguably the single most important factor in determining the success of orthodontic treatment.[48] The importance of compliance becomes even more significant when asking patients to wear a removable retainer long term. Most research seems to suggest that patients prefer to wear clear plastic retainers rather than traditional Hawley retainers.[31,49] But how much do patients actually wear their retainers? Asking patients tends to result in an overestimation of compliance, but monitoring compliance with retainer wear can now be undertaken more accurately using microelectronic monitors. These sensors can be incorporated within the clear plastic and used to measure the actual amount of retainer wear.[50] At the present time, the size and cost of these sensors may prevent their routine use, but in future developments in this technology will help inform retainer research, allow orthodontists to monitor their patients' compliance, and perhaps act as a motivator to the patient to wear their retainers, if they know they are being monitored.

Long-term research into retainer compliance typically involves recalling the patient to collect records, such as photos, impressions, or 3D scans. In the future, retainers may be monitored remotely using information captured by patients on their own smart devices, utilizing artificial intelligence.

7.21 The Future

Improvements in material science, greater understanding of relapse, and the results of clinical research has improved our knowledge about the use of clear plastic appliances as retainers. However, there are a number of areas where further research is required:

- Which cases are unsuitable for clear plastic retainers?
- How do clear plastic retainers compare with other types of retainers in terms of stability, patient satisfaction, survival, safety, and cost-effectiveness?
- How do we monitor and improve our patients' compliance with clear plastic retainers?
- Due to long-term potential for relapse, how do we improve the longevity of clear plastic retainers, or ensure there is a process in place for appropriate replacements in the future?

It is over 50 years since clear plastic appliances were first suggested as retainers. It will be interesting to see whether we will continue to prescribe clear plastic retainers over the next 50 years.

References

[1] Nahoum HI. The vacuum formed dental contour appliance. N Y State Dent J. 1964;9:385–390

[2] Ponitz RJ. Invisible retainers. Am J Orthod. 1971;59 (3):266–272

[3] Sheridan JJ, LeDoux W, McMinn R. Essix retainers: fabrication and supervision for permanent retention. J Clin Orthod. 1993;27(1):37–45

[4] Ab Rahman N, Low TF, Idris NS. A survey on retention practice among orthodontists in Malaysia. Korean J Orthod. 2016;46(1):36–41

[5] Al-Jewair TS, Hamidaddin MA, Alotaibi HM, et al. Retention practices and factors affecting retainer choice among orthodontists in Saudi Arabia. Saudi Med J. 2016;37(8):895–901

[6] Valiathan M, Hughes E. Results of a survey-based study to identify common retention practices in the United States. Am J Orthod Dentofacial Orthop. 2010;137(2):170–177, discussion 177

[7] Vandevska-Radunovic V, Espeland L, Stenvik A. Retention: type, duration and need for common guidelines. A survey of Norwegian orthodontists. Orthodontics (Chic). 2013;14(1):e110–e117

[8] Pratt MC, Kluemper GT, Hartsfield JK, Jr, Fardo D, Nash DA. Evaluation of retention protocols among members of the American Association of Orthodontists in the United States. Am J Orthod Dentofacial Orthop. 2011;140(4):520–526

[9] Singh P, Grammati S, Kirschen R. Orthodontic retention patterns in the United Kingdom. J Orthod. 2009;36(2):115–121

[10] Lai CS, Grossen JM, Renkema AM, Bronkhorst E, Fudalej PS, Katsaros C. Orthodontic retention procedures in Switzerland. Swiss Dent J. 2014;124(6):655–661

[11] Meade MJ, Millett D. Retention protocols and use of vacuum-formed retainers among specialist orthodontists. J Orthod. 2013;40(4):318–325

[12] Wong PM, Freer TJ. A comprehensive survey of retention procedures in Australia and New Zealand. Aust Orthod J. 2004;20(2):99–106

[13] Littlewood SJ. Evidence-based retention – where are we now? Semin Orthod. 2017;23:229–236

[14] Raja TA, Littlewood SJ, Munyombwe T, Bubb NL. Wear resistance of four types of vacuum-formed retainer materials: a laboratory study. Angle Orthod. 2014;84(4):656–664

[15] Gardner GD, Dunn WJ, Taloumis L. Wear comparison of thermoplastic materials used for orthodontic retainers. Am J Orthod Dentofacial Orthop. 2003;124(3):294–297

[16] Moshkelgosha V, Shomali M, Nomeni M. Comparison of wear resistance of Hawley and vacuum formed retainers: An in-vitro study. J Dent Biomater. 2016;3(2):248–253

[17] Ahn HW, Kim KA, Kim SH. A new type of clear orthodontic retainer incorporating multi-layer hybrid materials. Korean J Orthod. 2015;45(5):268–272

[18] Fernandez Sanchez J, Pernia Ramirez I, Martin Alonso J. Osamu active retainer for correction of mild relapse. J Clin Orthod. 1998;32(1):26–28

[19] Zhu Y, Lin J, Long H, et al. Comparison of survival time and comfort between 2 clear overlay retainers with different thicknesses: A pilot randomized controlled trial. Am J Orthod Dentofacial Orthop. 2017;151(3):433–439

[20] Chua J. Short-Term Effects of Various Removable Orthodontic Retainers on Clinical and Microbiological Parameters [dissertation]. Singapore: Discipline of Orthodontics and Paediatric Dentistry, National University of Singapore;2007

[21] Low B, Lee W, Seneviratne CJ, Samaranayake LP, Hägg U. Ultrastructure and morphology of biofilms on thermoplastic orthodontic appliances in 'fast' and 'slow' plaque formers. Eur J Orthod. 2011;33(5):577–583

[22] Hourfar J, Kanavakis G, Ludwig B. Acrylic removable retainers. In: Katsaros C, Eliades T, eds. Stability, Retention, and Relapse in Orthodontics. London: Quintessence Publishing Co.;2017:147–175

[23] Littlewood SJ, Millett DT, Doubleday B, Bearn DR, Worthington HV. Retention procedures for stabilising tooth position after treatment with orthodontic braces. Cochrane Database Syst Rev. 2016(1):CD002283

[24] Thickett E, Power S. A randomized clinical trial of thermoplastic retainer wear. Eur J Orthod. 2010;32(1):1–5

[25] Gill DS, Naini FB, Jones A, Tredwin CJ. Part-time versus full-time retainer wear following fixed appliance therapy: a randomized prospective controlled trial. World J Orthod. 2007;8(3):300–306

[26] Littlewood SJ. Responsibilities and retention. APOS Trends Orthod.. 2017;7:211–214

[27] Johnston CD, Littlewood SJ. Retention in orthodontics. Br Dent J. 2015;218(3):119–122

[28] Sauget E, Covell DA, Jr, Boero RP, Lieber WS. Comparison of occlusal contacts with use of Hawley and clear overlay retainers. Angle Orthod. 1997;67(3):223–230

[29] Sackett DL, Rosenberg WM, Gray JA, Haynes RB, Richardson WS. Evidence based medicine: what it is and what it isn't. BMJ. 1996;312(7023):71–72

[30] Rowland H, Hichens L, Williams A, et al. The effectiveness of Hawley and vacuum-formed retainers: a single-center randomized controlled trial. Am J Orthod Dentofacial Orthop. 2007;132(6):730–737

[31] Hichens L, Rowland H, Williams A, et al. Cost-effectiveness and patient satisfaction: Hawley and vacuum-formed retainers. Eur J Orthod. 2007;29(4):372–378

[32] Rohaya MAW, Shahrul Hisham ZA, Doubleday B. Randomised clinical trial: comparing the efficacy of vacuum-formed and Hawley retainers in retaining corrected tooth rotations. Malays Dent J. 2006;27:38–44

[33] Sun J, Yu YC, Liu MY, et al. Survival time comparison between Hawley and clear overlay retainers: a randomized trial. J Dent Res. 2011;90(10):1197–1201

[34] Kumar AG, Bansal A. Effectiveness and acceptability of Essix and Begg retainers: a prospective study. Aust Orthod J. 2011;27(1):52–56

[35] Storey M, Forde K, Littlewood SJ, Scott P, Luther F, Kang J. Bonded versus vacuum-formed retainers: a randomized controlled trial. Part 2: periodontal health outcomes after 12 months. Eur J Orthod. 2018;40(4):399–408

[36] Forde K, Storey M, Littlewood SJ, Scott P, Luther F, Kang J. Bonded versus vacuum-formed retainers: a randomized controlled trial. Part 1: stability, retainer survival, and patient satisfaction outcomes after 12 months. Eur J Orthod. 2018;40(4):387–398

[37] O'Rourke N, Albeedh H, Sharma P, Johal A. Effectiveness of bonded and vacuum-formed retainers: A prospective randomized controlled clinical trial. Am J Orthod Dentofacial Orthop. 2016;150(3):406–415

[38] Al-Moghrabi D, Johal A, O'Rourke N, Donos N, Gonzales-Marin C, Fleming PS. Effects of fixed vs removable orthodontic retainers on stability and periodontal health: 4-year follow-up of a randomized controlled trial. Am J Orthod Dentofacial Orthop. 2018;154:167–174

[39] McDermott P, Millett DT, Field D, Van den Heuvel A, Erfid I. Lower incisor retention with fixed or vacuum formed retainers. IADR Conference Abstract 0642. Toronto, 2008

[40] McDermott P, Field D, Erfida I, Millett DT. Operator and patient experiences with fixed or vacuum formed retainers. Irish Division IADR Conference Abstract 0017. Cork, 2007

[41] Aslan BI, Dinçer M, Salmanli O, Qasem MAM. Comparison of the effects of modified and full-coverage thermoplastic retainers on occlusal contacts. Orthodontics (Chic). 2013;14(1):e198–e208

[42] Jung WS, Kim H, Park SY, Cho EJ, Ahn SJ. Quantitative analysis of changes in salivary mutans streptococci after orthodontic treatment. Am J Orthod Dentofacial Orthop. 2014;145(5):603–609

[43] Türköz C, Canigür Bavbek N, Kale Varlik S, Akça G. Influence of thermoplastic retainers on Streptococcus mutans and Lactobacillus adhesion. Am J Orthod Dentofacial Orthop. 2012;141(5):598–603

[44] Birdsall J, Robinson S. A case of severe caries and demineralisation in a patient wearing an essix-type retainer. Prim Dent Care. 2008;15(2):59–61

[45] Eliades T, Pratsinis H, Athanasiou AE, Eliades G, Kletsas D. Cytotoxicity and estrogenicity of Invisalign appliances. Am J Orthod Dentofacial Orthop. 2009;136(1):100–103

[46] Kotyk MW, Wiltshire WA. An investigation into bisphenol-A leaching from orthodontic materials. Angle Orthod. 2014;84(3):516–520

[47] Pascual AL, Beeman CS, Hicks EP, Bush HM, Mitchell RJ. The essential work of fracture of thermoplastic orthodontic retainer materials. Angle Orthod. 2010;80(3):554–561

[48] Klaus K, Stark P, Serbesis TSP, Pancherz H, Ruf S. Excellent versus unacceptable orthodontic results: influencing factors. Eur J Orthod. 2017;39(6):615–621

[49] Mirzakouchaki B, Shirazi S, Sharghi R, Shirazi S. Assessment of factors affecting adolescent patients' compliance with Hawley and vacuum formed retainers. J Clin Diagn Res. 2016;10(6):ZC24–ZC27

[50] Schott TC, Göz G. Applicative characteristics of new microelectronic sensors Smart Retainer® and TheraMon® for measuring wear time. J Orofac Orthop. 2010;71(5):339–347

8 Digital Workflow in Aligner Therapy

Marc Schätzle and Raphael Patcas

Summary

Digital workflow in orthodontics must be assessed for its potential benefits and shortfalls, and must convince when being compared to the norm it aims to replace. If the digital workflow is to be advocated, each step of the process must be methodologically scrutinized and weighted. This chapter focuses on the digital workflow involving the dental arches with particular emphasis on the use of electronic dental casts in aligner orthodontic therapy. It further explores the evidence base of a digital workflow in orthodontics, considering dental records, data acquisition, diagnosis, planning, outcome simulation, designing aligners, management portals, and manufacturing aligners.

Keywords: orthodontic aligners, digital workflow, dental records, data acquisition, outcome simulation, orthodontic treatment

8.1 Introduction

The term workflow, first introduced in 1921,[1] is usually defined as procedural sequences of steps involved to accomplish a working process. In aligner orthodontics, the standardized procedure from the initial data acquisition to the start of treatment clearly conforms to the definition of a workflow. Aiming to digitalize this workflow would mean transferring the entire working process to a virtual level (▶Fig. 8.1).

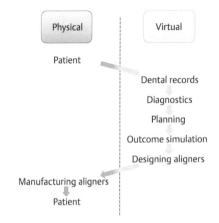

Fig. 8.1 Digital workflow in orthodontics for aligners.

A workflow is commonly defined as processing a piece of work from initiation *to completion.*[2] It is therefore worthy of mention that in contrast to other fields, digital workflow in orthodontics remains restricted to sequences *preceding* the actual therapy. Thus, manufacturing the device, and not the treatment, is seen as completion.

Since the introduction of CEREC (Chairside Economical Restoration of Esthetic Ceramics/CEramic REConstroction),[3] digitalization in dentistry has been extensively discussed, and its rising popularity has also increasingly influenced orthodontics. It is therefore rather surprising that scientific investigations on digital workflow in orthodontics are practically nonexistent. As for any introduction of a novel workflow, digital workflow in orthodontics must nevertheless be assessed for its potential benefits and deficiencies, and must persuade when being compared to the norm it aims to replace. If the digital workflow is to be encouraged, each step of the process must be methodologically scrutinized and weighted.

8.2 Dental Records

The initial step comprises the acquisition of patient data required to perform the intended treatment, and its digitalization. In basic terms, physical entities (e.g., dental arches, facial appearance, or skeletal cranial composition) are being collected and visualized as 2D or 3D imaging, while further pieces of vital information (e.g., patient history and expectations, functional diagnostic findings) are being digitally filed.

This chapter focuses on the digital workflow related to the dental arches, although the same questions would arise for the other collected dental records as well. As an example, digital radiographic imaging must similarly be reviewed for its accuracy of measurements, its reliability as diagnostic tool, and its validity concerning an outcome simulation.

8.3 Data Acquisition

Intraoral 3D data can be collected in many ways (▶Fig. 8.2). Impressions (▶Fig. 8.3) or casts (▶Fig. 8.4) of patients can be scanned with

Digital workflow: encoding the dental arch

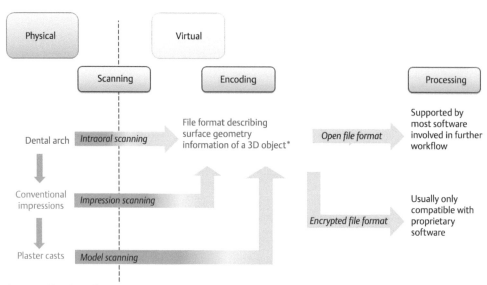

*E.g., STL files. These files contain only the surface geometry of the object without any representation of color, texture or other attributes. STL files define unstructured raw triangulated surfaces based on a 3D Cartesian coordinate system, and are widely used in computer-aided manufacturing.

Fig. 8.2 Data acquisition workflow.

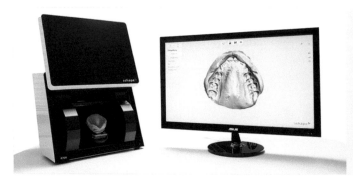

Fig. 8.3 Impression scanner.

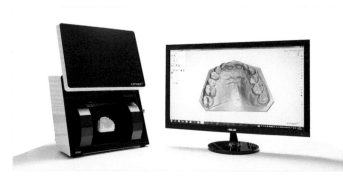

Fig. 8.4 Cast scanner.

desktop scanners and digital study models can subsequently be created, either for diagnostic purposes or to produce orthodontic appliances.

Although this path is incontestably possible, one of the reasons for a digital workflow would be to avoid taking impressions and model fabrication; hence, this option seems mainly suitable for eliminating larger quantities of already produced study models. The storage of models is often a burden for larger orthodontic practices, as regulations related to medicolegal records often disallow clinicians from discarding these.

Intraoral scanning has opened new avenues for planning, designing, and executing orthodontic treatment for our patients. Any orthodontic treatment needs dental casts for a series of treatment steps: planning, appliance production, progress review, treatment analysis, and archiving. Recent technological advances have made intraoral scans and digital models a promising alternative to conventional alginate impressions. As with any new technology, accuracy must be assessed by comparison with the existing standard—in the present case, digital model acquisition with alginate impressions.[4,5] The superimposition of full-arch digital models created by direct intraoral scanning technology on digitalized conventional casts indeed discloses a high relative accuracy of digital models made from intraoral scans.[6] Similarly, the few other studies that have addressed the accuracy of models derived from full-arch intraoral scans generally found that these models were clinically acceptable for diagnosis, treatment planning, and manufacturing of removable orthodontic appliances.[7,8,9] Yet all of the digitalization approaches presented suffer from several inherent sources of error. For instance, in digital models obtained from alginate impressions, fine details of tooth anatomy might be lost because of the limited ability of the impression material to flow into areas with undercuts, and potential shrinkage upon desiccation can compound the problem.[10,11,12] Additional loss of information may be related to the scanning process since the accuracy of a digital model is limited by the resolution of the scanner. For intraoral scans, there may be an additional decline in accuracy if the scanning sequence diverges from the manufacturer's recommendation.[13] On the whole, intraoral scanning is considered to provide digital models that more accurately represent the intraoral situation owing to the fewer sources of error. It is logical to assume that when processing steps are eliminated in the production of digital models, the models will be more accurate.[6] Grünheid and coworkers have shown that the chairside time required for impressions was significantly shorter than that for intraoral scans, a consideration that may outweigh the gain of greater accuracy[14] When processing time was however included (i.e. disinfection, packaging of impressions, and scan submission) the time expenditure did not differ significantly between the two procedures. Strictly relating to the total time requirement, neither method is surpassed by the other.

Regarding patient's acceptance, no conclusive statements are possible, as patient satisfaction is dependent on scanning time, scan area, and dimensions of the scanning tip and the interference with the patient's coronoid process.[14,15]

The requirements for digital orthodontic impression are a reproduction of the entire dentition with a precise bite registration. This is in contrast to more often used quadrant dental impressions, which were proven to be more accurate.[16,17]

In the last few years, the availability of intraoral scanning devices has increased considerably. The quality of the data set produced by these devices has impressively improved, while at the same time speed, the size and costs of the device have been downscaled. Several of the intraoral scanners are now able to produce study and working models in color, thereby increasing the diagnostic and treatment planning options.[18] Furthermore, using photographs or an intraoral color scan may help the patient and the orthodontist determine which aspects need to be included in the treatment plan to ensure that the concerns of the patients have been addressed. However, the marketing claims of a better patient experience, improved patient satisfaction, and a general patient preference of intraoral scans over traditional impressions that have been made by several manufacturers of oral scanners, but could not always be substantiated.[14]

A major drawback is certainly the fact that no software exists that is able to archive and process all acquired data together (dental arch scanning, radiographic images including cephalometric projections, patient history, etc.), and the clinician is forced to use several, often incompatible proprietary software.

8.4 Diagnostics

Having a 3D model available for analysis can help the clinician obtain an array of data points in a very short period of time. Arch length, arch width, crowding, spacing, tooth size discrepancies, and occlusal plane assessments can be calculated with minimal effort (►Fig. 8.5). Software packages are available to help the orthodontist or technician produce diagnostic setups that can be reviewed with the patient in order to discuss different options for the orthodontic therapy and their likely visual outcomes. This can be particularly helpful if there are treatments options that require restorative or prosthodontic elements. Traditionally, orthodontists took alginate impressions of the patient's teeth and cast these into stone models. Tooth widths would be measured using calipers and a Bolton analysis performed manually. Various studies have demonstrated that calipers are accurate and reliable.[19,20] They have therefore been widely regarded as the gold standard for tooth-width measurements.[21,22]

The literature seems to indicate that a statistically significant difference between mean tooth widths from the digital method and the caliper might exist. Generally, the tooth width measurements made on digital models tend to be larger than those made on physical models. However, the practical significance of this discrepancy is questionable since it varies from 0 to 0.384 mm in the literature.[8,21,23,24]

Possible reasons for the difference between the physical and digital recordings include the following: (1) there is no physical obstacle to the placement of measurement points with virtual models, thus allowing the operator to measure the maximum mesiodistal diameter of the tooth without the restrictions inherent in physical calipers when considering inaccessible landmarks; (2) the difficultly in scanning contact points often resulting in small amounts of missing data, and virtual construction of the missing surface based on interpolations and asumptions made by a computer algorithm. This too, can cause slight variations in contact point locations between the stone and digital models; (3) shrinkage of the alginate impressions occurring during transportation despite rapid processing within 24 hours,[25] possibly explaining the smaller recordings made on the stone casts. However, reliability and reproducibility of the digital method is excellent.[23]

The tooth width discrepancy resulted also in an overestimation of the Bolton ratio by the digital method.[21,24] Yet tooth-size discrepancies of less than 1.5 mm are rarely clinically significant and remain therefore clinically acceptable. With regard to occlusal indices, since the Peer Assessment Rating (PAR) analysis and its constituent measurements are not significantly different between plaster and e-model media, digital models are an accceptable replacement for assessing malocclusion and do not compromise diagnosis, treatment planning, and outcome assessment.[24]

Nevertheless, scientific evidence so far collected on intraoral scanning is neither exhaustive nor authoritative. Data from full-arch scans performed in children are still missing and should be collected. For a meaningful assessment of time efficiency, agreement should be reached on the procedural steps to be included in the computation of scanning time.[26]

8.5 Planning

Traditionally, orthodontics has been a field with heavy emphasis on treatment planning based on physical records. Most orthodontists have been trained to plan their cases without virtual tools but by measuring gypsum casts and tracing lateral cephalometric radiographs. Encouraging the planning of cases based solely on digital data is indeed tempting and might allow new avenues to be used. At the same time, the clinician must be cognizant that a possible lack of training could affect the planning, and at the very least, a learning curve must be respected. Several studies have in the past highlighted the fact that personal preferences affect the treatment plan.[27] It is therefore surprising that no research has been published on whether the specific modality of the models (digital vs. physical) affects the decisions concerning the treatment planning.

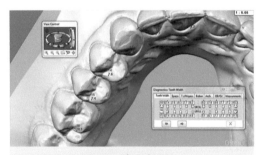

Fig. 8.5 Measurement with OrthoCAD.[23]

8.6 Outcome Simulation

The benefits of a digital setup are obvious. First, the communication between the dental laboratory and the clinician is immensely facilitated. Second, a virtual outcome simulation is unquestionably a major improvement in patient education. The traditional way to produce a dental setup requires time-consuming physical segmentation of gypsum teeth subsequently positioned in wax.

Virtual setups, however, present several advantages, such as digital storage; the same model can undergo several treatment simulations, and communication between dental and surgical professionals and between dental professionals and patients is facilitated. Despite these advantages, considerable time and training are needed for dental professionals to master and adopt the general use of digital models and virtual setups in dentistry.[28]

So far there is no study analyzing the treatment outcome to the initially, intended aligner treatment result. So, strictly speaking a "treatment objective" rather than a "treatment outcome" is being simulated.

Moreover, two caveats must be mentioned. On the one hand, there is still a lack of scientific proof for the validity of the simulated outcome. Many assumptions are being made, and while some may be more predictable, others are still best described as "learned guesses." The simulation will often contain many assumptions, such as equaling positional changes of teeth (from one aligner to the next) to a certain (acceptable) force, or estimating the response of teeth, intra- and extraoral soft tissues to the applied forces. Most of these assumptions are better considered imprecise expectations, since the simulations are not based on biological data. Thus, tooth protrusion can be simulated without bearing in mind the possibility of dehiscences, and sagittal corrections are being

calculated without any knowledge of skeletal and dental responses of the mandible and maxilla.

Second, transferring patient data back and forth to a dental laboratory or even to the patient can be legally problematic. Although this is often touted as a great and wonderful advancement, it does carry with it certain administrative responsibilities.[29] To whom do the digital data belong? If the simulation outcome is to be considered an intellectual property, who holds the rights?

Cloud services providers are separate entities from those that provide health care services and business associates who transact with these entities. Once a health care provider engages the services of a cloud service provider to create, receive, maintain, or transmit electronic protected health information, the cloud services provider becomes a business associate and is thus obligated to enter into a business associate agreement with the health care provider. It is up to the care service provider and its respective associates to secure total data integrity so that neither unauthorized viewing nor processing is possible by any of the business entities involved. From a legal point of view, cloud services must clearly differentiate between transmission service, data processing and storing.[29] A final question remains: how long must the cloud provider retain electronic health information after the provided service has been completed? Clinicians must be made aware that laws specific to retention of patient records may vary according to location and time.

8.7 Designing Aligners and Management Portals

The 3D data can be exported to laboratories for the production of appliances (▶Fig. 8.6). Many of the companies offering appliances have portals

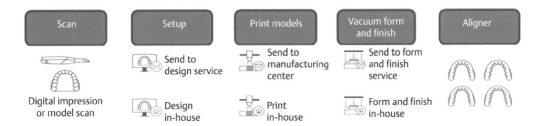

Fig. 8.6 Workflow for laboratory aligner processing and production.

helping the clinicians transfer the data securely through the Internet. Once received and accepted by the provider, the proposed treatment plan by the aligner system might be reviewed, modified if necessary during the designing process by the clinician, and subsequently manufactured.

There are several aligner suppliers who can now receive 3D dataset and produce the requested setups and aligners from the respective data.

8.8 Manufacturing Aligners

To conform to a truly digital workflow, the aligners should also be manufactured without physical models. To date, most aligner companies produce the aligners based on printed models. A welcome optimization of the digital workflow would therefore be the production of aligners without the creation of unnecessary models, thus minimizing the consumption of resources. Other fields in dentistry have already mastered this final step,[30] and even in orthodontics novel methods of digitally constructed orthodontic appliances have recently been introduced.

References

[1] Journal of the Institute of Transport 1921;1:148

[2] Oxford English Dictionary. Workflow. OED online. 2018. Available at: http://www.oed.com/view/Entry/400203

[3] Mörmann WH. The evolution of the CEREC system. J Am Dent Assoc. 2006;137(Suppl):7S–13S

[4] Bland JM, Altman DG. Statistical methods for assessing agreement between two methods of clinical measurement. Lancet. 1986;1(8476):307–310

[5] Bland JM, Altman DG. Measuring agreement in method comparison studies. Stat Methods Med Res. 1999;8(2):135–160

[6] Grünheid T, McCarthy SD, Larson BE. Clinical use of a direct chairside oral scanner: an assessment of accuracy, time, and patient acceptance. Am J Orthod Dentofacial Orthop. 2014;146(5):673–682

[7] Ender A, Mehl A. Full arch scans: conventional versus digital impressions--an in-vitro study. Int J Comput Dent. 2011;14(1):11–21

[8] Cuperus AM, Harms MC, Rangel FA, Bronkhorst EM, Schols JG, Breuning KH. Dental models made with an intraoral scanner: a validation study. Am J Orthod Dentofacial Orthop. 2012;142(3):308–313

[9] Vasudavan S, Sullivan SR, Sonis AL. Comparison of intraoral 3D scanning and conventional impressions for fabrication of orthodontic retainers. J Clin Orthod. 2010;44(8):495–497

[10] Rudd KD, Morrow RM, Strunk RR. Accurate alginate impressions. J Prosthet Dent. 1969;22(3):294–300

[11] Miller MW. Syneresis in alginate impression materials. Br Dent J. 1975;139(11):425–430

[12] Sakaguchi RL, Powers JM, eds. Craig's Restorative Dental Materials. St. Louis, MO: Mosby;2012

[13] Ender A, Mehl A. Influence of scanning strategies on the accuracy of digital intraoral scanning systems. Int J Comput Dent. 2013;16(1):11–21

[14] Grünheid T, Patel N, De Felippe NL, Wey A, Gaillard PR, Larson BE. Accuracy, reproducibility, and time efficiency of dental measurements using different technologies. Am J Orthod Dentofacial Orthop. 2014;145(2):157–164

[15] Burzynski JA, Firestone AR, Beck FM, Fields HW, Jr, Deguchi T. Comparison of digital intraoral scanners and alginate impressions: Time and patient satisfaction. Am J Orthod Dentofacial Orthop. 2018;153(4):534–541

[16] Ender A, Zimmermann M, Attin T, Mehl A. In vivo precision of conventional and digital methods for obtaining quadrant dental impressions. Clin Oral Investig. 2016;20(7):1495–1504

[17] Ender A, Attin T, Mehl A. In vivo precision of conventional and digital methods of obtaining complete-arch dental impressions. J Prosthet Dent. 2016;115(3):313–320

[18] Zimmermann M, Mehl A, Mörmann WH, Reich S. Intraoral scanning systems - a current overview. Int J Comput Dent. 2015;18(2):101–129

[19] Quimby ML, Vig KW, Rashid RG, Firestone AR. The accuracy and reliability of measurements made on computer-based digital models. Angle Orthod. 2004;74(3):298–303

[20] Schirmer UR, Wiltshire WA. Manual and computer-aided space analysis: a comparative study. Am J Orthod Dentofacial Orthop. 1997;112(6):676–680

[21] Naidu D, Scott J, Ong D, Ho CT. Validity, reliability and reproducibility of three methods used to measure tooth widths for bolton analyses. Aust Orthod J. 2009;25(2):97–103

[22] Santoro M, Galkin S, Teredesai M, Nicolay OF, Cangialosi TJ. Comparison of measurements made on digital and plaster models. Am J Orthod Dentofacial Orthop. 2003;124(1):101–105

[23] Naidu D, Freer TJ. Validity, reliability, and reproducibility of the iOC intraoral scanner: a comparison of tooth widths and Bolton ratios. Am J Orthod Dentofacial Orthop. 2013;144(2):304–310

[24] Stevens DR, Flores-Mir C, Nebbe B, Raboud DW, Heo G, Major PW. Validity, reliability, and reproducibility of plaster vs digital study models: comparison of peer assessment rating and Bolton analysis and their constituent measurements. Am J Orthod Dentofacial Orthop. 2006;129(6):794–803

[25] Coleman RM, Hembree JH, Jr, Weber FN. Dimensional stability of irreversible hydrocolloid impression material. Am J Orthod. 1979;75(4):438–446

[26] Goracci C, Franchi L, Vichi A, Ferrari M. Accuracy, reliability, and efficiency of intraoral scanners for full-arch impressions: a systematic review of the clinical evidence. Eur J Orthod. 2016;38(4):422–428

[27] Markic G, Katsaros C, Pandis N, Eliades T. Temporary anchorage device usage: a survey among Swiss orthodontists. Prog Orthod. 2014;15(1):29

[28] Camardella LT, Rothier EK, Vilella OV, Ongkosuwito EM, Breuning KH. Virtual setup: application in orthodontic practice. J Orofac Orthop. 2016;77(6):409–419

[29] Jerrold L. Cloudy. Am J Orthod Dentofacial Orthop. 2017;151(3):616–618

[30] Joda T, Brägger U. Complete digital workflow for the production of implant-supported single-unit monolithic crowns. Clin Oral Implants Res. 2014;25(11):1304–1306

III

9 Outcome Assessment and Evidence on the Clinical Performance of Orthodontic Aligners

Spyridon N. Papageorgiou and Theodore Eliades

Summary

In the last decade several systematic reviews of clinical studies comparing orthodontic aligners with fixed appliances have emerged. However, they all present methodological issues that can introduce bias and hamper their ability to draw robust evidence-based recommendations, including among others: assessment of oral hygiene but not efficacy, lack of an a priori design/pre-registered protocol, language bias, inclusion of nonrandomized studies with uncontrolled confounding, inadequate handing of the studies' risk of bias, lack of quantitative data synthesis (meta-analysis), improper data synthesis methods, and being outdated. This chapter presents a critical appraisal on the clinical performance of orthodontic aligners based on currently available studies founded on the principles of evidence-based medicine. According to currently existing clinical evidence from randomized trials and matched nonrandomized studies on mostly adult patients with mild to severe malocclusions treated with or without extractions it seems that orthodontic treatment with aligners is associated with inferior treatment outcome compared to fixed appliances. Treatment duration is not directly influenced by choice of appliance alone and patient-related or treatment-related factors might come into play.

Keywords: orthodontics, aligners, treatment outcome, treatment duration.

9.1 Background

The use of sequential clear aligners has seen a remarkable surge in the last decades and, following considerable technical developments, has been widely adopted by both orthodontic specialists and general dentists alike. Fueled by aggressive marketing campaigns from various manufacturers of aligner systems, a growing interest has been reported, especially among adult patients, for such methods of invisible orthodontics.[1,2] A survey of Australian orthodontists in 2013 indicated that 73% of responders had used aligners to treat at least one case in the last year, with a median of 8 aligner cases/year.[3] A similar survey among Irish orthodontists in 2014 reported that 19% of them often used aligners to treat adult patients.[4] A large 2014 survey among orthodontists in the United States[5] revealed that 89% of them had treated at least one case with aligners (compared to 76% in 2008) and treated a median of 22 cases/year with aligners (compared to 12 cases/year in 2008). Responding orthodontists who used aligners employed them in a variety of cases, with the most common diagnostic category for aligner treatment being: Class I with moderate crowding (94%), space closure (78%), Class II (68%), lower incisor extraction (47%), Class I with severe crowding (37%), and Class III (49%), while only few orthodontists used aligners for premolar extraction cases (9–18%). Interestingly, responders in 2014 considered 90% of their aligner cases successful (compared to 80% in 2008), but also saw about 10% of aligner cases with relapse (same as 10% in 2008). Additionally, another survey among members of the European Aligner Society indicated that 45% of orthodontists believed that aligners limit orthodontic treatment outcomes (even though the respective percentage among general dentists was only 5%).[6] These data might indicate that the initial surge of aligner treatment during its early years of fame might have now given its place to a more mature evaluation of this treatment modality, based on long-term evaluations of previously treated patients.

In any case, it is imperative that any treatment modality offered to orthodontic patients as an alternative is based on both the doctor's clinical expertise and solid evidence on the clinical performance on this modality. Unfortunately, contrary to many medical fields, it is commonly seen in orthodontics that novel marketed products and treatment approaches are clinically adopted based on advertisement without the appropriate clinical evidence to back any claims made by the manufacturers.[7,8] Good clinical practice, however, obligates that any treatment decision between the treating orthodontist and the patient is done after meticulous discussion of all available treatment options and evidence-based notions about their efficacy and adverse effects. Ideally, these should be based on well-designed and well-reported comparative clinical trials on human patients and systematic reviews/meta-analyses thereof.[9,10] Ample empirical evidence has now been gathered about the importance of proper study design and the role that various methodological characteristics can play in introducing bias.[11,12,13,14,15,16,17]

In the last decade, several systematic reviews of clinical studies comparing orthodontic aligners with fixed appliances have emerged.[18,19,20,21,22,23,24,25,26,27] However, they all present methodological issues that can introduce bias and hamper their ability to draw robust evidence-based recommendations, including among others: assessment of oral hygiene but not efficacy,[18,23,24] lack of an a priori design/preregistered protocol,[19,18,19,20,21,22,26,27] language bias,[20,22,25] inclusion of nonrandomized studies with uncontrolled confounding,[19,20,22,25,26,27] inadequate handing of the studies' risk of bias,[19,20,21,22,25,26,27] lack of quantitative data synthesis (meta-analysis),[19,20,22,25,27] outdated data synthesis methods,[21,26] and outdated literature searches.[19,20,21] Therefore, clinical practice ought to be informed by a critical appraisal of currently available studies according to the principles of evidence-based medicine.

9.2 Appraisal of Evidence from Existing Clinical Studies

To this end, a systematic review was designed a priori based on the Cochrane guidelines,[28] registered in PROSPERO (CRD42019131589), and is reported according to the PRISMA statement.[29] Eight databases (MEDLINE through PubMed, Cochrane Database of Systematic Reviews, Cochrane Central Register of Controlled Trials, Cochrane Database of Abstracts of Reviews of Effects, Scopus, Virtual Health Library, and Web of Knowledge) were searched up to April 25, 2019, without any restrictions for publication date, language, or type with the following search strategy: *(orthodon* OR malocclusion* OR "tooth movement" OR "fixed appliances") AND (aligner* OR "clear aligner" OR "clear aligners" OR "ClearCorrect" OR "Invisalign" OR "Orthocaps" OR "TwinAligner").*

Eligible for inclusion were randomized trials comparing adolescent/adult patients with any kind of malocclusion receiving full-arch comprehensive treatment with either orthodontic aligners or any kind of fixed appliances. Due to the scarcity of randomized trials on the subject, nonrandomized studies were also included, with the requirement that the populations to be compared were matched regarding baseline malocclusion severity with objective measures such as the Peer Assessment Rating (PAR) index[30] or the Discrepancy Index (DI)[31] from the American Board of Orthodontics (ABO). The PAR index uses seven criteria: tooth alignment (referring to dental crowding), right and left buccal segment relationship (sagittal, vertical, and transverse assessments), overjet, overbite, and centerline (midline discrepancies). Each difference from the norm has points attributed to the severity of the discrepancy. Once tabulated and weighted according to the United States or United Kingdom weightings, an overall score for the malocclusion is calculated. The ABO DI scores 12 target disorders: overjet, overbite, anterior open bite, lateral open bite, crowding, occlusal relationship, lingual posterior cross-bite, buccal posterior cross-bite, ANB angle, mandibular plane inclination, lower incisor inclination, and a category "other" that includes complexes such as Bolton discrepancy, shortened roots, deep curve of Spee, traumatic injuries, bimaxillary protrusion cases with critical anchorage need, and craniofacial dysmorphologies. Similarly to the PAR index, scores are assigned and tabulated to reflect the malocclusion severity. Matching was judged adequate when the Cohen's d for PAR or ABO DI between aligner and fixed appliance group at baseline was up to 0.3. The primary outcome for this review was the outcome of comprehensive orthodontic treatment judged with objective and reliable measures such as the PAR index and the ABO's Objective Grading System (ABO-OGS) for dental casts and panoramic radiographs.[32] The ABO-OGS rates the final occlusion after appliance removal with eight criteria that contribute to ideal intercuspation and function: alignment, marginal ridges, buccolingual inclination, overjet, occlusal contacts, occlusal relationships, interproximal contacts, and root angulation. Best occlusion and alignment receive a score of 0 points, while for each parameter that deviates from the ideal, 1 or 2 penalty points are added. The greater the posttreatment ABO-OGS score, the more the final treatment result deviates from ideal occlusion, while a case can also be classified as "successful" or "failed" according to their ABO criteria for score lower or higher than 30 points. Secondary outcomes included treatment duration, as well as adverse effects such as loss of periodontal support, external apical root resorption (EARR), gingival recession, and uncontrolled proclination of the lower incisors during treatment.

Study selection, data extraction, and risk of bias assessment were performed by three independent assessors. The risk of bias of included studies was assessed according to Cochrane guidelines with the RoB 2.0 tool for randomized trials[33] and the ROBINS-I ("Risk Of Bias In Nonrandomised Studies—of Interventions") tool for nonrandomized studies.[34] Mean differences (MDs) for continuous outcomes and relative risks (RRs) for binary outcomes and their corresponding 95% confidence intervals (CIs) were pooled with random-effects meta-analysis (using a restricted maximum likelihood variance estimator[35]), with $p < 0.05$ considered significant, and presented in contour-enhanced forest plots.[36] Relative/absolute heterogeneity was assessed with I^2 and tau,[2] respectively, and incorporated into random-effects 95% predictions to quantify expected treatment effects in a future clinical setting.[37] The overall quality of clinical recommendations (confidence in effects estimates) for each of the main outcomes was rated using the Grades of Recommendation, Assessment, Development, and Evaluation (GRADE) approach[38] using an improved Summary of Findings table format[39] and guidance on how to combine randomized and nonrandomized studies.[40]

9.3 Characteristics of Existing Clinical Studies Comparing Aligners to Fixed Appliances

The electronic literature search up to April 2019 yielded 1,376 hits, while 7 additional studies were manually identified through checking of the reference or citation lists of identified reports (▶Fig. 9.1). After applying the review's eligibility criteria, 11 publications pertaining to 11 unique studies (4 randomized and 7 retrospective nonrandomized)[41,42,43,44,45,46,47,48,49,50,51] published as journal papers or dissertation/theses were included (▶Table 9.1). The included studies were conducted in university clinics ($n = 6$; 55%), private practices ($n = 4$; 36%), or hospitals ($n = 1$; 9%) and originated from six different countries (Canada, China, Ireland, Italy, South Korea, and the United States). A total of 446 and 443 patients were treated with aligners and fixed appliances, respectively, with a median total sample of 66 patients per included study (range 19–200 patients per study). Out of the 7 studies reporting on patient sex, 215 of the 661 patients in total were male (33%), while the mean patient age out of the 9 studies reporting this was 28.0 years.

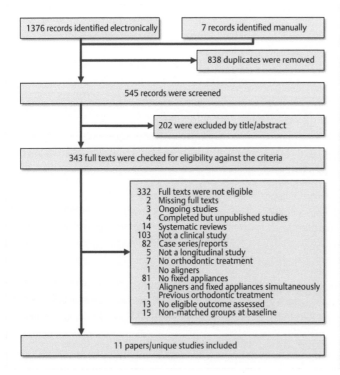

Fig. 9.1 PRISMA flow diagram for the identification and selection of eligible studies in this review.

As far as complexity of the treated cases is concerned, only six studies (55%) reported this with either the PAR index (n = 3; 27%) or the ABO DI (n = 3; 27%). Eight of the studies (73%) performed nonextraction treatment, one study (9%) both extraction and nonextraction treatment, and one study (9%) extraction treatment. The majority of studies (9/11 studies; 82%) reported on conventional comprehensive treatment, while 1 study (9%) reported on orthodontic treatment of patients with history of periodontal disease and 1 study (9%) reported on combined orthodontic/orthognathic treatment. Details of the aligner treatment were only partly reported among the included studies, with only two studies (18%) reporting the number of aligners, four studies (36%) reporting on "refinement" rate (i.e., the midcourse re-evaluation and planning of additional aligners), and two studies (18%) on the actual amount of interproximal enamel reduction performed during treatment in both groups.

The included randomized trials presented several issues that increased their risk for bias (▶Table 9.2).

Two trials were in high risk of bias due to problems in the randomization process, deviations from intended interventions, missing outcome data, and outcome measurement. The remaining two trials were in low risk of bias, except for the fact that no a priori trial protocol could be found to rule out selective reporting. The included nonrandomized studies were in considerably higher risk of bias, with five of them presenting moderate risk of bias, one of them serious risk of bias, and one of them critical risk of bias (▶Table 9.3). Their main shortcomings pertained to confounding, selection of participants into the study, deviations from intended interventions, outcome measurement, and selection of the reported result.

The included studies reported on a wide spectrum of treatment outcomes, with only three studies[41,45,47] reporting on the complete ABO-OGS score including all eight components, as well as failure of the case to pass the ABO criteria for adequate occlusal results (ABO-OGS score < 30 points). One study reported on the ABO-OGS score of seven out of eight components (excluding

Table 9.1 Characteristics of included studies

Study	Design; setting; country[a]	Patients (M/F); age[b]	Malocclusion/ Tx	Appliance	Aligners/ refinement/ IPR	FU (mo)	Outcome
Abbate 2015	RCT; Uni; ITA	AL: 25 (NR); (10–18) FX: 22 (NR); (10–18)	Non-Ex	AL: Invisalign FX: Labial CLB	NR/NR/NR	BL, 3.0, 6.0, 9.0, 12.0 mo in Tx	PPD
Djeu 2005	rNRS; Pract; USA	AL: 48 (NR); 33.6 FX: 48 (NR); 23.7	DI: 19.3; Ex/ Non-Ex	AL: Invisalign FX: Labial CLB (TE)	NR/NR/ allowed	BL, END	ABO-OGS$_8$; TxDur
Fetouh 2008	rNRS; Pract; USA	AL: 33 (NR); NR FX: 33 (NR); NR	Mild crowding; DI: 3.22/ Non-Ex	AL: Invisalign FX: Labial CLB	NR/NR/NR	BL, END	ABO-OGS$_7$
Gu 2017	rNRS; Pract; USA	AL: 48 (16/32); 26.0 FX: 48 (18/30); 22.1	PAR: 21.8; compliant/ Non-Ex	AL: Invisalign FX: Labial CLB (SW)	NR/38%/NR	BL, END	PAR; TxDur
Han 2015	rNRS; Uni; KOR	AL: 10 (NR); 51.2 FX: 9 (NR); 47.3	Previous PerioDis; DI: 4.4/Non-Ex	AL: NR FX: Labial CLB	NR/NR/ allowed	BL, END	PB; ABL TxDur
Hennessy 2016	RCT; Hosp; IRL	AL: 20 (6/14); 29.1 FX: 20 (7/13); 23.7	Mild crowding/ Non-Ex	AL: Invisalign FX: Labial SLB (MBT)	18 ALs/ allowed/ AL:FX 1.9:1.5	BL, END	IMPA; TxDur

(Continued)

Table 9.1 (*Continued*) Characteristics of included studies

Study	Design; setting; country[a]	Patients (M/F); age[b]	Malocclusion/ Tx	Appliance	Aligners/ refinement/ IPR	FU (mo)	Outcome
Lanteri 2018	rNRS; Pract; ITA	AL: 100 (30/70); 28.0 FX: 100 (30/70); 25.0	PAR: 23.3/ Non-Ex	AL: Invisalign FX: Labial SLB (MBT)	43 ALs[c]/37%/ AL:FX 1.3:1.5	BL, END, 24.0 mo Post-Tx	PAR; RetFail; GingRec
Li 2015	RCT; Uni; CHN	AL: 76 (27/45); 35.2 FX: 76 (27/45); 32.2	DI: 27.4/Ex	AL: Invisalign FX: Labial CLB	NR/NR/ allowed (AL)	BL, END	ABO-OGS$_8$; TxDur
Preston 2017	RCT; Uni; USA	AL: 22 (10/12); 27.8 FX: 22 (7/15); 25.4	Mild crowding/ Non-Ex	AL: Invisalign FX: Labial CLB (ALX)	100% (2 refinements)	BL, END, 1.0, 6.0 mo Post-Tx	ABO-OGS$_2$; TxDur; con- tact areas
Robitaille 2016	rNRS; Uni; CAN	AL: 24 (11/13); 29.8 FX: 25 (6/19); 23.4	DI: 31.5/ orthognathic surgery	AL: Invisalign FX: Labial CLB	NR/NR/NR	BL, END	ABO-OGS$_8$; TxDur
Yi 2018	rNRS; Uni; CHN	AL: 40 (9/31); 21.8 FX: 40 (11/29); 23.3	PAR: 22.6/ Non-Ex	AL: NR FX: Labial CLB	NR/65%/NR	BL, END	PAR; TxDur; EARR

Abbreviations: ABL, alveolar bone level; ABO-OGS, American Board of Orthodontics Objective Grading System (number of components assessed given in subscript); AL, aligner; ALX, Alexander technique; BL, baseline; CLB, conventionally ligated brackets; DI, discrepancy index; EARR, external apical root resorption; END, end of comprehensive treatment; Ex, extraction; FU, follow-up; FX, fixed appliance; GingRec, gingival recession; Hosp, hospital; IMPA, inclination of lower incisors to mandibular plane; IPR, interproximal enamel reduction; M/F, male/female; MBT, MacLaughlin-Bennet-Trevisi prescription; mo, month; NR, not reported; PAR, peer assessment rating; PPD, periodontal probing depth; Pract, private practice/clinic; RCT, randomized clinical trial; SLB, self-ligating bracket; SW, straightwire; TE, Tip-Edge; Tx, treatment; TxDur, treatment duration; Uni, university clinic.
[a]Countries given with their alpha-3 codes.
[b]Patient age is given either as mean (one value in without parenthesis) or, if mean is not reported, as range (two values in parenthesis).
[c]Including refinement aligners.

root angulation)[42] and also excluded scoring the second molars without any justification. One study also reported solely on two of the eight ABO-OGS components[49]—namely, marginal ridges and buccolingual inclination. Three studies used the PAR index[48,50,51] and reported either posttreatment PAR scores or PAR reductions. Eight studies reported on treatment duration,[41,46,47,48,49,50,51] though considerable variation in the reported results was seen. Finally, single studies reported on periodontal probing depth, alveolar bone loss, EARR, lower incisor inclination, and gingival recessions.

9.4 Treatment Efficacy in Terms of Occlusal Outcome

The ABO-OGS enables the objective and precise evaluation of the outcome of comprehensive orthodontic treatment including the fine details of a balanced ideal occlusion. The meta-analysis combining the results of the three existing studies measuring the total ABO-OGS score at debond is presented in ▶ Fig. 9.2. On average, meta-analysis of three studies indicated that orthodontic treatment with aligners was associated with a

Table 9.2 Risk of bias of included randomized clinical trials with the RoB 2.0 tool

Study	Randomization process	Deviations from intended interventions	Missing outcome data	Measurement of the outcome	Selection of the reported result	Overall	Comments
Abbate 2015	High	High	Low	Low	Some concerns	High	Additionally, incomplete reporting is seen for all continuous outcomes
Hennessy 2016	Low	High	High	High	Some concerns	High	Also, incomplete reporting of treatment duration
Li 2015	Low	Low	Low	Low	Some concerns	Some concerns	Incomplete reporting for treatment duration, due to missing standard deviations, but these were provided by the authors after contacting them
Preston 2017	Low	Low	Low	Low	Some concerns	Some concerns	–

Table 9.3 Risk of bias of included nonrandomized studies with the ROBINS-I tool

	Bias due to/in							
	Confounding	Selection of participants into the study	Classification of interventions	Deviations from intended interventions	Missing data	Measurement of outcomes	Selection of the reported result	Overall
Djeu 2005	Moderate	NI	Low	NI	NI	Moderate	Low	Moderate
Fetouh 2008	Moderate	NI	Low	NI	NI	Moderate	Low	Moderate
Gu 2017	Moderate	Critical	Low	NI	NI	Low	Low	Critical
Han 2015	Moderate	NI	Low	NI	NI	Low	Moderate	Moderate
Lanteri 2018	Moderate	NI	Low	Low	NI	Moderate	Low	Moderate
Robitaille 2016	Moderate	NI	Low	NI	NI	Moderate	Low	Moderate
Yi 2018	Moderate	NI	Low	Serious	NI	Low	Moderate	Serious

Abbreviation: NI, no information.

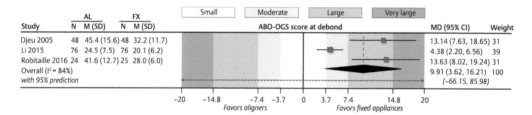

Fig. 9.2 Contour-enhanced forest plot on the comparison of total ABO-OGS scores posttreatment between aligners and fixed appliances. ABO-OGS, American Board of Orthodontics Objective Grading System; AL, aligner; CI, confidence interval; FX, fixed appliance; M, mean; MD, mean difference; N, number of patients; SD, standard deviation. Contours correspond to different effect magnitude and the *red dotted line* corresponds to 95% random-effects prediction.

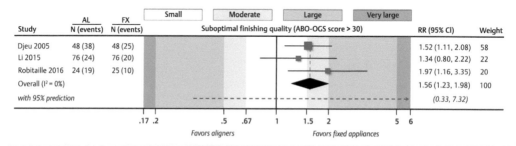

Fig. 9.3 Contour-enhanced forest plot on the comparison of proportion of "passing" cases according to the ABO examination (cases with ABO-OGS score lower than 30 points) posttreatment between aligners and fixed appliances. ABO-OGS, American Board of Orthodontics Objective Grading System; AL, aligner; CI, confidence interval; FX, fixed appliance; N, number of patients; RR, relative risk. Contours correspond to different effect magnitude and the red dotted line corresponds to 95% random-effects prediction.

statistically significant reduction in the finishing quality according to ABO-OGS compared to fixed appliances (MD: 9.9 points; 95% CI: 3.6–16.2 points; p = 0.002). Considerable heterogeneity was seen among the three included studies (I^2 = 84%), which meant that several patient- or treatment-related factors might play a role in the actual final occlusal result. However, existing heterogeneity influenced only the precise calculation of the difference between aligners and fixed appliances, as one study indicated a moderate difference and the other two indicated a large one. It did not, however, influence the direction of the effect, as all three studies showed that fixed appliances were significantly associated with better treatment results than aligners.

The same conclusion was drawn when looking at the proportion of cases being finished to an acceptable quality according to the ABO standards—i.e., the proportion of patients having less than 30 ABO-OGS points at debond (▶ Fig. 9.3). Meta-analysis of

three studies indicated that treatment with aligners was associated with significantly increased probability for the case to be considered a "failure" according to the ABO standards (i.e., that the case has an ABO-OGS score more than 30) compared to fixed appliances (RR: 1.6; 95% CI: 1.2–2.0; p < 0.001). No considerable heterogeneity across studies was seen, which reported a small to moderate increase in the rate of suboptimal finishing quality. On absolute terms, this is translated to a 60.6% "failing" grade according to ABO for the aligner group compared to a 38.9% rate for the fixed appliance group (▶ Fig. 9.4). This is in turn translated to a number needed to treat of 5, which means that every fifth case treated with aligners instead of fixed appliances would fail the ABO examination, but would get a "passing" grade if it was treated with fixed appliances, which is a potentially clinically relevant effect.

Looking at the comparative performance for each separate component of ABO-OGS between

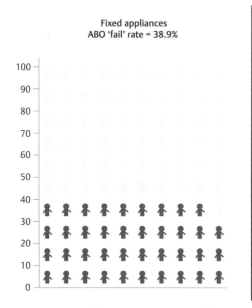

Fixed appliances
ABO 'fail' rate = 38.9%

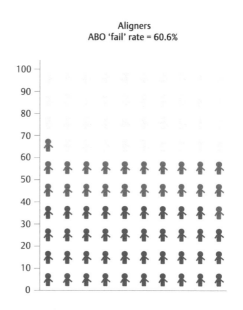

Aligners
ABO 'fail' rate = 60.6%

Fig. 9.4 Illustration of the expected absolute risk for a case to have an ABO-OGS score of over 30 post debond when treated with aligners or fixed appliances, according to the results of the meta-analysis. ABO, American Board of Orthodontics.

aligners and fixed appliances gives a more precise image about the occlusal aspects mostly affected by the treatment modality (▶ Fig. 9.5). Overall, meta-analyses of three studies indicated that five of the eight aspects of the occlusion were significantly better finished with fixed appliances than with aligners: buccolingual inclination (MD: 0.8 point; 95% CI: 0.5–1.1 point; $p < 0.001$), occlusal contacts (MD: 3.1 points; 95% CI: 0.6–5.6 points; $p = 0.02$), occlusal relationship (MD: 1.0 point; 95% CI: 0.6–1.4 points; $p < 0.001$), overjet (MD: 1.8 points; 95% CI: 0.6–3.0 points; $p = 0.002$), and root angulation (MD: 0.8 point; 95% CI: 0.5–.1 point; $p < 0.001$). It has been reported that it is considerably more difficult to control root movement with aligners compared to fixed appliances, especially without the use of attachments.[2,51,52] The third generation of aligners presumably allows for improved movement of this type by adding ellipsoid precision attachments that are able to produce couples creating root movement,[2] which remains to be tested experimentally. On the other side, three ABO-OGS components (alignment, marginal ridges, and interproximal contacts) gave very similar results for both modalities. This is not surprising, since aligners are known to consistently produce adequate space closure of up to

6 mm by progressively tipping teeth into spaces in small increments and can successfully straighten dental arches by derotating teeth, especially when composite attachments are bonded.[52,53,54] Looking carefully at the effect magnitude, it is obvious that the clinical relevance for each separate criterion is questionable, as small to moderate differences between aligners and fixed appliances are seen on average. However, when adding all these differences for each criterion, a clinically relevant worse finishing outcome is seen with aligners overall (as seen in ▶ Fig. 9.2 and ▶ Fig. 9.3).

Looking at the occlusal outcome of treatment through meta-analyses of two studies using the PAR index gives a slightly different picture (▶ Table 9-4). Overall, no statistically significant difference in the posttreatment PAR scores between aligners and fixed appliances was seen (MD: 0 points; 95% CI: −2.0 to 2.0 points; $p = 0.98$). Contrary to that, treatment with orthodontic aligners was associated with a significantly smaller reduction in PAR scores (significantly worse treatment efficacy) compared to fixed appliances (MD: −2.9 points; 95% CI: −5.0 to −0.8 points; $p = 0.007$). However, even though the effect was statistically significant, the magnitude of this difference was small, which

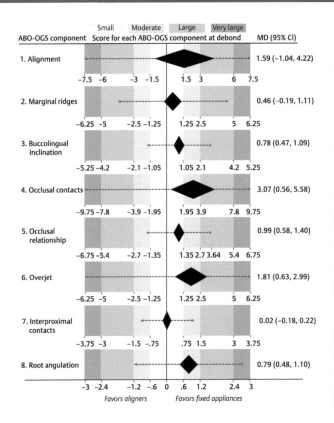

Fig. 9.5 Composite contour-enhanced forest plot illustrating the summary results of eight meta-analyses (each with three studies and 297 patients) for the comparison of each separate ABO-OGS component between orthodontic aligners and fixed appliances. ABO-OGS, American Board of Orthodontics Objective Grading System; CI, confidence interval; MD, mean difference. Contours correspond to different effect magnitude and the *red dotted lines* correspond to 95% random-effects predictions.

makes its clinical relevance questionable. Results of a single study[48] indicated that aligners were worse in terms of reduction for the PAR component for upper anteriors (MD: –1.0 point; 95% CI: –1.9 to –0.1 point; p = 0.02) and overbite (MD: –1.0 point; 95% CI: –1.9 to –0.2 points; p = 0.02) compared to fixed appliances (▶Table 9.5). Again, differences between aligners and fixed appliances for these outcomes might be statistically significant, but probably are not clinically relevant. On the other side, the proportion of patients experiencing a great improvement in their PAR scores through treatment (PAR reduction of at least 22 points or PAR score of 0 posttreatment) was significantly smaller with aligners than with fixed appliances (RR: 0.5; 95% CI: 0.3–0.9; p = 0.02; ▶Table 9.5). This corresponds to absolute risk for great PAR improvement of 22.9 and 45.8% for aligners and fixed appliance, respectively (▶Fig. 9.6). The number needed to treat is again 5, which is translated as every fifth case treated with aligners

instead of fixed appliances not experiencing a great reduction in PAR scores through treatment, which would be seen if the case had been treated with fixed appliances, and denotes a potentially clinically relevant effect. This discrepancy between the results of the ABO-OGS and the PAR index can be explained by obvious differences between the two tools. The PAR index was developed to assess in a systematic manner the outcome of orthodontic treatment in order to be incorporated in both quality assessment measures of orthodontic care and scientific research. It, however, provides a vague assessment of the occlusion and disregards aspects such as tooth inclination, remaining spaces, and alignment of the posterior dental arch, which are important variable for board examination cases.[32] It does not provide a detailed assessment of the position of each tooth and relationship with its neighbors within an ideal dental arch as the ABO-OGS does, which was developed in order to assess the fine details expected to be seen in a

Table 9.4 Results of random-effects meta-analyses for eligible outcomes with at least two contributing studies

Outcome	n	Effect	p	I^2 (95% CI)	tau² (95% CI)	95% prediction
ABO-OGS total score	3	MD: 9.91 (3.62, 16.21)	0.002[a]	84% (38%, 99%)	25.52 (3.01, 507.80)	−66.15, 85.98
ABO-OGS failure (score>30)	3	RR: 1.56 (1.23, 1.98)	<0.001[a]	0% (0%, 91%)	0 (0, 0.55)	0.33, 7.32
ABO-OGS component 1: alignment	3	MD: 1.59 (−1.05, 4.22)	0.24	91% (60%, 100%)	4.93 (0.71, 95.19)	−31.38, 34.55
ABO-OGS component 2: marginal ridges	3	MD: 0.46 (−0.18, 1.10)	0.16	0% (0%, 88%)	0 (0, 2.52)	−3.68, 4.61
ABO-OGS component 3: buccolingual inclination	3	MD: 0.78 (0.46,1.09)	<0.001[a]	0% (0%, 94%)	0 (0, 3.77)	−1.26, 2.81
ABO-OGS component 4: occlusal contacts	3	MD: 3.07 (0.57, 5.57)	0.02[a]	79% (19%, 99%)	3.78 (0.24, 79.63)	−26.47, 32.61
ABO-OGS component 5: occlusal relationship	3	MD: 0.99 (0.58, 1.40)	<0.001[a]	0% (0%, 94%)	0 (0, 7.24)	−1.66, 3.64
ABO-OGS component 6: overjet	3	MD: 1.81 (0.64, 2.98)	0.002[a]	50% (0%, 97%)	0.54 (0, 17.35)	−10.25, 13.87
ABO-OGS component 7: interproximal contacts	3	MD: 0.02 (−0.16, 0.21)	0.82	0% (0%, 89%)	0 (0, 0.74)	−1.18, 1.22
ABO-OGS component 8: root angulation	3	MD: 0.79 (0.49, 1.10)	<0.001[a]	0% (0%, 89%)	0 (0, 0.65)	−1.18, 2.76
PAR post-Tx	2	MD: −0.03 (−2.02, 1.96)	0.98	83% (0%, 100%)	1.72 (0, 258.55)	NC
PAR reduction via Tx	2	MD: −2.92 (−5.02, −0.81)	0.007[a]	0% (0%, 98%)	0 (0, 126.05)	NC
Treatment duration (months)	7	MD: −0.55 (−3.73, 2.63)	0.73	94% (82%, 99%)	16.25 (4.74, 73.67)	−11.72, 10.62

Abbreviations: ABO-OGS, American Board of Orthodontics Objective Grading System; CI, Confidence Interval; MD, Mean Difference;
n, number of contributing studies; NC, Noncalculable; PAR, Peer Assessment Rating; RR, Relative Risk.
Note: Meta-analyses that are both statistically significant and clinically relevant are given in bold, judged as having an effect being at least equal to the average standard deviation of the control (fixed appliance) group across included studies.
[a]Statistically significant findings at the 5% level.

meticulously finished case in all three planes (first, second, and third order). Reported limitations of the PAR index[55] include, among others, a low weighting for overbite scores and high weighting for overjet scores.[56] Indeed, posttreatment PAR scores do not correlate significantly with posttreatment ABO-OGS scores.[57,58] Subsequently, the PAR index has been widely used to also assess the baseline severity of a case. However, the PAR index to this end does not take into account aspects such as skeletal discrepancies/cephalometric values, developmental tooth anomalies, ectopic teeth, or soft-tissues relationships and again does not correlate well with the ABO DI.[57]

Table 9.5 Results of eligible outcomes assessed by only single studies

Outcome	Effect	P
PAR reduction per month	MD: 0.39 (0.09,0.69)	0.01[a]
PAR component 1: upper anteriors	MD: −1.00 (−1.86, −0.14)	0.02[a]
PAR component 2: lower anteriors	MD: −0.4 (−1.42,0.53)	0.38
PAR component 3: anteroposterior relationship	MD: −0.33 (−0.84,0.18)	0.20
PAR component 4: transverse relationship	MD: −0.17 (−0.42,0.08)	0.18
PAR component 5: vertical relationship	MD:0.04 (−0.02,0.10)	0.16
PAR component 6: overjet	MD:0.12 (−2.12,2.36)	0.92
PAR component 7: overbite	MD: −1.03 (−1.90, −0.16)	0.02[a]
PAR component 8: midline deviation	MD: −0.58 (−1.34,0.18)	0.14
PAR great improvement (reduction>30)	**RR:0.50 (0.27,0.91)**	**0.02[a]**
Mandibular alignment not perfect	RR:0.67 (0.29,1.56)	0.35
EARR (total)	MD: −1.84 (−2.35, −1.33)	<0.001[a]
EARR (maxillary central incisors)	MD: −1.13 (−2.20, −0.06)	0.04[a]
EARR (maxillary lateral incisors)	MD: −1.76 (−2.84, −0.68)	0.001[a]
EARR (mandibular central incisors)	MD: −1.15 (−2.07, −0.23)	0.02[a]
EARR (mandibular lateral incisors)	**MD: −3.30 (−4.24, −2.36)**	**<0.001[a]**
Lower incisor inclination to mandibular plane	MD: −1.90 (−4.14,0.34)	0.10
Gingival recession	RR:0.90 (0.31,2.68)	0.86

Abbreviations: CI, confidence interval; EARR, external apical root resorption; MD, mean difference; NC, noncalculable; PAR, Peer Assessment Rating; RR, relative risk.
Note: Results that are both statistically significant and clinically relevant are given in bold, judged as having an effect being at least equal to the average standard deviation of the control (fixed appliance) group of the included study.
[a]Statistically significant findings at the 5% level.

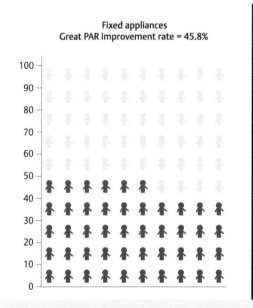
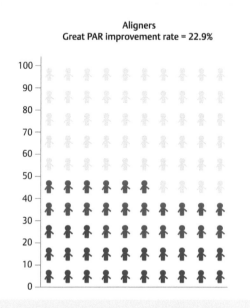

Fig. 9.6 Illustration of the expected absolute risk for a case to experience a great improvement in its PAR score (PAR reduction of at least 22 points or PAR score of 0 posttreatment) when treated with aligners or fixed appliances, according to the results of a single included study. PAR, peer assessment rating.

9.5 Treatment Efficiency in Terms of Duration and Adverse Effects

Considerable variation was seen in the effect of treatment modality on treatment duration. Meta-analysis of seven studies indicated that on average no definite conclusions can be drawn regarding treatment duration with either aligners or fixed appliances (MD: −0.6 month; 95% CI: −3.7 to 2.6 months; $p = 0.73$). Extreme heterogeneity was seen across studies ($I^2 = 94\%$), which makes the ability to synthesize existing studies questionable (▸ Fig. 9.7). Specifically, two studies reported statistically significant reduction in treatment duration with aligners and two studies reported statistically significant increase in treatment duration with aligners, while the remaining three studies did not find statistically significant differences. Furthermore, exclusion of a study assessing combined orthodontic/orthognathic treatment[47] instead of only orthodontic treatment did not improve the results (six studies; MD: −0.1 month; 95% CI: −3.5 to 3.4 months; $I^2 = 95\%$). Nor was the situation improved by limiting the meta-analysis to only randomized trials (two studies; MD: 2.69 months; 95% CI: −5.0 to 10.4 months; $I^2 = 96\%$) or to only studies with nonextraction treatment (five studies; MD: 0.6 month; 95% CI: −3.2 to 4.4 months; $I^2 = 96\%$). Therefore, it is logical to assume that treatment duration is influenced by many other confounding variables and that the choice of appliance alone does not show a consistent effect on treatment duration.

Additionally, results of a single study[48] indicated that aligners were more efficient in terms

of PAR reduction/month of treatment compared to fixed appliances (MD: 0.4 point/month; 95% CI: 0.1–0.7 point/month; $p = 0.01$). However, as the same study reported that aligners were overall associated with smaller reductions in the PAR scores than fixed appliances, looking at the PAR reduction/month outcome might be misleading.

As far as adverse effects of treatment are concerned, a single identified study on EARR[51] reported that significantly smaller percentage of the incisors' root was resorbed during aligner treatment compared to fixed appliances (MD: −1.8%; 95% CI: −2.4 to −1.3%; $p < 0.001$; ▸ Table 9.5). The same was seen for the various subgroups according to tooth type (central vs. lateral incisor) and jaw (maxilla vs. mandible), but the effect magnitude was on average very small and probably of no clinical relevance. It must be stressed here also that evaluation of EARR during treatment is complicated, since many risk factors come into play, including the patient's genetic predisposition toward EARR,[59] the chosen mechanotherapy,[60] the duration of treatment,[61] and the actual amount of tooth movement (and especially apical movement).[59] A carefully conducted retrospective nonrandomized study taking confounders such as baseline severity through ABO DI, genetic polymorphisms, and absolute apical displacement into account concluded that treatment with orthodontic aligners results in similar amounts of EARR compared to fixed appliances. Therefore, it might be prudent to check if any significant differences in EARR reported in the literature are not rather due to actually teeth being moved less around with aligners.

Additionally, treatment with aligners was not associated, in a single included study[46] with

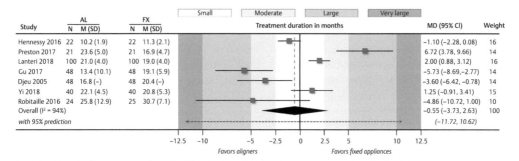

Fig. 9.7 Contour-enhanced forest plot on the comparison of treatment duration in months between aligners and fixed appliances. AL, aligner; CI, confidence interval; FX, fixed appliance; M, mean; MD, mean difference; N, number of patients; SD, standard deviation. Contours correspond to different effect magnitude and the red dotted line corresponds to 95% random-effects prediction.

significantly lower proclination of the lower incisors compared to fixed appliances (MD: –1.9°; 95% CI: –4.1 to 0.3°; p = 0.10). However, it must be noted that a very small sample was included, which makes the study probably underpowered to identify such a small difference of 1.9° between groups, if this really exists.

Furthermore, no significant difference in the development of gingival recessions 2 years after treatment with aligners or fixed appliances was seen in another single study (MD: 0.9; 95% CI: 0.3–2.7; p = 0.86).[50] It might be expected that choice of appliance alone might not directly influence the development of gingival recession. Even if appliance choice was associated with increased anterior anchorage loss/incisor proclination (which was not seen), this would not necessarily translate to increased risk of gingival recession.[62,63] Although orthodontic treatment on average increases the risk for gingival recessions,[64] its precise etiology is multifactorial with risk factors including periodontal disease, mechanical trauma, patient age, smoking, and induction of bone dehiscences by positioning the teeth beyond the alveolar plate.[65,66,67,68,69,70,71,72]

Finally, limited evidence on the effect of appliance choice on loss of periodontal attachment was provided by a single identified study,[44] which assessed orthodontic alignment of anterior teeth in adult patients with previous history of treated periodontal disease. After retrieving raw data from the author and matching the study's groups for baseline status, no differences between aligners and fixed appliances were seen for periodontal probing depth (MD: 0 mm; 95% CI: –0.4 to 0.4 mm; p = 1.00) or alveolar bone levels (MD: 0.1 mm; 95% CI: –0.4 to 0.6 mm; p = 0.69). On the other side, fixed appliances were significantly quicker in repositioning the patients' migrated anterior teeth compared to aligners (3.9 vs. 6.0 months; MD: –2.1 months; 95% CI: –3.7 to –0.5 months; p = 0.01). It must be noted here that although previous systematic reviews of mostly compromised studies have reported that aligners might be associated with facilitation of better oral hygiene than fixed appliances,[18,23,45] a recent randomized clinical trial[73] found no significant consistent advantage in terms of plaque index, gingival index, or periodontal bleeding index between patients treated with aligners and fixed appliances. It seems, therefore, that fixed appliances also can be compatible with proper oral hygiene.

9.6 Strength of Current Recommendations and Threats to Their Validity

Our confidence in the clinical recommendations that can be formulated based on the quality of evidence using the GRADE framework is presented in ▶Table 9.6. We can say with moderate certainty that compared to treatment with fixed appliances, treatment with orthodontic aligners: (1) leads to worse finishing quality (higher ABO-OGS scores), (2) leads to greater proportion of treated cases that would not pass the ABO examination criteria (ABO-OGS score > 30 points), and (3) makes little to no difference in the development of gingival recessions. This means that future research could have an important impact, which might change current estimates of effect. The main reason for downgrading the quality of evidence pertained to the inclusion of nonrandomized studies that (although being matched) had methodological issues that could introduce some bias. Therefore, even though a potentially large clinical difference in posttreatment ABO-OGS scores between aligners and fixed appliances was seen, this cannot be used as basis to upgrade our confidence in these estimates, as heterogeneity across studies precludes precise effect quantification (▶Fig. 9.2).

We can say with low confidence that compared to treatment with fixed appliances treatment with orthodontic aligners: (1) leads to lower treatment efficacy (smaller PAR reduction through treatment), (2) leads to greater proportion of treated cases seeing a great improvement (PAR reduction of at least 22 points or PAR score of 0 posttreatment), (3) leads to greater EARR, and (4) makes little to no difference in proclination of the lower incisors during treatment. The main reason for downgrading the quality of evidence pertained to the inclusion of nonrandomized studies with serious/critical methodological issues that most probably introduce bias. This was especially seen in the retrospective study of Gu et al[48] that selectively reported data from what might be regarded as "good" cases, while excluding patients with issues of compliance or oral hygiene. This means that further research in terms of well-designed studies is very likely to have an important impact, which is likely to change our current estimates of effect.

Finally, we have very low confidence on the currently observed effect of treatment modality

Table 9.6 Summary of findings table according to the GRADE approach

Outcome [follow-up] Studies (patients)	Relative effect (95% CI)	Anticipated absolute effects (95% CI)			Quality of the evidence (GRADE)[b]	What happens with aligners
		Fixed appliance[a]	Aligners	Difference with aligners		
ABO-OGS score [post Tx] 297 patients (3 studies)	–	26.7 pts	–	9.9 pts greater (3.6 to 16.2 greater)	⊕⊕⊕O moderate[c,d,e] due to bias	Probably leads to worse finishing quality (higher ABO-OGS scores)
Unacceptable finishing quality (ABO-OGS score>30 pts) [post Tx] 297 patients (3 studies)	RR 1.6 (1.23 to 1.98)	38.9%	60.6% (47.8%–77.0%)	21.7% more (8.9% to 38.0% more)	⊕⊕⊕O moderate[c] due to bias	Probably leads to more patients with unacceptable finishing quality
PAR reduction [post Tx] 176 patients (2 studies)	–	19.6 pts	–	2.9 pts less (0.8 to 5.0 less)	⊕⊕OO low[f] due to bias	Might lead to lower treatment efficacy (smaller reduction in PAR scores)
Great improvement in PAR (PAR reduction>30 pts) [post Tx] 96 patients (1 study)	RR 0.5 (0.27 to 0.91)	45.8%	22.9% (12.4%–41.7%)	22.9% less (4.1% to 33.4% less)	⊕⊕OO low[f] due to bias	Might lead to less patients with great improvement in PAR scores
Treatment duration [post Tx] 759 patients (7 studies)	–	19.6 mo	–	0.6 mo shorter (3.7 shorter to 2.6 longer)	⊕OOO very low[g,h] due to bias, inconsistency	Too heterogenous response to synthesize across studies
EARR as % of anteriors' root length [post Tx] 80 patients/640 teeth (1 study)	–	7.0%	–	1.8% less (1.3% to 2.4% less)	⊕⊕OO low[f] due to bias	Might lead to greater EARR
Inclination of lower incisors [near Tx end] 44 patients (1 study)	–	5.3°	–	1.9° less (4.1° less to 0.3° more)	⊕⊕OO low[i,j] due to bias, imprecision	Little to no difference in lower incisor inclination
Gingival recession [2 years post Tx] 158 patients (1 study)	RR 0.9 (0.31 to 2.68)	8.0%	7.2% (2.5%–21.4%)	0.8% less (5.5% less to 13.4% more)	⊕⊕⊕O moderate[c] due to bias	Little to no difference in gingival recession

Abbreviations: ABO-OGS, American Board of Orthodontics Objective Grading System; CI, confidence interval; EARR, external apical root resorption; GRADE, Grading of Recommendations Assessment, Development and Evaluation; PAR, peer assessment rating; pt, point; Tx, treatment.

Note: Intervention: comprehensive orthodontic treatment with thermoplastic aligners versus fixed appliances. Population: adolescent or adult patients with any kind of malocclusion. Setting: university clinics, private practice, hospital (Canada, China, Ireland, Italy, United States).

[a]Response in the control group is based on average response of included studies (random-effects meta-analysis).

[b]Starts from "high."

[c]Downgraded by one level for bias due to the inclusion of nonrandomized studies with moderate risk of bias.

[d]No downgrading for inconsistency (even though $I^2 > 75\%$), as it affects only our estimate about the difference between treatment modalities, but not our decision (all studies are on the right side of forest plot and show significant effects).

[e]Potentially great effect observed (larger than one average standard deviation), but no upgrading due to residual confounding.

[f]Downgraded by two levels for bias due to the inclusion of nonrandomized studies with critical/serious risk of bias.

[g]Downgraded by two levels for bias due to the inclusion of randomized trials with high risk of bias and nonrandomized studies with serious/critical risk of bias.

[h]Downgraded by one level due to inconsistency; great variability is seen among included studies with significant studies arranged on both sides of the forest plot (confident signs of heterogeneity that influence our decision about which treatment is shorter, which precludes calculating an average effect).

[i]Downgraded by one level for bias due to the inclusion of a randomized trial with high risk of bias.

[j]Downgraded by one level for imprecision due to the inclusion of an inadequate sample.

choice (aligners vs. fixed appliances) on treatment duration. This has to do with the fact that very heterogeneous results were seen across existing studies that could not be explained by either clinical heterogeneity, study design, or incorporation of extractions in the treatment plan. Therefore, any estimate about the average difference in duration between aligners and fixed appliances is very uncertain and future well-designed studies should be based on careful selection of cases matched for baseline severity and take into account potential confounders such as case severity, incorporation of extractions, amount of interproximal enamel reduction, and quality of the final occlusal outcome.

Nevertheless, it is important to point out that several threats to the validity of currently available clinical recommendations exist. For one, methodological issues existed for all included studies that might influence conclusions, and this is especially the case for included retrospective nonrandomized studies.[11–14] Furthermore, most meta-analyses were based predominantly on small trials, which might affect their results.[74] Additionally, the small number of trials that were ultimately included in the meta-analyses and their incomplete reporting of results and potential confounders such as level of case severity, oral hygiene, compliance, use of bonded attachments, number of aligners, rate of refinement need, or amount of interproximal enamel reduction precluded the conduct of many analyses for subgroups and meta-regressions that might enable identification of patient subgroups for which aligners might be equally or even more appropriate treatment alternative compared to fixed appliances.

9.7 Conclusion

According to currently existing clinical evidence from randomized trials and matched nonrandomized studies on mostly adult patients with mild to severe malocclusions treated with or without extractions, it seems that orthodontic treatment with aligners is associated with worse treatment outcome compared to fixed appliances. On the other side, aligners might be associated with a small decrease in EARR during treatment, while there seems to be little to no difference on proclination of lower incisors and development of gingival recessions. Treatment duration is not defined

by choice of appliance alone and patient- or treatment-related factors might come into play.

Note

Since the preparation and submission of this chapter, additional data were made available, which explains small differences in the results of this chapter compared to the subsequent journal paper,[75] and a publication notice was issued.[76] However, the study's results and final conclusions in all instances remain practically the same with no threat to their validity.

References

[1] Boyd RL, Miller RJ, Vlaskalic V. The Invisalign system in adult orthodontics: mild crowding and space closure cases. J Clin Orthod. 2000;34:203–212

[2] Hennessy J, Al-Awadhi EA. Clear aligners generations and orthodontic tooth movement. J Orthod. 2016;43(1):68–76

[3] Miles P. 2013 survey of Australian orthodontists' procedures. Aust Orthod J. 2013;29(2):170–175

[4] McMorrow SM, Millett DT. Adult orthodontics in the Republic of Ireland: specialist orthodontists' opinions. J Orthod. 2017;44(4):277–286

[5] Keim RG, Gottlieb EL, Vogels DS, III, Vogels PB. 2014 JCO study of orthodontic diagnosis and treatment procedures, Part 1: results and trends. J Clin Orthod. 2014;48(10):607–630

[6] d'Apuzzo F, Perillo L, Carrico CK, et al. Clear aligner treatment: different perspectives between orthodontists and general dentists. Prog Orthod. 2019;20(1):10

[7] O'Brien K, Sandler J. In the land of no evidence, is the salesman king? Am J Orthod Dentofacial Orthop. 2010;138(3):247–249

[8] Seehra J, Pandis N, Fleming PS. Clinical evaluation of marketed orthodontic products: are researchers behind the times? A meta-epidemiological study. Prog Orthod. 2017;18(1):14

[9] Pandis N. Randomized Clinical Trials (RCTs) and Systematic Reviews (SRs) in the context of Evidence-Based Orthodontics (EBO). Semin Orthod. 2013;19:142–157

[10] Papageorgiou SN, Eliades T. Evidence-based orthodontics: Too many systematic reviews, too few trials. J Orthod. 2019;46(1_suppl, suppl 1):9–12

[11] Papageorgiou SN, Kloukos D, Petridis H, Pandis N. Publication of statistically significant research findings in prosthodontics & implant dentistry in the context of other dental specialties. J Dent. 2015;43(10):1195–1202

[12] Papageorgiou SN, Xavier GM, Cobourne MT. Basic study design influences the results of orthodontic clinical investigations. J Clin Epidemiol. 2015;68(12):1512–1522

[13] Papageorgiou SN, Höchli D, Eliades T. Outcomes of comprehensive fixed appliance orthodontic treatment: A systematic review with meta-analysis and methodological overview. Korean J Orthod. 2017;47(6):401–413

[14] Papageorgiou SN, Koretsi V, Jäger A. Bias from historical control groups used in orthodontic research: a meta-epidemiological study. Eur J Orthod. 2017;39(1):98–105

[15] Papageorgiou SN, Xavier GM, Cobourne MT, Eliades T. Registered trials report less beneficial treatment effects than unregistered ones: a meta-epidemiological study in orthodontics. J Clin Epidemiol. 2018;100:44–52

[16] Sideri S, Papageorgiou SN, Eliades T. Registration in the international prospective register of systematic reviews (PROSPERO) of systematic review protocols was associated with increased review quality. J Clin Epidemiol. 2018;100:103–110

[17] Papageorgiou SN, Antonoglou GN, Martin C, Eliades T. Methods, transparency and reporting of clinical trials in orthodontics and periodontics. J Orthod. 2019;46(2):101–109

[18] Rossini G, Parrini S, Castroflorio T, Deregibus A, Debernardi CL. Periodontal health during clear aligners treatment: a systematic review. Eur J Orthod. 2015;37(5):539–543

[19] Rossini G, Parrini S, Castroflorio T, Deregibus A, Debernardi CL. Efficacy of clear aligners in controlling orthodontic tooth movement: a systematic review. Angle Orthod. 2015;85(5):881–889

[20] Elhaddaoui R, Qoraich HS, Bahije L, Zaoui F. Orthodontic aligners and root resorption: A systematic review. Int Orthod. 2017;15(1):1–12

[21] Zheng M, Liu R, Ni Z, Yu Z. Efficiency, effectiveness and treatment stability of clear aligners: A systematic review and meta-analysis. Orthod Craniofac Res. 2017;20(3):127–133

[22] Aldeeri A, Alhammad L, Alduham A, Ghassan W, Shafshak S, Fatani E. Association of orthodontic clear aligners with root resorption using three-dimension measurements: A systematic review. J Contemp Dent Pract. 2018;19(12):1558–1564

[23] Jiang Q, Li J, Mei L, et al. Periodontal health during orthodontic treatment with clear aligners and fixed appliances: A meta-analysis. J Am Dent Assoc. 2018;149(8):712–720.e12

[24] Lu H, Tang H, Zhou T, Kang N. Assessment of the periodontal health status in patients undergoing orthodontic treatment with fixed appliances and Invisalign system: A meta-analysis. Medicine (Baltimore). 2018;97(13):e0248

[25] Galan-Lopez L, Barcia-Gonzalez J, Plasencia E. A systematic review of the accuracy and efficiency of dental movements with Invisalign®. Korean J Orthod. 2019;49(3):140–149

[26] Ke Y, Zhu Y, Zhu M. A comparison of treatment effectiveness between clear aligner and fixed appliance therapies. BMC Oral Health. 2019;19(1):24

[27] Papadimitriou A, Mousoulea S, Gkantidis N, Kloukos D. Clinical effectiveness of Invisalign® orthodontic treatment: a systematic review. Prog Orthod. 2018;19(1):37

[28] Higgins J, Green S. Cochrane Handbook for Systematic Reviews of Interventions. Version 5.1.0 (updated March 2011). The Cochrane Collaboration. 2011. Available at: http://www.cochr aneha ndbook.org

[29] Liberati A, Altman DG, Tetzlaff J, et al. The PRISMA statement for reporting systematic reviews and meta-analyses of studies that evaluate health care interventions: explanation and elaboration. J Clin Epidemiol. 2009;62(10):e1–e34

[30] Richmond S, Shaw WC, O'Brien KD, et al. The development of the PAR Index (Peer Assessment Rating): reliability and validity. Eur J Orthod. 1992;14(2):125–139

[31] Cangialosi TJ, Riolo ML, Owens SE, Jr, et al. The ABO discrepancy index: a measure of case complexity. Am J Orthod Dentofacial Orthop. 2004;125(3):270–278

[32] Casko JS, Vaden JL, Kokich VG, et al;American Board of Orthodontics. Objective grading system for dental casts and panoramic radiographs. Am J Orthod Dentofacial Orthop. 1998;114(5):589–599

[33] Sterne JAC, Savović J, Page MJ, et al. RoB 2: a revised tool for assessing risk of bias in randomised trials. BMJ. 2019;366:l4898

[34] Sterne JA, Hernán MA, Reeves BC, et al. ROBINS-I: a tool for assessing risk of bias in non-randomised studies of interventions. BMJ. 2016;355:i4919

[35] Langan D, Higgins JPT, Jackson D, et al. A comparison of heterogeneity variance estimators in simulated random-effects meta-analyses. Res Synth Methods. 2019;10(1):83–98

[36] Papageorgiou SN. Meta-analysis for orthodontists: Part II--Is all that glitters gold? J Orthod. 2014;41(4):327–336

[37] IntHout J, Ioannidis JP, Rovers MM, Goeman JJ. Plea for routinely presenting prediction intervals in meta-analysis. BMJ Open. 2016;6(7):e010247

[38] Guyatt GH, Oxman AD, Schünemann HJ, Tugwell P, Knottnerus A. GRADE guidelines: a new series of articles in the Journal of Clinical Epidemiology. J Clin Epidemiol. 2011;64(4):380–382

[39] Carrasco-Labra A, Brignardello-Petersen R, Santesso N, et al. Improving GRADE evidence tables part 1: a randomized trial shows improved understanding of content in summary of findings tables with a new format. J Clin Epidemiol. 2016;74:7–18

[40] Schünemann HJ, Cuello C, Akl EA, et al;GRADE Working Group. GRADE guidelines: 18. How ROBINS-I and other tools to assess risk of bias in nonrandomized studies should be used to rate the certainty of a body of evidence. J Clin Epidemiol. 2019;111:105–114

[41] Djeu G, Shelton C, Maganzini A. Outcome assessment of Invisalign and traditional orthodontic treatment compared with the American Board of Orthodontics objective grading system. Am J Orthod Dentofacial Orthop. 2005;128(3):292–298, discussion 298

[42] Fetouh O. Comparison of Treatment Outcome of Invisalign® and Traditional Fixed Orthodontics by Model Analysis Using ABO Objective Grading System. New York, NY: State University of New York at Buffalo;2009

[43] Abbate GM, Caria MP, Montanari P, et al. Periodontal health in teenagers treated with removable aligners and fixed orthodontic appliances. J Orofac Orthop. 2015;76(3):240–250

[44] Han JY. A comparative study of combined periodontal and orthodontic treatment with fixed appliances and clear aligners in patients with periodontitis. J Periodontal Implant Sci. 2015;45(6):193–204

[45] Li W, Wang S, Zhang Y. The effectiveness of the Invisalign appliance in extraction cases using the the ABO model grading system: a multicenter randomized controlled trial. Int J Clin Exp Med. 2015;8(5):8276–8282

[46] Hennessy J, Garvey T, Al-Awadhi EA. A randomized clinical trial comparing mandibular incisor proclination produced by fixed labial appliances and clear aligners. Angle Orthod. 2016;86(5):706–712

[47] Robitaille P. Traitement combiné d'orthodontie et de chirurgie orthognatique avec Invisalign®: revue de la durée de traitement et des résultats obtenus [MSc thesis]. Montreal: University of Montreal;2016

[48] Gu J, Tang JS, Skulski B, et al. Evaluation of Invisalign treatment effectiveness and efficiency compared with conventional fixed appliances using the Peer Assessment Rating index. Am J Orthod Dentofacial Orthop. 2017;151(2):259–266

[49] Preston KA. Treatment and Post-treatment Posterior Occlusal Changes in Invisalign® and Traditional Braces: A Randomized Controlled [MSc thesis]. College Station, TX: Texas A&M University;2017

[50] Lanteri V, Farronato G, Lanteri C, Caravita R, Cossellu G. The efficacy of orthodontic treatments for anterior crowding with Invisalign compared with fixed appliances using the Peer Assessment Rating Index. Quintessence Int. 2018;49(7):581–587

[51] Yi J, Xiao J, Li Y, Li X, Zhao Z. External apical root resorption in non-extraction cases after clear aligner therapy or fixed orthodontic treatment. J Dent Sci. 2018;13(1):48–53

[52] Simon M, Keilig L, Schwarze J, Jung BA, Bourauel C. Treatment outcome and efficacy of an aligner technique--regarding incisor torque, premolar derotation and molar distalization. BMC Oral Health. 2014;14:68

[53] Kravitz ND, Kusnoto B, BeGole E, Obrez A, Agran B. How well does Invisalign work? A prospective clinical study evaluating the efficacy of tooth movement with Invisalign. Am J Orthod Dentofacial Orthop. 2009;135(1):27–35

[54] Chisari JR, McGorray SP, Nair M, Wheeler TT. Variables affecting orthodontic tooth movement with clear aligners. Am J Orthod Dentofacial Orthop. 2014;145(4, Suppl):S82–S91

[55] Fox NA. The first 100 cases: a personal audit of orthodontic treatment assessed by the PAR (peer assessment rating) index. Br Dent J. 1993;174(8):290–297

[56] Hamdan AM, Rock WP. An appraisal of the Peer Assessment Rating (PAR) Index and a suggested new weighting system. Eur J Orthod. 1999;21(2):181–192

[57] Deguchi T, Honjo T, Fukunaga T, Miyawaki S, Roberts WE, Takano-Yamamoto T. Clinical assessment of orthodontic outcomes with the peer assessment rating, discrepancy index, objective grading system, and comprehensive clinical assessment. Am J Orthod Dentofacial Orthop. 2005;127(4):434–443

[58] Hong M, Kook YA, Baek SH, Kim MK. Comparison of treatment outcome assessment for Class I malocclusion patients: Peer Assessment Rating versus American Board of Orthodontics - Objective Grading System. J Korean Dent Sci. 2014;7:6–15

[59] Iglesias-Linares A, Sonnenberg B, Solano B, et al. Orthodontically induced external apical root resorption in patients treated with fixed appliances vs removable aligners. Angle Orthod. 2017;87(1):3–10

[60] Iliadi A, Koletsi D, Eliades T. Forces and moments generated by aligner-type appliances for orthodontic tooth movement: A systematic review and meta-analysis. Orthod Craniofac Res. 2019;22(4):248–258

[61] Samandara A, Papageorgiou SN, Ioannidou-Marathiotou I, Kavvadia-Tsatala S, Papadopoulos MA. Evaluation of orthodontically induced external root resorption following orthodontic treatment using cone beam computed tomography (CBCT): a systematic review and meta-analysis. Eur J Orthod. 2019;41(1):67–79

[62] Artun J, Grobéty D. Periodontal status of mandibular incisors after pronounced orthodontic advancement during adolescence: a follow-up evaluation. Am J Orthod Dentofacial Orthop. 2001;119(1):2–10

[63] Renkema AM, Navratilova Z, Mazurova K, Katsaros C, Fudalej PS. Gingival labial recessions and the post-treatment proclination of mandibular incisors. Eur J Orthod. 2015;37(5):508–513

[64] Papageorgiou SN, Eliades T. Clinical evidence on the effect of orthodontic treatment on the periodontal tissues. In: Eliades T, Katsaros C, eds. The Ortho-Perio Patient: Clinical Evidence and Therapeutic Guidelines. Chicago, IL: Quintessence Publishing;2019

[65] Wennström JL, Lindhe J, Sinclair F, Thilander B. Some periodontal tissue reactions to orthodontic tooth movement in monkeys. J Clin Periodontol. 1987;14(3):121–129

[66] Löe H, Anerud A, Boysen H. The natural history of periodontal disease in man: prevalence, severity, and extent of gingival recession. J Periodontol. 1992;63(6):489–495

[67] Smith RG. Gingival recession. Reappraisal of an enigmatic condition and a new index for monitoring. J Clin Periodontol. 1997;24(3):201–205

[68] Albandar JM, Streckfus CF, Adesanya MR, Winn DM. Cigar, pipe, and cigarette smoking as risk factors for periodontal disease and tooth loss. J Periodontol. 2000;71(12):1874–1881

[69] Kassab MM, Cohen RE. The etiology and prevalence of gingival recession. J Am Dent Assoc. 2003;134(2):220–225

[70] Litonjua LA, Andreana S, Bush PJ, Cohen RE. Toothbrushing and gingival recession. Int Dent J. 2003;53(2):67–72

[71] Rawal SY, Claman LJ, Kalmar JR, Tatakis DN. Traumatic lesions of the gingiva: a case series. J Periodontol. 2004;75(5):762–769

[72] Levin L, Zadik Y, Becker T. Oral and dental complications of intra-oral piercing. Dent Traumatol. 2005;21(6):341–343

[73] Chhibber A, Agarwal S, Yadav S, Kuo CL, Upadhyay M. Which orthodontic appliance is best for oral hygiene? A randomized clinical trial. Am J Orthod Dentofacial Orthop. 2018;153(2):175–183

[74] Cappelleri JC, Ioannidis JP, Schmid CH, et al. Large trials vs meta-analysis of smaller trials: how do their results compare? JAMA. 1996;276(16):1332–1338

[75] Papageorgiou SN, Koletsi D, Iliadi A, Peltomaki T, Eliades T. Treatment outcome with orthodontic aligners and fixed appliances: a systematic review with meta-analyses. Eur J Orthod. 2020;46(4):297–310

[76] Papageorgiou SN, Koletsi D, Iliadi A, Peltomaki T, Eliades T. Comment on: Treatment outcome with orthodontic aligners and fixed appliances: a systematic review with meta-analyses. Eur J Orthod. 2020;42(3):344–346

10 Forces and Moments Generated by Aligner-Type Appliances for Orthodontic Tooth Movement

Anna Iliadi, Despina Koletsi, and Theodore Eliades

Summary

Notwithstanding the wide clinical use of aligner treatments, forces and moments generated by such thermoplastic appliances on teeth remain largely unknown to clinicians. Also, clinical behavior of this type of aligner-type appliances does not remain unaffected by occlusal forces and/or wear-related properties. This chapter provides information on the existing evidence from three different perspectives regarding aligner thickness, generated tooth movement, and aligner material. It also addresses the importance of the internal validity of the existing scientific evidence. Review of all relevant studies concludes that laboratory investigations are the sole source of evidence on aligner mechanics and tooth movement–related conditions. Use of fabrication material of the aligners has been currently confined to different types of PETG. Aligner thickness does not appear to play a significant role over initial forces and moments generated by thermoplastic aligners, given specific tooth movements and aligner design. The most widely examined tooth movements are tipping and rotation, with rotational forces ascending to a much higher level. However, the existing evidence and findings may be applicable to specific conditions and tooth movements in laboratory settings. Therefore, data acquired cannot be directly transferred to biologic mechanisms of tooth movement within the periodontal ligament. In addition, tooth movement mechanics that have been studied across existing studies on a single-tooth specific frame, without consideration of adjacent teeth, elastic modulus of the ligament, occlusal/mastication forces, or soft-tissue considerations.

Keywords: thermoplastic aligner-type appliances, aligner thickness, tooth movement, aligner material, PETG

10.1 Introduction

The concept of fabricating aligners on setup casts for orthodontic tooth movement dates back to 1945 when Kesling introduced the use of positioners during the final stages of orthodontic treatment to facilitate tooth settling.[1] Nowadays, the increasing demand for invisible orthodontics and esthetic considerations, primarily across adult patients, has made the use of thermoplastic aligners quite popular. By the end of the 1990s, two novel thermoplastic aligner systems were introduced, allowing for a wide range of tooth movement. The Clear-Aligner system[2,3] (Scheu Dental GmbH, Iserlohn, Germany) implemented setups comprising tooth displacements between 0.5 and 1 mm.[2] This required a sequence of three aligners per setup step, with increasing thickness from 0.5 to 0.625 and 0.75 mm, respectively. The Invisalign system[3] (Align Technology, Santa Clara, California, United States), on the contrary, allowed for setup steps to be reduced to approximately 0.2 mm, so that stiffer aligners could be employed. Stereolithographic models and digital setups were implemented, allowing for only one initial impression.

Notwithstanding the wide clinical use of these treatment methods, forces and moments generated by such aligner-type appliances on teeth remain largely unknown to clinicians. A number of studies compared the force-delivery properties of thermoplastic orthodontic aligners in terms of setup magnitude. It has been stated that setup increments should preferably range between 0.2 and 0.5 mm, depending on the type of thermoplastic material used.[4] Other studies investigated the forces and moments applied on teeth by thermoplastic aligners in a series of movements. During mesiodistal rotation, forces were exceeding the suggested load of 20 N mm.[5] Similar findings were confirmed for intrusion, tipping, and bodily movement.[6,7,8]

Clinical behavior of thermoplastic aligner-type appliances is not unaffected by occlusal forces and/or wear-related properties. The former has been associated with load increases when it comes to rotational moments or intrusive forces.[9] The latter may lead to a considerable force decay and deactivation, which may reach approximately 50% after a 2-week period of aligner use.[10]

The importance of setup increments in conjunction with the selection of the appropriate thermoplastic foil thickness during aligner manufacturing is pivotal to avoid overloading of teeth during orthodontic movement. A number of studies have attempted to quantify the effect of setup increments and thermoplastic material thickness on aligner mechanics.

10.2 Existing Evidence

Evidence on forces and moments generated by aligner adjuncts stems from experimental laboratory studies published during the last decade. A range of different types of tooth movement has been produced by various aligner materials (Biolon, Erkodur, Ideal Clear, Duran, All-In, Invisalign) with foil thickness from 0.3 to 1 mm. The characteristics and outcomes of the identified literature studies are summarized in ▶ Table 10.1, based on the most recent systematic review.[11]

The existing evidence has been examined from three different perspectives regarding aligner thickness, generated tooth movement, and aligner material. This arbitrary categorization was implemented simply to facilitate data comprehension.

10.2.1 Aligner Thickness

The thickness of plastic foil used for thermoforming PETG aligners ranges from 0.3 to 1 mm. The forces generated by the thinnest commercially available aligners of 0.5 mm result in significant overloading of the periodontal structures.[7] When PETG aligners of reduced thickness, namely of 0.4 and 0.3 mm are used, the aforementioned forces decrease by 35 and 71%, respectively.[7] It has been reported that aligner thickness of 0.3 mm may reduce rotational stiffness by 76%.[13] Despite the fact that 0.3-mm PETG aligners seem to exert ideal forces, they are considered unsuitable for clinical use due to deformation.[7,13] Thus, a sequence of aligners including 0.4, 0.5, and 0.75 mm has been proposed[7,13,14] in order to achieve low initial stiffness combined with a steady load. As for 0.625- and 0.75-mm PETG foils, findings indicate that both present similar mechanical behavior with respect to rotational moments during mandibular canine and maxillary central incisor rotation,[13,14] as well as labiolingual tipping and bodily movement.[6–8] Three studies examined the behavior of 1-mm PETG aligners and concluded that forces

and moments generated were higher than those recommended.[9,15,16] Finally, forces applied by 0.7-mm Invisalign system aligners have been reported to lie within the range of acceptable orthodontic forces.[20]

No differences between the thinnest commercially available aligners of 0.5 mm and its counterparts of either 0.625 or 0.75 mm in terms of moment-to-force (M/F) ratio have been reported. Material of increased thickness may reach higher levels of rigidity; however, this does not result in higher levels of effectively exerted forces that may translate to clinical implications.[11] It has been suggested that the intermediate stage thickness of these adjuncts such as 0.625 mm may be questionable or even unnecessary in the clinical context.[8] This is in contrast with the existing recommendations for clinical use of three consecutive aligners of increasing thickness very close to one another.[2] In any case, for any detected variations or similarities in terms of forces and moments generated by materials of different aligner thickness, gingival width extension of the aligner appears as a significant predictor.[11]

10.2.2 Type of Tooth Movement

Tipping of upper central incisors[12] and lower canine intrusion[18] is feasible with the use of PETG aligners. On the contrary, three studies indicated that bodily movement and torque are the most demanding movements to achieve since plain aligners without modifications cannot establish the force couple required.[7,16,17] Upper incisor rotation movement with aligners has been frequently coupled with an intrusive force, which may present an increase in magnitude when combined with simulated occlusal forces.[9,13,15] Hahn and coworkers[15] found that only a slight activation of ±0.17 mm or 0.5 degrees per step during rotation could produce ideal forces which have been estimated to range between 0.35 and 0.6 N.[21] Finally, Simon and coworkers stated that Invisalign aligners bear the potential to deliver force levels of such magnitude, which may produce premolar derotation, bodily movement, molar distalization, and torque when combined with appropriate attachment setups.[20]

Special attention has been given to palatal tipping movement of the upper incisor across different types of aligner thickness. Based on the most recent systematic review,[11] no differences were detected between any of the retrieved

Table 10.1 Characteristics of the existing studies

	Author and year of publication	Study design	Sample size/teeth type	Groups under comparison	Interventions	Outcomes
1	Brockmeyer et al 2017[12]	In vitro	Total $n = 45$ aligners, same thickness 1-mm Biolon uncut $n = 5$, z11 $n = 5$, z12–21 $n = 5$ Erkodur uncut $n = 5$, z11 $n = 5$, z12–21 $n = 5$ IdealClear uncut $n = 5$, z11 $n = 5$, z12–21 $n = 5$ upper central incisor	Material vs. cut, deflection distance vs. material, deflection distance vs. cut	Thermoplastic aligners modified by incisal cuts	Horizontal force component magnitude, vertical force component magnitude in labial and palatal translation of upper central incisors
2	Elkholy et al 2015[6]	In vitro	Total $n = 27$ aligners Duran 0.5 mm ($n = 3$), 0.625 mm ($n = 3$), 0.75 mm ($n = 3$) Erkodur 0.5 mm ($n = 3$), 0.6 mm ($n = 3$), Track-A 0.5 mm ($n = 3$), 0.63 mm ($n = 3$), 0.8 mm ($n = 3$) upper central incisors	Forces delivered aligner/thickness	Different aligner thickness and material Duran 0.5 mm ($n = 3$), 0.625 mm ($n = 3$), 0.75 mm ($n = 3$) Erkodur 0.5 mm ($n = 3$), 0.6 mm ($n = 3$), 0.8 mm ($n = 3$) Track-A 0.5 mm ($n = 3$), 0.63 mm ($n = 3$), 0.8 mm ($n = 3$)	Forces and moments magnitude to upper central incisor for labial and palatal translation
3	Elkholy et al 2016[7]	In vitro	Total $n = 15$ Duran 0.3 mm ($n = 3$) 0.4 mm ($n = 3$) 0.5 mm ($n = 3$) 0.625 mm ($n = 3$) 0.75 ($n = 3$) upper central incisors	Forces delivered aligner/thickness	Reduced thickness aligners Duran 0.3 mm ($n = 3$) 0.4 mm ($n = 3$) 0.5 mm ($n = 3$) 0.625 mm ($n = 3$) 0.75 mm ($n = 3$)	Forces and moments delivered during labiopalatal movement of upper central incisor
4	Elkholy et al 2017[13]	In vitro	Total $n = 15$ Duran 0.5 mm ($n = 3$), 0.625 mm ($n = 3$), 0.75 mm ($n = 3$) vs. 0.3 mm ($n = 3$), 0.4 mm ($n = 3$) upper central incisors	Forces applied by 0.3/0.4 mm aligners vs. conventional >0.5 mm	Reduced thickness aligners 0.4, 0.3 mm Duran 0.5 mm ($n = 3$), 0.625 mm ($n = 3$), 0.75 mm ($n = 3$) vs. 0.3 mm ($n = 3$), 0.4 mm ($n = 3$)	Forces and moments delivered during mesiodistal derotation of upper central incisor
5	Elkholy et al 2017[14]	In vitro	Total $n = 9$ Duran 0.5 mm ($n = 3$), 0.625 mm ($n = 3$), 0.75 mm ($n = 3$) mandibular canine	Forces delivered aligner/thickness	Duran 0.5 mm ($n = 3$), 0.625 mm ($n = 3$), 0.75 mm ($n = 3$)	Forces and moments delivered during mesial and distal derotation of mandibular canine

(Continued)

Table 10.1 (*Continued*) Characteristics of the existing studies

	Author and year of publication	Study design	Sample size/teeth type	Groups under comparison	Interventions	Outcomes
6	Gao et al 2017[8]	In vitro	Total n = 27 × 2 = 54? Duran 0.5 mm/0–1 width n = 3 Duran 0.5 mm/3–4 width n = 3 Duran 0.5 mm/6–7 width n = 3 Duran 0.625 mm/0–1 width n = 3 Duran 0.625 mm/3–4 width n = 3 Duran 0.625 mm/6–7 width n = 3 Duran 0.75 mm/0–1 width n = 3 Duran 0.75 mm/3–4 width n = 3 Duran 0.75 mm/6–7 width n = 3 upper central incisor	Edge width comparison/aligner thickness	Different aligner thickness width Duran 0.5 mm/0–1 width n = 3 Duran 0.5mm/3–4 width n=3 Duran 0.5 mm/6–7 width n = 3 Duran 0.625 mm/0–1 width n = 3 Duran 0.625 mm/3–4 width n = 3 Duran 0.625 mm/6–7 width n = 3 Duran 0.75 mm/0–1 width n = 3 Duran 0.75 mm/3–4 width n = 3 Duran 0.75 mm/6–7 width n = 3	Forces and moments delivered during maxillary central incisor palatal tipping and intrusion
7	Hahn et al 2010[15]	In vitro	n = 15 Ideal Clear 1 mm n = 5 Erkodur 1 mm n = 5 Biolon 1 mm n = 5 upper central incisor	Forces delivered aligner material	Different aligner material	Force system and moments produced by three different types of plastic aligners during rotation
8	Hahn et al 2010[16]	In vitro	n = 15 Ideal Clear 1 mm n = 5 Erkodur 1 mm n = 5 Biolon 1 mm n = 5 upper central	Forces delivered aligner material	Different aligner material	Force system and moments produced by three different types of plastic aligners during torque
9	Hahn et al 2011[9]	In vitro	n = 20 Biolon 0.75 mm n = 5 Biolon 1 mm n = 5 Erkodur 0.8 mm n = 5 Erkodur 1 mm n = 5 upper central	Forces delivered material/with and without simulated occlusal forces	Different aligner material + occlusal forces	Forces produced by two different types of aligners with and without simulated occlusal forces during rotation of upper central incisors

(*Continued*)

Table 10.1 (*Continued*) Characteristics of the existing studies

	Author and year of publication	Study design	Sample size/teeth type	Groups under comparison	Interventions	Outcomes
10	Li et al 2016[17]	In vitro	$n = 5$, Erkodur 1 mm activation 0.2 mm $n = 1$ activation 0.3 mm $n = 1$ activation 0.4 mm $n = 1$ activation 0.5 mm $n = 1$ activation 0.6 mm $n = 1$ upper central	Forces delivered between various amounts of activation aligners	Aligners with various amounts of activation	Forces delivered between various amounts of activation aligners and attenuation during lingual bodily movement of upper central incisor
11	Liu and Hu 2018[18]	In vitro	$n = 55$, Duran 0.8 mm thickness G0 control $n = 5$ G1 intrude mand canines by 0.2 mm $n = 5$ G2 intrude 4 mand incisors by 0.2 mm $n = 5$ G3 intrude canines and inc by 0.2 mm $n = 5$ G4 intrude can 0.1 mm, lat inc 0.15 mm, centr inc 0.2 mm plus attachments on 1st and 2nd premolars and 1st molars	G0, G1, G2, G3, G4	Aligners with different activation	Forces delivered between various types/amount of aligner activation during intrusion of lower anterior
12	Mencattelli et al 2015[19]	In vitro	All in, Micerium $n = 3$ • Aligner with no forces $n = 1$ • Aligner without divot $n = 1$ • aligner with divot $n = 1$ maxillary central incisor	With divot/without divot	Aligner with divot	Forces delivered from aligner with divot during rotation
13	Simon et al 2014[20]	In vitro	$n = 970$ aligners (60 series/30 patients) Invisalign incisor torque, $n = 10$ patients (split mouth torque < 10 degrees + attachment); premolar derotation, $n = 10$ patients (split mouth derotation <10 degrees + attachment); molar distalization, $n = 10$ patients (split mouth distalization <1.5mm + attachment; 20 tooth movements (2 per patient)	With/without attachments in specific movements: torque, derotation, distalization	With/without attachments	Initial force systems that are delivered by an individual aligner, force systems generated by a series of aligners, influence of auxiliaries (attachments, power ridges) on the force transfer

145

aligner thickness comparisons with regard to M/F ratio. More specifically, for aligner thickness of 0.5 mm compared to that of 0.75 mm, the pooled estimate was a standardized mean difference (SMD) of –3.33 (95% confidence interval [CI]: –9.63 to 2.96; *p*-value = 0.30; I^2 = 82.0%) (▶Fig. 10.1). Accordingly, no differences to M/F ratio were detected for comparisons between 0.5- and 0.625-mm thickness (SMD = –0.43; 95% CI: –4.16 to 3.29; *p*-value = 0.82; I^2 = 84.1%), or 0.625 to 0.75 mm (SMD = –0.98; 95% CI: –7.41 to 5.46; *p*-value = 0.77; I^2 = 89.9%), as well.

In vitro studies in laboratory conditions may effectively represent initial tooth movement mechanics. As such, the reported levels of forces or moments are the highest that may have been generated overall. Force decay produced by thermoplastic aligners over a 2-week period has been documented between 50% of the initial magnitude[10] and a fivefold decrease[22] (▶Fig. 10.2). Tooth movement is described by an interaction of forces and moments exerted and, as such, the metric "moment-to-force ratio" is the one that better represents the simulated tooth movement conditions,

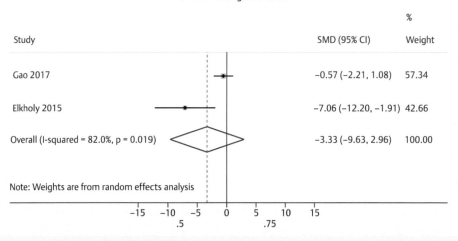

Fig. 10.1 Random effects meta-analysis for the effect of aligner thickness on moment-to-force (M/F) ratio, for palatal tipping of the upper central incisor (aligner thickness: 0.5 vs. 0.75 mm).

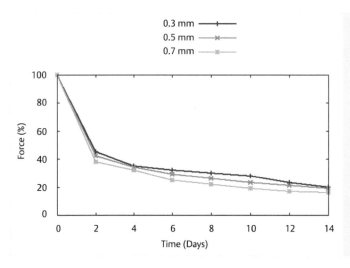

Fig. 10.2 Force decay over a 2-week period for materials of different aligner thickness.

for tipping and translational movements, irrespective of the anticipated magnitude of the movement. However, gingival edge width of the aligner has been identified as a significant predictor of at least the initial moments/forces generated by the aligners. Intrusive movements have been reported to be particularly prone to edge width configuration than tipping movements, while edgeless aligners have been associated with decreased force levels.[8]

10.2.3 Aligner Material

Studies comparing different PETG aligner materials of 1-mm thickness report that aligners vacuum-formed with Biolon (Dreve Dentamid GmbH, Unna, Germany) deliver the highest forces and moments ranging from 1.15 to 6.19 N during tipping[12,16] and 35.3 to 71.8 N mm during rotation,[9,15] respectively, depending on the activation magnitude. The only exception was observed during rotation at low rotation range of ±0.17 mm where the Ideal Clear appliance (Dentsply GAC, Gräfelfing, Germany) exerted the highest values (18.3–20.2 N mm).[15] The lowest forces and rotational moments have been reported for Erkodur (Erkodent Erich Kopp GmbH, Pfalzgrafenweiler, Germany) at all activation ranges.[9,12,15,16]

Friction phenomena, deformations created at the contact areas during thermoforming, and polymer material may explain the differences on mechanical behavior between Biolon and Erkodur.[12,15] The former appliances are thermoformed with a pressure of 6 bars, whereas the latter with 0.8 bars.[9] Moreover, according to the manufacturers' instructions, a spacing foil of 0.05-mm thickness placed between tooth and appliance should be used during thermoforming of Erkodur appliances.[12,15] Although this foil would experience a certain amount of shrinkage after thermoforming, one can assume that its final thickness could be comparable to one activation step.

Aligner modifications such as divots have also been described by manufacturers and clinicians in an attempt to achieve the desired tooth rotation.[12,19,20] The use of divots corresponding to the tooth to be treated was found to increase rotational forces by 58%,[19] whereas the placement of attachments in teeth with short crowns and few undercuts facilitated as well the delivery of the necessary force system.[12]

10.2.4 Internal Validity of the Existing Evidence

Reporting of studies on aligner mechanics in vitro has been positive overall. Experimental conditions are the most well-reported parts of the existing publications and are comparable between the tested groups of aligners.[6,8,9,13,14,15,16,17,18,20] However, no information about blinding of the investigators is provided overall. Losses or noninclusion of specimens is not frequent, precluding attrition bias, while selective outcome reporting has not been suspected. In general, efforts should be directed in optimizing laboratory conditions that would allow researchers to remain blinded when feasible during the assessment of the efficiency of different types of aligners in terms of biomechanical considerations. Moreover, it should be noted that although the risk of selective outcome reporting has been considered minimum given the adequate matching of the reported variables within the methodology section and the results or the retrieved studies, a priori registration of studies is missing.

In vitro studies may suffer from inherent bias due to the lack of standardization of procedures followed to determine the desired effects. In general, specific measuring devices connected to mounted tooth models via a group of sensors and complying with a coordinate system allowing for tooth mobility and simulation of the periodontal ligament have been used. Apparently, any variation within the described laboratory setup across individual studies may result in heterogeneous results. As such and following guidelines from clinical research, there is an overriding need for the development of consistent study protocols prior to the commencement of research, as well as for the agreement on the experimental settings and the most valuable core outcome sets to be universally used.[23]

10.3 Conclusion

It is clear that laboratory studies are identified as the sole source of evidence on aligner mechanics and tooth movement–related conditions. Use of fabrication material of the aligners has been currently confined to different types of PETG. Aligner thickness does not appear to play a significant role over initial forces and moments generated by thermoplastic aligners, given specific tooth movements and aligner design. Foils have been typically reported to range between 0.5 and 1 mm. The most widely examined tooth movements are tipping and rotation, with rotational forces ascending to a much higher level. However, the existing evidence and findings may be applicable to specific conditions and tooth movements in laboratory settings. Overall, there is a need for standardized protocols, types of movements, or design of the aligners in order to inform the current evidence with more conclusive outcomes.

Between-study heterogeneity and apparent differences in settings, aligner material and type, tooth type, and type of movement preclude concrete comparisons between aligner types. Data acquired from the existing studies are based on laboratory simulation conditions and cannot be directly transferred to biologic mechanisms of tooth movement within the periodontal ligament. In addition, tooth movement mechanics that have been studied across included studies on a single-tooth specific frame, without consideration of adjacent teeth, elastic modulus of the ligament, occlusal/mastication forces, or soft-tissue considerations.

References

[1] Kesling HD. The philosophy of the tooth positioning appliance. Am J Orthod Oral Surg. 1945;31:297–304
[2] Kim TW, Echarri P. Clear aligner: an efficient, esthetic, and comfortable option for an adult patient. World J Orthod. 2007;8(1):13–18
[3] Boyd RL, Miller RJ, Vlaskalic V. The Invisalign system in adult orthodontics: mild crowding and space closure cases. J Clin Orthod. 2000;34:203–212
[4] Kwon JS, Lee YK, Lim BS, Lim YK. Force delivery properties of thermoplastic orthodontic materials. Am J Orthod Dentofacial Orthop. 2008;133(2):228–234, quiz 328.e1
[5] Proffit WR. Contemporary Orthodontics. St Louis, MO: Mosby;2007;359–394
[6] Elkholy F, Panchaphongsaphak T, Kilic F, Schmidt F, Lapatki BG. Forces and moments delivered by PET-G aligners to an upper central incisor for labial and palatal translation. J Orofac Orthop. 2015;76(6):460–475
[7] Elkholy F, Schmidt F, Jäger R, Lapatki BG. Forces and moments delivered by novel, thinner PET-G aligners during labiopalatal bodily movement of a maxillary central incisor: An in vitro study. Angle Orthod. 2016;86(6):883–890
[8] Gao L, Wichelhaus A. Forces and moments delivered by the PET-G aligner to a maxillary central incisor for palatal tipping and intrusion. Angle Orthod. 2017;87(4):534–541
[9] Hahn W, Engelke B, Jung K, et al. The influence of occlusal forces on force delivery properties of aligners during rotation of an upper central incisor. Angle Orthod. 2011;81(6):1057–1063
[10] Vardimon AD, Robbins D, Brosh T. In-vivo von Mises strains during Invisalign treatment. Am J Orthod Dentofacial Orthop. 2010;138(4):399–409
[11] Iliadi A, Koletsi D, Eliades T. Forces and moments generated by aligner-type appliances for orthodontic tooth movement: A systematic review and meta-analysis. Orthod Craniofac Res. 2019;22(4):248–258
[12] Brockmeyer P, Kramer K, Böhrnsen F, et al. Removable thermoplastic appliances modified by incisal cuts show altered biomechanical properties during tipping of a maxillary central incisor. Prog Orthod. 2017;18(1):28
[13] Elkholy F, Schmidt F, Jäger R, Lapatki BG. Forces and moments applied during derotation of a maxillary central incisor with thinner aligners: An in-vitro study. Am J Orthod Dentofacial Orthop. 2017;151(2):407–415
[14] Elkholy F, Mikhaiel B, Schmidt F, Lapatki BG. Mechanical load exerted by PET-G aligners during mesial and distal derotation of a mandibular canine : An in vitro study. J Orofac Orthop. 2017;78(5):361–370
[15] Hahn W, Engelke B, Jung K, et al. Initial forces and moments delivered by removable thermoplastic appliances during rotation of an upper central incisor. Angle Orthod. 2010;80(2):239–246
[16] Hahn W, Zapf A, Dathe H, et al. Torquing an upper central incisor with aligners--acting forces and biomechanical principles. Eur J Orthod. 2010;32(6):607–613
[17] Li X, Ren C, Wang Z, Zhao P, Wang H, Bai Y. Changes in force associated with the amount of aligner activation and lingual bodily movement of the maxillary central incisor. Korean J Orthod. 2016;46(2):65–72
[18] Liu Y, Hu W. Force changes associated with different intrusion strategies for deep-bite correction by clear aligners. Angle Orthod. 2018;88(6):771–778
[19] Mencattelli M, Donati E, Cultrone M, Stefanini C. Novel universal system for 3-dimensional orthodontic force-moment measurements and its clinical use. Am J Orthod Dentofacial Orthop. 2015;148(1):174–183
[20] Simon M, Keilig L, Schwarze J, Jung BA, Bourauel C. Forces and moments generated by removable thermoplastic aligners: incisor torque, premolar derotation, and molar distalization. Am J Orthod Dentofacial Orthop. 2014;145(6):728–736
[21] Proffit WR. Contemporary Orthodontics. 3rd ed. St Louis, MO: Mosby Inc;2000:304–305, 313–315
[22] Barbagallo LJ, Shen G, Jones AS, Swain MV, Petocz P, Darendeliler MA. A novel pressure film approach for determining the force imparted by clear removable thermoplastic appliances. Ann Biomed Eng. 2008;36(2):335–341
[23] Tsichlaki A, O'Brien K, Johal A, et al. Development of a core outcome set for orthodontic trials using a mixed-methods approach: protocol for a multicentre study. Trials. 2017;18(1):366

11 Aligners and the Oral Microbiome

William Papaioannou, Iosif Sifakakis, Dimitrios Kloukos, and Theodore Eliades

Summary

This chapter provides information on the effect of orthodontic aligners on the oral microbiome, which might have a direct influence on both caries and periodontal disease. Although it is clear that the scientific literature concerning the impact of orthodontic aligners on the oral microbiome is still limited, this chapter addresses various aspects of oral hygiene during orthodontic treatment, the effect of orthodontic treatment on the oral microbiome, and issues relating aligner treatment with the cariogenic and periodontopathic bacteria. Despite having various shortcomings in their design, the studies available tend to suggest that orthodontic aligners allow for a better clinical condition, from both the standpoint of caries and that of periodontal disease. The impact of better, unhindered, oral hygiene is the clear differentiating factor of aligners from the classic fixed orthodontic treatment protocols. This may be the key factor toward safeguarding the periodontal health of adults, who may also be more susceptible to disease and present as the most significant target group for this more innovative treatment option.

Keywords: aligners, fixed orthodontic appliances, oral microbiome, cariogenic bacteria, periodontopathic bacteria

11.1 Introduction

Fixed orthodontic appliances have revolutionized contemporary therapies and treatment planning; nevertheless, at the same time, they can be considered a risk factor primarily to the integrity of tooth enamel but also periodontal tissues due to plaque accumulation and their colonization by oral microbes.[1] The placement of fixed orthodontic appliances complicates the use of standard oral hygiene procedures and causes alterations in the oral microflora by reducing pH, as well as by increasing plaque accumulation and the affinity of bacteria to metallic surfaces due to electrostatic reactions.[2] The insertion of these appliances creates new retentive areas that favor the local growth of *streptococci*, which in turn increase the levels of these organisms in saliva and around the appliances.[3]

In more recent years, the popularity of orthodontic treatment with thermoplastic aligners has grown due to increased demand for esthetic orthodontic appliances. Traditionally, these materials have been used extensively in the form of vacuum-formed retainers after the completion of orthodontic treatment. It has been reported that these retainers influence the adhesion of *Streptococcus mutans* and *Lactobacillus spp.*, whose numbers of colonies may increase 2 months after debonding.[4] However, microbiological information on the use of thermoplastic aligners as an alternative to fixed appliances is scarce. There is some evidence that recessed and sheltered areas of the aligner, such as the cusp tips and attachment dimples, harbor more biofilm than their flat surfaces.[5] A recent systematic review of the literature published up to 2014 indicated that orthodontic treatment with thermoplastic aligners might be superior in terms of periodontal health, as well as quantity and quality of plaque, compared to conventional fixed appliances.[6] In addition, a relevant retrospective study indicated that the periodontal parameters of patients treated with thermoplastic aligners might be better than those treated with lingual fixed appliances.[7] On the other side, a recent randomized trial[8] found that although patients treated with thermoplastic aligners had initially better periodontal parameters than patients treated with conventional or self-ligating fixed appliances, ultimately appliance choice had no significant effect overall on periodontal health during treatment.

Several appliance-related factors might influence the intraoral performance of thermoplastic aligners. The material most widely used for the fabrication of the thermoplastic aligners and retainers is usually the clear transparent PET-G (polyethylenterephthalat-glycol copolyester). The material used for the Invisalign (Align Technology, Santa Clara, California, United States) aligners is polyurethane-based and seems to have higher hardness and modulus values, a slightly higher brittleness, and lesser creep resistance compared to PETG-based products.[9] It has been suggested that the surface morphology of the aligner might contribute to bacterial adhesion and thereby to salivary bacteria levels. The surface of aligners is not completely smooth but exhibits microabrasions and irregularities, and this configuration with its furrowed corrugated facade makes the appliance more conducive to bacterial and biofilm accumulation.[5]

Classic orthodontic appliances, especially fixed, which are placed in close proximity to the gingival margin, often initiate adverse changes in the gingiva and impact the overall periodontal health of the patient. This is especially true of orthodontic bands' placement, which by their nature are next to the gingiva or even extending into the sulcus, especially in interdental areas. Inflammation will usually ensue, due to the plaque-retentive properties in combination with inadequate oral hygiene and the focal irritation they may cause. Appliances with the propensity for higher plaque accumulation provide the necessary conditions in which it is easier for the balance in the plaque composition to move toward a more complex configuration. In time, more gram-negative, anaerobic, and periodontopathic bacteria can be found within this complex biofilm, bacteria which, if allowed to overgrow, will in turn cause a further inflammatory reaction of the gingival tissues.[10] This has been found to be true especially in interdental regions, where the bacteria are even further protected from removal forces.

Although the orthodontic aligners do not provide new fixed retentive zones for bacterial accumulation, per se, they may affect periodontal health in an indirect manner. The gingival coverage of an aligner, which differs across the various systems, could directly influence periodontal parameters and microbial colonization. Although Invisalign aligners have no significant gingival coverage, other aligner systems are trimmed to overlap the attached gingiva, in order to improve retention. This method is claimed to provide improved aligner retention, which might, however, come at the cost of periodontal implications. Furthermore, the manufacturing process may also play an important role in the aligner's surface, as pressure-forming involves higher pressures than vacuum-forming, which might affect up to a limit the detail of the inner, fitting surface of the aligner.[11]

Caries and periodontal disease are indeed of an infectious nature for which specific pathogens have been implicated. *S. mutans* and *S. sobrinus* have been identified as the main contributors in the pathogenesis of dental caries, and their presence contributes to the risk for

enamel demineralization.[12] Increased levels of *S. mutans* and *Lactobacillus* species have also been reported to be detected in the oral cavity after bonding orthodontic attachments, and some studies have reported that there is a positive correlation between dental caries and the degree of infection with these bacterial species. On the other hand, the periodontal pathogens responsible for inflammation of the gingiva and periodontal breakdown constitute a much more diverse group of bacteria consisting of primarily gram-negative anaerobes, the most notable being *Porphyromonas gingivalis*, *Prevotella intermedia*, *Tannerella forsythia*, *Aggregatibacter actimomycetemcomitans*, and *Treponema denticola*.[13,14]

The aim of this chapter is to present the most recent data on the effect of orthodontic aligners on the oral microbiome, which might have a direct influence on both caries and periodontal disease.

11.2 Oral Hygiene during Orthodontic Treatment

When considering the oral microbiome and its composition, several factors are of special significance: the presence of the hard nonshedding surfaces (primarily those of the teeth, but also other prosthetic or restorative surfaces), dietary habits (most importantly the frequency of sugar consumption), and daily oral hygiene regimen (including tooth-brushing and interdental cleaning).

The placement of brackets on the tooth crowns will affect the amount and balance of specific bacteria. The key bacterial types adhering and forming the plaque biofilm primarily push toward a more cariogenic composition. Indeed, increases in *S. mutans* and *Lactobacilli* spp., which are the primary cariogenic bacteria, are usually detected in patients undergoing orthodontic therapy.[15,16] These bacteria are responsible for the increase in the demineralization of the enamel around the brackets and cause early caries lesions in the form of white spots. Of course, this situation, if left unchecked, can lead to cavitation of the lesions.

Treatment with fixed appliances in adolescents may also transitionally increase the values of all periodontal indices, but without destructive effects on deep periodontal tissues.[10] It was demonstrated that regular patient motivation sessions and mechanical tooth cleaning by a professional dental hygienist help in maintaining good oral hygiene during orthodontic therapy with fixed appliances.[17] In addition, if patient compliance with oral hygiene is reduced, facilitation of regular professional tooth cleaning appointments improves the periodontal condition of adolescents with fixed appliances so that it does not differ from that in untreated patients.[18] An orthodontic oral health promotion program for patients undergoing fixed appliance orthodontic treatment produced a short-term reduction (up to 5 months) in plaque and improvement in gingival health.[19] A recent systematic review demonstrated that only one out of nine randomized controlled trials (RCTs) investigating the periodontal health during orthodontic treatment with manual versus powered toothbrushes showed a statistically significant benefit of powered over manual toothbrushes with regard to gingival index and bleeding. These RCTs did not provide quantified measurements regarding caries activity. The authors conclude that better study standardization and longer follow-up studies are necessary in order to elucidate the clinical relevance of these findings.[20] A smartphone application was developed for preventing dental caries through improved oral-health behavior and oral hygiene in adolescents with fixed orthodontic appliances.[21]

Patients wearing lingual appliances had more plaque retention and gingival inflammation as well as more *S. mutans* counts 2 months after bonding, in comparison with patients wearing conventional labial appliances. No differences were found between the two groups regarding the *Lactobacillus* counts, the salivary flow rate, and saliva buffer capacity.[22] Another study compared patients wearing lingual appliances or aligners. Oral hygiene with lingual appliances is more difficult and this fact is reflected in the lingual patients' indices scores, which were almost twice as high as those of the aligner's wearers. Accordingly, the periodontal risk is considered lower than that associated with fixed lingual appliances, since the aligners are removable, permitting unimpeded oral hygiene.[7] A recent systematic review demonstrated that patients with lingual orthodontic appliances have more problems in maintaining adequate oral hygiene, although no differences in caries risk were identified. However, larger sample sizes and longer follow-up periods are needed in further prospective studies to confirm these results.[23]

Several studies compared oral hygiene and periodontal parameters during orthodontic treatment with conventional appliances versus removable aligners. Aligners do not limit the ability of patients to perform proper oral hygiene. Therefore, adolescents who wore aligners presented better periodontal health and more improvement in oral hygiene than their peers with fixed appliances after 1 year of orthodontic treatment.[24] A statistically significant but clinically insignificant decrease in mean average papillary bleeding score was found during treatment with hard or soft aligners.[25] Patients that are highly aware of oral health maintain gingival inflammation and plaque indices at the same level during the first 8 months of orthodontic treatment with aligners.[26]

Another study in adults demonstrated a decrease in the periodontal status during treatment with fixed labial orthodontic appliances versus removable orthodontic aligners over 1 year of active therapy. The authors used clinical indices and the hydrolysis of N-benzoyl-DL-arginine-naphthylamide (BANA) test. The treatment with fixed appliances was associated with increased levels of periodontopathic bacteria.[27] The same results were obtained from another study with a shorter observational period: patients treated with aligners had better periodontal health during orthodontic treatment than patients treated with fixed appliances. However, mean age differed between the two study groups: adolescents were included in the fixed appliance group and adults in the aligner group.[28] Two other systematic reviews provided the same results.[6,29] The former concluded that these appliances should be considered as the first treatment option in patients with risk of developing periodontal disease.[6] However, the authors of the most recent review downgraded the level of the evidence because of the risk of bias and inconsistency. High-quality studies in this area are still required.[29]

A recent randomized clinical trial found no evidence of differences in oral hygiene levels among clear aligners, self-ligated brackets, and conventional elastomeric ligated brackets after 18 months of active orthodontic treatment.[8]

When visualized at high magnification, the aligner surfaces are not completely smooth but exhibit microabrasions and irregularities, which may contribute to bacterial adhesion (▶ Fig. 11.1). The overall surface configuration, with its furrowed corrugated facade, would appear to make the appliance more conducive to bacterial and

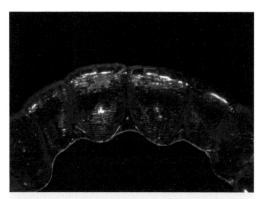

Fig. 11.1 The aligner surfaces are not completely smooth but exhibit microabrasions and irregularities, which may contribute to bacterial adhesion.

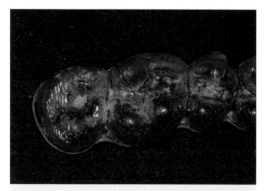

Fig. 11.2 The overall surface configuration, with its furrowed corrugated facade, makes the appliance more conducive to calculus accumulation.

biofilm accumulation (▶Fig. 11.2). Thus, it may be surmised that the composition of the salivary proteins adsorbed onto the surface of aligners is compositionally different from that on enamel surfaces, leading to differing flora in the subsequent biofilm.[5] However, a recent report noted that the use of a vibrating bath with cleaning solution protocol reduced biofilm adherence more than regular brushing or immersion of the aligner in chlorhexidine mouthwash.[30] The use of a low-dose chlorhexidine solution in patients that are highly aware of oral health was deemed unnecessary.[26]

Some plaque indices are inappropriate for patients under orthodontic treatment with fixed appliances. The original Silness and Löe plaque index and the papillary bleeding index have been used in most orthodontic trials. Some of them included measurements of the sulcus probing depth[7,24] and the attachment level.[31] However, if a categorical index is chosen, the modified Silness and Löe index may be considered the most valid and discriminatory. Direct digital measurement of percentage plaque coverage is likely to prove more valid and more reproducible than categorical indices but unfortunately is more complex.[32] Trial periods implemented in the relevant studies usually did not exceed 12 months.

11.3 Effect of Orthodontic Treatment on the Oral Microbiome

As already mentioned, after insertion of fixed orthodontic appliances, adverse effects may ensue in the short- and long-term. Current evidence

suggested that the plaque accumulation caused by orthodontic appliances and improper orthodontic force may alter the equilibrium of the microbial ecosystem and increase the potential for pathogenicity.[33] As a result of ecological changes after bracket insertion, an increase in the amount, composition, metabolic activity, and pathogenicity of the oral microflora,[31,34,35] followed by a worsening of periodontal parameters and an increase of incipient caries lesions, has been observed.[1,35,36] Indeed, adult patients are considered to have a higher risk of periodontal diseases compared with adolescent patients.[33]

Researchers have observed significantly higher prevalence primarily of cariogenic bacterial species, such as the mutans streptococci (*S. mutans* and *S. sobrinus*) and *Lactobaccili* species,[13,14,35] but also of many of the more important periodontal pathogens such as *A. actinomycetemcomitans*, *P. gingivalis*, and *P. intermedia*.[31,37] Therefore, bracket bonding affects the oral microflora not only by the higher plaque accumulations in general, but also by allowing the increase in specific pathogenic bacteria.

The placement of fixed appliances hinders good oral hygiene, and the appliance components can cause alterations in the oral microflora by reducing pH as well as by increasing plaque accumulation, either by their complex plaque retentive design and/or due to affinity of bacteria to the metallic surface because of electrostatic reactions.[2] This indicates that orthodontic brackets could be a potential risk for enamel demineralization. Enamel demineralization has been demonstrated around orthodontic brackets after only 1 month of treatment.[38] However, the changes in the local microbiota around orthodontic appliances and their close proximity to the gingival tissues lead to an increased risk for inflammation of the gingiva.[39] A common reaction is the hyperplastic form of gingivitis, especially in patients with fixed orthodontic appliances that include the use of brackets. This in turn may create the necessary ecological conditions for the predominance of periodontopathic species, further aggravating the periodontal condition.

Questions arise, however, concerning the use of removable appliances, such as thermoplastic aligners. The fact that these devices are in fact removable clearly allows the patient to overcome the difficulties that are present when attempting to exercise proper oral hygiene with the various fixed orthodontic appliances in the mouth. This is proposed as a significant advantage that the removable devices have over the conventional fixed appliances. On the other hand, they do completely cover the tooth surfaces and in some cases areas of the soft tissues surrounding the teeth, for almost the whole day (20–22 hours),[40] preventing to a significant degree the flow of saliva over these areas and protecting bacteria from removal forces.

Nevertheless, clear aligner treatment (CAT) has been suggested in the orthodontic treatment planning of patients at risk for periodontitis.[6,27] Compared with fixed appliances, clear aligners were associated with a better periodontal status and decreased amounts of periodontopathic bacteria, as measured by the metabolic activity of anaerobic bacteria.[27] Although clear aligner patients have lower periodontal indices, such as bleeding on probing and plaque index, than fixed appliance patients, others have reported that the periodontal indices during CAT are slightly higher than those before CAT.[28] Considering that teeth and keratinized gingiva are covered almost all day long by aligners, it is important from a clinical perspective to have a sound judgment regarding the periodontal effects of CAT.

A clear aligner is a protective environment that limits the flow of saliva, negating saliva's natural cleansing, buffering, and remineralizing properties. Additionally, the usual cleansing activities of the lips, cheeks, and tongue are interrupted, allowing further entrapment and development of plaque under the appliances. Some patients may drink liquids without removing their aligners, providing the opportunity for pooling of these liquids beneath the trays. If these factors are compounded by poor oral hygiene, a rapid demineralization—often in areas not normally considered to be prone to caries—can result in greater dental damage than might be found in a noncompliant brusher with fixed appliances.[41] In contrast to these findings, it was reported that orthodontic treatment with CAT showed a low incidence of newly developed white spot lesions.[42]

Concerning the effect on the specific pathogenic bacterial species, either the cariogenic or periodontopathic, the available information is scarce.

11.4 Cariogenic Bacteria

Although the demineralization of the tooth surfaces, by specific bacteria, is a relatively common unwanted occurrence during orthodontic therapy, there are very little data concerning this matter when thermoplastic aligners are used.

The only available clinical research data are from a recent prospective comparative cohort study.[43] It specifically aimed to answer the question: whether there is a difference in the prevalence of cariogenic bacteria (specifically *S. mutans*, *L. acidophilus*, and *S. sanguinis*) among adolescent patients (12–18-year-old) treated orthodontically with thermoplastic aligners or fixed appliances (self-ligating brackets), for an initial short period. The oral levels of these bacteria were examined, specifically in the saliva, by quantitative polymerase chain reaction (PCR) in 30 patients that were divided into two groups according to the two different treatment protocols. Comparisons were also made between baseline, 2 weeks and 1 month after placement/initiation of treatment. No significant difference was found between the two groups concerning the cariogenic bacteria *S. mutans*, while almost no *L. acidophilus* were identified in either group. However, significantly lower levels of *S. sanguinis* were found in the aligner group. *S. sanguinis* has an antagonistic role toward *S. mutans* in the oral cavity, inhibiting its colonization of the tooth surface.[44] Thus, lower levels of this organisms could signify an increase in susceptibility to demineralization over time, in the aligner group. However, this is more significantly offset by the higher levels of plaque control and removal that is possible when fixed appliances are removed. This outcome was obvious in this report by the fact that the aligner group had significantly less plaque than the group with the brackets. Although this investigation does provide some information on the microbiological effect of orthodontic aligners, it has limitations, the most important of which is the short term of 1 month that the patient were followed.

11.5 Periodontopathic Bacteria

The use of thermoplastic aligners has shown that they allow better compliance in oral hygiene resulting in lower plaque levels and gingival inflammation. Abbate and coworkers showed this to be true in adolescent patients, in which they also looked for specific periodontopathogens (*P. intermedia, P. gingivalis, T. forsythia,* and *A. actimycetemcomitans*). None of the patients, neither those with fixed orthodontic appliances (brackets, archwires) nor those with aligners, were positive for their presence over the 12-month evaluation period.[24]

However, the demand for esthetic orthodontic treatment protocols with lingual appliances or clear aligners is significantly higher in adult patients. These are in turn the patients that are at a higher risk for periodontal disease. However, adults are generally more amenable to following instructions on daily oral hygiene than adolescent patients.[45] It is thus of important interest to examine older patients concerning the effects on the oral microbiota in terms of the periodontopathic species.

As already mentioned above, Karkhanechi and coworkers followed two groups of adults, one with aligners and one with fixed labial appliances, for over a year. After 6 months, the fixed orthodontic group showed significantly higher plaque and gingival indices along with increased probing pocket depth and bleeding on probing. These conditions, which continued over the whole year, are conducive for the establishment of periodontopathic bacteria. The authors looked for their presence by collecting plaque and assessing its ability to hydrolyze N-benzoyl-DL-arginine-naphthylamide using a commercial test (BANA test). This is considered a semi-quantitative test for the presence of *P. gingivalis, T. forsythia,* and *T. denticola.* Indeed, their findings were that the fixed orthodontic group had a much higher risk for higher BANA scores (i.e., more pathogens). They concluded that aligners are associated with better periodontal and bacterial conditions.[27]

Modern microbiology relies more and more on newer techniques in molecular diagnostics. With modern PCR, bacteria can be more readily detected but also enumerated, either as total bacterial load or as specific levels of pathogens. A recent study, utilizing real-time PCR examined the bacteria of sulci of two specific teeth (upper right first molar and upper left central incisor) in three groups of individuals (aligner, fixed orthodontic, and control groups) over three time periods (beginning of treatment, 1 month, and 3 months later). This was a mixed group of 77 adolescents and adults (16–30 years old) with a mean age of 24.3 years. Overall, the aligner patients showed better periodontal health (with statistically significant differences for all periodontal indices examined) and reduced total biofilm mass compared to fixed, over the initial 3-month evaluation period. Although the authors mentioned the use of specific primers and probes for four primary periodontopathogens (*A. actinomycetemcomitans, P. gingivalis, P. intermedia,* and *T. forsythia*), the specific information is missing, and they mention only that they detected *A. actinomycetemcomitans* in one fixed orthodontic patient at 1 and 3 months. It is not clear if the other pathogens were detected or not and at what levels.[46]

More recently, Guo and coworkers evaluated 10 aligner patients with high throughput 16S rRNA gene sequencing, which examines in depth the complexity of the microbiome in question. They found no significant differences in the relative abundance of periodontal pathogens at the genus and species level after 3 months of therapy when compared with baseline. They concluded that "clear aligners induced nonpathogenic changes of the subgingival microbiome in the first 3 months of treatment."[47]

11.6 Conclusion

It is clear that the scientific literature concerning the impact of orthodontic aligners on the oral microbiome is still quite poor. There is definitely a need for more comparative studies on their impact on the oral cavity, especially considering their proposed advantages, i.e., the opportunity they offer for a more efficient oral hygiene, over a longer time period—keeping in perspective that they are in further intimate contact with more of the tooth structures and the periodontal tissue by nature of their design. This restricts the flow and beneficial influence of saliva over these tissues which may have a detrimental effect over the long term.

The studies available, however, despite having various shortcomings in their design (group characteristics, sampling of the oral microbiome, target bacteria, etc.), do show an important tendency. This is that orthodontic aligners allow for a better clinical condition, both from the standpoint of caries and that of periodontal disease. The impact of better, unhindered, oral hygiene is the clear differentiating factor of aligners from the classic fixed orthodontic treatment protocols. This may be the key factor toward safeguarding the periodontal health of adults, who may also be more susceptible to disease and present as the most significant target group for this more innovative treatment option. Moreover, adults are generally more amenable to following instructions on daily oral hygiene than adolescent patients and thus more in a position to benefit from the aforementioned benefits of CAT therapy.

References

[1] Zachrisson BU. Oral hygiene for orthodontic patients: current concepts and practical advice. Am J Orthod. 1974;66(5):487–497

[2] Ahn SJ, Lee SJ, Lim BS, Nahm DS. Quantitative determination of adhesion patterns of cariogenic streptococci to various orthodontic brackets. Am J Orthod Dentofacial Orthop. 2007;132(6):815–821

[3] Øgaard B, Rølla G, Arends J. Orthodontic appliances and enamel demineralization. Part 1. Lesion development. Am J Orthod Dentofacial Orthop. 1988;94(1):68–73

[4] Türköz C, Canigür Bavbek N, Kale Varlik S, Akça G. Influence of thermoplastic retainers on Streptococcus mutans and Lactobacillus adhesion. Am J Orthod Dentofacial Orthop. 2012;141(5):598–603

[5] Low B, Lee W, Seneviratne CJ, Samaranayake LP, Hägg U. Ultrastructure and morphology of biofilms on thermoplastic orthodontic appliances in 'fast' and 'slow' plaque formers. Eur J Orthod. 2011;33(5):577–583

[6] Rossini G, Parrini S, Castroflorio T, Deregibus A, Debernardi CL. Periodontal health during clear aligners treatment: a systematic review. Eur J Orthod. 2015;37(5):539–543

[7] Miethke RR, Brauner K. A comparison of the periodontal health of patients during treatment with the Invisalign system and with fixed lingual appliances. J Orofac Orthop. 2007;68(3):223–231

[8] Chhibber A, Agarwal S, Yadav S, Kuo CL, Upadhyay M. Which orthodontic appliance is best for oral hygiene? A randomized clinical trial. Am J Orthod Dentofacial Orthop. 2018;153(2):175–183

[9] Alexandropoulos A, Al Jabbari YS, Zinelis S, Eliades T. Chemical and mechanical characteristics of contemporary thermoplastic orthodontic materials. Aust Orthod J. 2015;31(2):165–170

[10] Ristic M, Vlahovic Svabic M, Sasic M, Zelic O. Clinical and microbiological effects of fixed orthodontic appliances on periodontal tissues in adolescents. Orthod Craniofac Res. 2007;10(4):187–195

[11] Weir T. Clear aligners in orthodontic treatment. Aust Dent J. 2017;62(Suppl 1):58–62

[12] Babaahmady KG, Challacombe SJ, Marsh PD, Newman HN. Ecological study of Streptococcus mutans, Streptococcus sobrinus and Lactobacillus spp. at sub-sites from approximal dental plaque from children. Caries Res. 1998;32(1):51–58

[13] Lundström F, Krasse B. Streptococcus mutans and lactobacilli frequency in orthodontic patients;the effect of chlorhexidine treatments. Eur J Orthod. 1987;9(2):109–116

[14] Lundström F, Krasse B. Caries incidence in orthodontic patients with high levels of Streptococcus mutans. Eur J Orthod. 1987;9(2):117–121

[15] Forsberg CM, Brattström V, Malmberg E, Nord CE. Ligature wires and elastomeric rings: two methods of ligation, and their association with microbial colonization of Streptococcus mutans and lactobacilli. Eur J Orthod. 1991;13(5):416–420

[16] Rosenbloom RG, Tinanoff N. Salivary Streptococcus mutans levels in patients before, during, and after orthodontic treatment. Am J Orthod Dentofacial Orthop. 1991;100(1):35–37

[17] Migliorati M, Isaia L, Cassaro A, et al. Efficacy of professional hygiene and prophylaxis on preventing plaque increase in orthodontic patients with multibracket appliances: a systematic review. Eur J Orthod. 2015;37(3):297–307

[18] Alstad S, Zachrisson BU. Longitudinal study of periodontal condition associated with orthodontic treatment in adolescents. Am J Orthod. 1979;76(3):277–286

[19] Gray D, McIntyre G. Does oral health promotion influence the oral hygiene and gingival health of patients undergoing fixed appliance orthodontic treatment? A systematic literature review. J Orthod. 2008;35(4):262–269

[20] Al Makhmari SA, Kaklamanos EG, Athanasiou AE. Short-term and long-term effectiveness of powered toothbrushes in promoting periodontal health during orthodontic treatment: a systematic review and meta-analysis. Am J Orthod Dentofacial Orthop. 2017;152(6):753–766.e7

[21] Scheerman JFM, van Meijel B, van Empelen P, et al. Study protocol of a randomized controlled trial to test the effect of a smartphone application on oral-health behavior and oral hygiene in adolescents with fixed orthodontic appliances. BMC Oral Health. 2018;18(1):19

[22] Lombardo L, Ortan YÖ, Gorgun Ö, Panza C, Scuzzo G, Siciliani G. Changes in the oral environment after placement of lingual and labial orthodontic appliances. Prog Orthod. 2013;14:28

[23] Ata-Ali F, Ata-Ali J, Ferrer-Molina M, Cobo T, De Carlos F, Cobo J. Adverse effects of lingual and buccal orthodontic techniques: a systematic review and meta-analysis. Am J Orthod Dentofacial Orthop. 2016;149(6):820–829

[24] Abbate GM, Caria MP, Montanari P, et al. Periodontal health in teenagers treated with removable aligners and fixed orthodontic appliances. J Orofac Orthop. 2015;76(3):240–250

[25] Clements KM, Bollen AM, Huang G, King G, Hujoel P, Ma T. Activation time and material stiffness of sequential removable orthodontic appliances. Part 2: Dental improvements. Am J Orthod Dentofacial Orthop. 2003;124(5):502–508

[26] Schaefer I, Braumann B. Halitosis, oral health and quality of life during treatment with Invisalign(®) and the effect of a low-dose chlorhexidine solution. J Orofac Orthop. 2010;71(6):430–441

[27] Karkhanechi M, Chow D, Sipkin J, et al. Periodontal status of adult patients treated with fixed buccal appliances and removable aligners over one year of active orthodontic therapy. Angle Orthod. 2013;83(1):146–151

[28] Azaripour A, Weusmann J, Mahmoodi B, et al. Braces versus Invisalign®: gingival parameters and patients'

satisfaction during treatment: a cross-sectional study. BMC Oral Health. 2015;15:69

[29] Jiang Q, Li J, Mei L, et al. Periodontal health during orthodontic treatment with clear aligners and fixed appliances: A meta-analysis. J Am Dent Assoc. 2018;149(8):712–720.e12

[30] Shpack N, Greenstein RB, Gazit D, Sarig R, Vardimon AD. Efficacy of three hygienic protocols in reducing biofilm adherence to removable thermoplastic appliance. Angle Orthod. 2014;84(1):161–170

[31] Paolantonio M, Pedrazzoli V, di Murro C, et al. Clinical significance of Actinobacillus actinomycetemcomitans in young individuals during orthodontic treatment. A 3-year longitudinal study. J Clin Periodontol. 1997;24(9 Pt 1):610–617

[32] Al-Anezi SA, Harradine NW. Quantifying plaque during orthodontic treatment. Angle Orthod. 2012;82(4):748–753

[33] Ong MM, Wang HL. Periodontic and orthodontic treatment in adults. Am J Orthod Dentofacial Orthop. 2002;122(4):420–428

[34] Diamanti-Kipioti A, Gusberti FA, Lang NP. Clinical and microbiological effects of fixed orthodontic appliances. J Clin Periodontol. 1987;14(6):326–333

[35] Chang HS, Walsh LJ, Freer TJ. The effect of orthodontic treatment on salivary flow, pH, buffer capacity, and levels of mutans streptococci and lactobacilli. Aust Orthod J. 1999;15(4):229–234

[36] van Gastel J, Quirynen M, Teughels W, Carels C. The relationships between malocclusion, fixed orthodontic appliances and periodontal disease. A review of the literature. Aust Orthod J. 2007;23(2):121–129

[37] Lee SM, Yoo SY, Kim HS, et al. Prevalence of putative periodontopathogens in subgingival dental plaques from gingivitis lesions in Korean orthodontic patients. J Microbiol. 2005;43(3):260–265

[38] Gorelick L, Geiger AM, Gwinnett AJ. Incidence of white spot formation after bonding and banding. Am J Orthod. 1982;81(2):93–98

[39] Ellis PE, Benson PE. Potential hazards of orthodontic treatment—what your patient should know. Dent Update. 2002;29(10):492–496

[40] Boyd RL, Miller R, Vlaskalic V. The Invisalign system in adult orthodontics: mild crowding and space closure cases. J Clin Orthod. 2000;34:203–212

[41] Moshiri M, Eckhart JE, McShane P, German DS. Consequences of poor oral hygiene during aligner therapy. J Clin Orthod. 2013;47(8):494–498

[42] Azeem M, Hamid W. Incidence of white spot lesions during orthodontic clear aligner therapy. J World Fed Orthod. 2017;6:127–130

[43] Sifakakis I, Papaioannou W, Papadimitriou A, Kloukos D, Papageorgiou SN, Eliades T. Salivary levels of cariogenic bacterial species during orthodontic treatment with thermoplastic aligners or fixed appliances: a prospective cohort study. Prog Orthod. 2018;19(1):25

[44] Caufield PW, Dasanayake AP, Li Y, Pan Y, Hsu J, Hardin JM. Natural history of Streptococcus sanguinis in the oral cavity of infants: evidence for a discrete window of infectivity. Infect Immun. 2000;68(7):4018–4023

[45] Ramsay DS. Patient compliance with oral hygiene regimens: a behavioural self-regulation analysis with implications for technology. Int Dent J. 2000;Suppl Creating A Successful:304–311

[46] Levrini L, Mangano A, Montanari P, Margherini S, Caprioglio A, Abbate GM. Periodontal health status in patients treated with the Invisalign(®) system and fixed orthodontic appliances: A 3 months clinical and microbiological evaluation. Eur J Dent. 2015;9(3):404–410

[47] Guo R, Zheng Y, Liu H, Li X, Jia L, Li W. Profiling of subgingival plaque biofilm microbiota in female adult patients with clear aligners: a three-month prospective study. PeerJ. 2018;6:e4207

12 Intraoral Aging and Changes on Aligner Mechanical Properties

Spiros Zinelis, T. Gerard Bradley, and Theodore Eliades

Summary

The aim of this chapter is to give information on the degradation of mechanical properties of orthodontic aligners after clinical use. The weakening of mechanical properties has significant clinical implications as it is deeply associated with the clinical efficacy of these appliances. Hardness, modulus of elasticity, creep, and relaxation are mechanical properties with significant clinical implications. Hardness is associated with wear resistance, while the rest three are associated with the extent and duration of exerted orthodontic forces. The chapter presents all the available data from the literature based on clinically aged aligners and discusses all the associated degradation mechanism that may be activated during clinical service.

Keywords: mechanical properties, instrumented indentation testing, retrieval analysis, orthodontic aligner, thermoplastic materials, in vivo aging

12.1 Introduction

All orthodontic appliances used for teeth movement is a "force reservoir" from a biomechanical standpoint of view. The exerted forces decay over time as teeth move and then they are activated using strain to fill force tank. Therefore, the efficacy of orthodontic therapy is strongly dependent on mechanical properties of materials involved and time-dependent response of mechanical properties themselves. Although metallic and ceramic materials have a long clinical record, the same is not true for the recently introduced thermoplastic aligners where their mechanical properties differ dramatically from both aforementioned categories.

Previous reports have found that the efficacy of orthodontic treatment with clear aligners varies from 41 to 59%.[1,2] In addition, the applied forces vary during therapy as forces exerted by successive aligners might differ significantly, resulting in a nonconstant tooth movement.[3] In first place,

the extent of orthodontic forces applied by a thermoplastic material depends on its elastic modulus for a given activation and appliance thickness.[4] On the other hand, increased hardness is a desirable property, enhancing the wear resistance and thus preserving the dimensional integrity of appliance itself. The aforementioned comments demonstrate that any possible difference in mechanical properties among different thermoplastic materials or mechanical degradation over intraoral aging time may have a significant effect on treatment outcome.[4] The differences in mechanical properties have already been thoroughly presented in previous chapter and thus the aim of this chapter is the review of mechanical properties degradation over intraoral aging based on clinical data. However, only a few papers for the mechanical properties of retrieved appliances are available,[5–7] while few have used a simulated oral environment.[8–12] The limited number of retrieval analysis studies is appended to analytical limitations as orthodontic appliances have thin thickness and irregular shape and thus it is impossible to prepare samples for typical mechanical test (i.e., tensile, bending, and others). Alternatively, a vast spectrum of mechanical properties can be determined by modern techniques (i.e., hardness, elastic modulus, ductility, creep, relaxation) employing instrumented indentation testing (IIT) using micro and nano indentations.[4,13] In addition, IIT overcomes the inherent limitation of Vickers testing related to the overestimation of hardness due to elastic recovery around tip after force removal as Martens hardness is estimated automatically from the data obtained from force indentation depth curve.[14,15] ▶Fig. 12.1 demonstrates a typical Vickers indentation with elastic relaxation (pointed by the *arrows*) and a force indentation depth curve where Martens hardness is directly derived by a formula dividing maximum force by surface below indenter. Maximum force is recorded by the load cell, while surface below tip is calculated based on indentation depth and geometrical features of indenter.

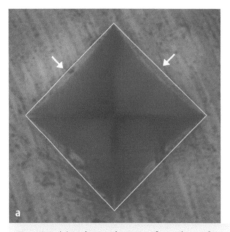
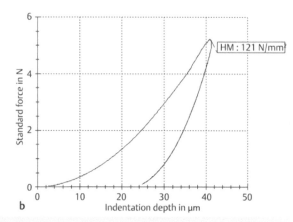

Fig. 12.1 (a) Vickers indentation from the surface of a thermoplastic orthodontic material with curved sides indicating elastic recovery around the tip. The *arrows* show the direction of elastic recovery. (b) Typical force indentation depth curve during loading unloading cycle of the same material. Martens hardness is directly calculated from the data of the curve and the geometry of indenter.

Table 12.1 Brand names, material identification, and Martens hardness (HM), indentation modulus (E_{IT}), elastic index (η_{IT}), and indentation creep (C_{IT}) for commercially available materials

Brand name	Material	HM (N/mm²)	E_{IT} (GPa)	η_{IT} (%)	C_{IT} (%)
A+ (Dentsply Raintree Essix, Sarasota, Florida, United States)	PETG	100.0 (0.7)[a]	2,256 (40)[a]	35.9 (0.6)[a]	2.2 (0.3)[a]
Clear Aligner (SCHEU-DENTAL GmbH, Iserlohn, Germany)	PETG	91.8 (0.8)[b]	2,112 (16)[b]	35.7 (0.2)[a]	2.6 (0.4)[a]
Essix ACE Plastic (Dentsply Raintree Essix, Sarasota, Florida, United States)	PETG	100.6(0.6)[a]	2,374 (4)[c]	34.0 (0.1)[b]	2.7 (0.5)[a]
Invisalign (Align Technology, San Jose, California, United States)	PUR	117.8 (1.1)[c]	2,467 (19)[d]	40.8 (0.2)[c]	3.7 (0.3)[b]

Abbreviations: PETG, polyethylene terephthalate glycol; PUR,polyurethane from methylene diphenyl diisocyanate and 1,6-hexanedial additives.
Note: Same superscripts denote mean values without statistical significant differences.

12.2 Mechanical Properties after In Vivo Aging

The majority of currently available orthodontic aligners are made of two different materials based on attenuated total reflectance Fourier-transformed infrared (ATR-FTIR) spectroscopy as shown in ▸Table 12.1. The first one is polyethylene terephthalate glycol (PETG)[16] and the other is a polyurethane-based material (PUR)[5,16,17] or more precisely a polyurethane from methylene diphenyl diisocyanate and 1,6-hexanedial additives as indicated by manufacturers' material safety data sheet.[8] Although the first three materials showed identical FTIR spectra, they demonstrated significant differences in their mechanical properties (▸Table 12.1). This finding was appended to two different reasons. The first one is that FTIR cannot identify possible differences in the molecular weight of the various PETG polymers. The second explanation is that thermoforming procedure has a significant effect on their mechanical properties[8,16] possible due to differences in thermoforming temperature, cooling rate, and developed residual stresses. Despite the fact that the material type is not enough by its own to characterize the mechanical properties of orthodontic aligners, the discrimination between PEGT and PUR will be adopted for the following text given that the relevant literature based on clinical data is limited and the effect of thermoforming procedure remains unknown.

12.3 Hardness

In a recent study, the Martens hardness of intact and clinically aged PUR appliances was tested by IIT and a significant decrease was allocated denoting that this property is significantly deteriorated during clinical aging.[7] ▶ Fig. 12.2 depicts representative force-indentation depth curves from both conditions.

The aforementioned finding denotes that PUR material is becoming more prone to wear phenomena during clinical service. Surface alterations after in vivo aging have been identified for both PUR and PETG materials,[5,6,17] implying that wear is a degradation mechanism which activated during clinical use. Although there are no reports for hardness changes of PETG materials after in vivo aging, it is anticipated that PETG cannot perform better than PUR due to their lower hardness values (▶ Table 12.1).

12.4 Elastic Modulus

Elastic modulus is strongly correlated with the capacity of thermoplastic appliances to deliver orthodontic forces.[4] Therefore, a higher value of elastic modulus benefits the appliances by exerting increased orthodontic forces or exerting the desired forces but with a thinner structure. All PETG materials tested showed inferior elastic modulus compared to PUR (▶ Table 12.1). Recent clinical data have pointed out that PUR showed a significant decrease after intraoral use for 1 or 2 months,[7] denoting a decrease in their efficacy to apply forces on dental arch. In contrast, an in vitro study did not find any difference in elastic modulus but the samples have been aged only for 1 day in water.[8] On the other hand, PETG showed an unexpected five time increase in modulus of elasticity after 2 weeks of intraoral ageing.[6] However, the authors stated that this increase is associated with the hard and tenacious attached biofilm which exhibited excessive mineralization rather than the material itself. An in vitro study depicted a slight increase in elastic modulus after 1 day of water aging.[8]

12.5 Tensile Strength

The tensile strength is a rarely tested property of orthodontic aligners due to its limited clinical implication. Both materials, PUR and PETG, demonstrate extensive plastic deformation (more than 100%),[8] meaning that they both double their length before fracture. However, in clinical practice even a slightly deformed aligner is discarded due to its inability to exert the desired orthodontic forces. There is only one report based on clinical data regarding the tensile strength of PETG showing that this property remains unchanged after 2 weeks intraoral aging.[6]

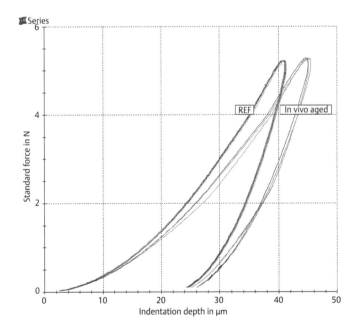

Fig. 12.2 Representative force-indentation depth curves from unused (REF) and clinically aged (in vivo aged) samples from Invisalign appliances. The deeper indentation depth denotes lower hardness.

12.6 Creep–Relaxation

Both creep and relaxation, two time-dependent properties, are critical for the clinical efficacy of orthodontic aligners. The former is defined as the increase in strain under constant stress, while the latter as the decay of stress under constant strain. Ideally, orthodontic aligners should withstand both scenarios successfully to avoid adverse consequences in their clinical efficacy. Orthodontic aligners exert an orthodontic force to teeth but they operate under the constant loading applied by teeth as a counteraction. Therefore, clear aligners operate under constant load and strain during orthodontic therapy. Thus, from a theoretical standpoint, both creep and relaxation are possible under clinical conditions and both have a detrimental effect on efficacy of orthodontic treatment.

A recent study used IIT to compare creep resistance between intact and in vivo aged PUR material.[7] The device applies a constant force and the indentation depth is recorded over time (▶ Fig. 12.3). The difference between final and initial indentation depth is indicative for the creep resistance and is called indentation creep after definition by ISO 14577.[13] Indeed, the retrieved material demonstrated higher creep, denoting that after aging PUR has decreased creep resistance. Therefore, it is rational to assume

that this property decreases during clinical aging, which implies that orthodontic forces are decayed too. However, until present there is no evidence that this degradation has adverse consequences on orthodontic therapy.

Unfortunately, there is no information for the creep behavior of PETG material after clinical aging; also, no information is available for relaxation of both PETG and PUR materials. However, PETG was found very sensitive to relaxation after testing in ambient and water environment for 4 hours. Two commercially available PETG materials (Erkodur, Erkodent Erich Kopp, Pfalzgrafenweiler, Germany, and Duran Scheu-dental, Iserlohn, Germany) retained only 66% (Erkodur) and 55% (Duran) of initial stresses after 4 hours in 37°C water and 5% constant strain.[12] Definitely, the study of creep and relaxation phenomena of orthodontic aligners requires further research to understand the time-dependent response of orthodontic aligners.

12.7 Mechanisms of Degradations of Mechanical Properties

Orthodontic aligners are made by thermoplastic viscoelastic materials and it is well known that

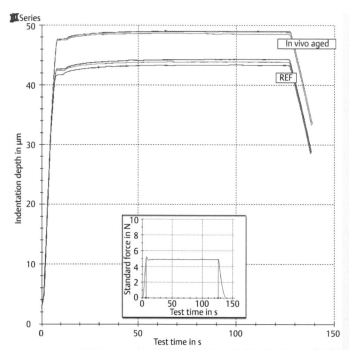

Fig. 12.3 Representative indentation creep curves of intact (REF) and retrieved after clinical aging (IN VIVO AGED) PUR material. The indentation depth increases over time under a constant loading and thus indentation creep can be measured. Inset: the applied force pulse.

their mechanical properties are influenced by three different factors including structural properties (crystalline-amorphous structure), thermoforming processes which affects structural properties, extent, and orientation of residual stresses, and environmental factors associated with in-service conditions, which, in dentistry, are related with water uptake, development of biofilm, loading under clinical conditions, and others.[6–8,16]

Different mechanisms have been proposed till today to explain the degradation of mechanical properties of orthodontic thermoplastic materials. The first explanation is associated with the structure of PUR and is named "polyurethane softening mechanism."[18] PUR shows a two-phase microstructure consisting of randomly segmented copolymers which are distinguished in hard and soft segments. The soft segments tends to create amorphous regions and the hard ones to develop into ordered domains. The proposed softening mechanism supports the orientation and fragmentation of hard domains perpendicular to the orientation of external stresses. This mechanism also facilitates the accommodation of further deformation.[18] Another proposed explanation is the leaching of plasticizers[5,7] during clinical aging, resulting in a more brittle structure as presented by the increase in elastic index of PUR (▶Table 12.1). The relaxation of residual stresses induced during thermoforming process has been also presented as a rational explanation at least for the decrease in hardness.[7] Other studies claim that water absorption may implicate the stress relaxation of matrix through plasticization.[9,10] It is proposed that water absorption breaks the intrachain and/or interchain hydrogen bonds, resulting in increased mobility of macromolecular segments.[12] Although all the aforementioned mechanisms may be activated intraorally, till today there is not any experimental proof for their existence under clinical conditions. Therefore, this is a promising area for further research as the understanding of degradation mechanism may help researchers and clinicians to enhance the clinical efficacy of clear aligners in every day practice.

References

[1] Kravitz ND, Kusnoto B, BeGole E, Obrez A, Agran B. How well does Invisalign work? A prospective clinical study evaluating the efficacy of tooth movement with Invisalign. Am J Orthod Dentofacial Orthop. 2009; 135(1):27–35

[2] Simon M, Keilig L, Schwarze J, Jung BA, Bourauel C. Treatment outcome and efficacy of an aligner technique—regarding incisor torque, premolar derotation and molar distalization. BMC Oral Health. 2014;14:68

[3] Simon M, Keilig L, Schwarze J, Jung BA, Bourauel C. Forces and moments generated by removable thermoplastic aligners: incisor torque, premolar derotation, and molar distalization. Am J Orthod Dentofacial Orthop. 2014;145(6):728–736

[4] Kohda N, Iijima M, Muguruma T, Brantley WA, Ahluwalia KS, Mizoguchi I. Effects of mechanical properties of thermoplastic materials on the initial force of thermoplastic appliances. Angle Orthod. 2013;83(3):476–483

[5] Schuster S, Eliades G, Zinelis S, Eliades T, Bradley TG. Structural conformation and leaching from in vitro aged and retrieved Invisalign appliances. Am J Orthod Dentofacial Orthop. 2004;126(6):725–728

[6] Ahn HW, Ha HR, Lim HN, Choi S. Effects of aging procedures on the molecular, biochemical, morphological, and mechanical properties of vacuum-formed retainers. J Mech Behav Biomed Mater. 2015;51:356–366

[7] Gerard Bradley T, Teske L, Eliades G, Zinelis S, Eliades T. Do the mechanical and chemical properties of InvisalignTM appliances change after use? A retrieval analysis. Eur J Orthod. 2016;38(1):27–31

[8] Ryokawa H, Miyazaki Y, Fujishima A, Miyazaki T, Maki K.The mechanical properties of dental thermoplastic materials in a simulated intraoral environment. Orthod Waves. 2006;65:64–72

[9] Boubakri A, Elleuch K, Guermazi N, Ayedi HF. Investigations on hygrothermal aging of thermoplastic polyurethane material. Mater Des. 2009;30:3958–3965

[10] Boubakri A, Haddar N, Elleuch K, Bienvenu Y. Impact of aging condition of mechanical properties of thermoplastic polyurethane. Mater Des. 2010;31:4194–4201

[11] Boubakri A, Haddar N, Elleuch K, Bienvenu Y. Influence of thermal aging on tensile and creep behavior of thermoplastic polyurethane. Comptes Rendus Mécanique. 2011;339:666–673

[12] Fang D, Zhang N, Chen H, Bai Y. Dynamic stress relaxation of orthodontic thermoplastic materials in a simulated oral environment. Dent Mater J. 2013;32(6):946–951

[13] International Organization for Standardization. ISO14577-1. Metallic materials - Instrumented indentation test for hardness and materials parameters. Geneva, Switzerland: International Organization for Standardization;2002

[14] Shahdad SA, McCabe JF, Bull S, Rusby S, Wassell RW. Hardness measured with traditional Vickers and Martens hardness methods. Dent Mater. 2007;23(9):1079–1085

[15] Zinelis S, Al Jabbari YS, Gaintantzopoulou M, Eliades G, Eliades T. Mechanical properties of orthodontic wires derived by instrumented indentation testing (IIT) according to ISO 14577. Prog Orthod. 2015;16:19

[16] Alexandropoulos A, Al Jabbari YS, Zinelis S, Eliades T. Chemical and mechanical characteristics of contemporary thermoplastic orthodontic materials. Aust Orthod J. 2015;31(2):165–170

[17] Gracco A, Mazzoli A, Favoni O, et al. Short-term chemical and physical changes in invisalign appliances. Aust Orthod J. 2009;25(1):34–40

[18] Qi H, Boyce M. Stress-strain behavior of thermoplastic polyurethanes. Mech Mater. 2005;37:817–839

13 Color Changes of Aligners and Thermoplastic Retainers during Intraoral Service

Anastasios A. Zafeiriadis, Athanasios E. Athanasiou, and Theodore Eliades

Summary

The use of aligners has grown in parallel with patients' demand for invisible esthetic orthodontic appliances. Thermoplastic aligners have high levels of patient acceptance due to their relatively better esthetics compared to conventional fixed appliances. Color stability and transparency of the thermoplastic material used for clear aligners worn full-time and for retainers used part-time constitute important parameters for both clinicians. Knowing the effects of the staining susceptibility of the surface of the thermoplastic aligner material could guide clinicians regarding the choice of the material used for their patients and the instructions given to patients about aligner insertion and cleaning, so that better long-term aligner and retainer maintenance and color stability are achieved. Discoloration of polymeric materials can result from a wide range of factors, external or internal. Updated literature indicates the relative in vivo discoloration potential of coffee, tea, and, to a lesser extent, red wine, on thermoplastic materials under investigations. This suggests the importance of patients avoiding drinking such staining beverages while the aligners or retainers are in the mouth. Further research on different materials or different modes of retainer use would be necessary to document the physical and optical properties of thermoplastic material when aligners or retainers are subjected to the hostile conditions of the oral cavity.

Keywords: orthodontic aligners, orthodontic retainers, discoloration, dental materials, spectrophotometry, staining agents, dental esthetics

13.1 Introduction

The use of aligners has grown in parallel with patients' demand for invisible esthetic orthodontic appliances. Thermoplastic aligners have high levels of patient acceptance due to their relatively better esthetic and removable characteristics compared to conventional fixed orthodontic appliances. From the appearance point of view, color stability and transparency of the thermoplastic material utilized for the fabrication of clear active aligners of full-time use and, more particularly, for the passive retainers to be worn for much longer period remain critical parameters for both clinicians and patients (►Fig. 13.1).

13.2 Mechanisms of Discoloration of Aligners and Thermoplastic Retainers

The discoloration of polymeric materials may arise from a wide array of sources. Color changes in aligner material may be caused both by factors intrinsic to the nature of the material and by external factors that adversely affect the optical properties of thermoplastic polymer. The stability of the chemical as well as optical properties, such as refraction, absorption, reflection, and light scattering, may be influenced by numerous factors presenting in the oral cavity including the continuous exposure to saliva, crevicular fluid, and other organic and inorganic constituents of the oral environment.

One specific factor is related to the extrinsic discoloration arising from the superficial absorption or adsorption of color pigments from food dyes, colored mouth rinses, plaque, the colored components formed in plaque by chromogenic bacteria, or from the chemical transformation of pellicle components.[1–3] In addition, phenomena such as the adsorption of proteinaceous substances and local calcification of inactive points known to occur in the surface of aligners can constitute factors affecting their color.[4,5]

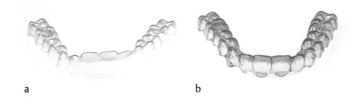

Fig. 13.1 Color difference evident to the naked eye between **(a)** an unused aligner and **(b)** an aligner retrieved after 2-week oral use by a nonsmoker patient. The company logo and patient serial number were digitally erased for anonymity.

Another extrinsic factor relates to the surface discoloration from the absorption or superficial penetration of staining agents passing through the oral cavity following chemical degradation of the surface of the material, or discoloration of the outer layers, caused by diffusion of hydrophilic colorings.[6] These factors can be exacerbated by the substantial changes in aligner morphology caused by swallowing, speech, and bruxism, which have been reported to alter the surface and structural characteristics of the material.[4,5] External staining of the aligners can occur as a function of time, pH, and temperature when the aligners are kept in the mouth while imbibing acidic soft drinks, coffee, tea, wine, or fruit juices.[7] Smoking or chewing tobacco and the oral use of various medications have also been shown to cause tooth discoloration,[8] although there is no current information about the possible impacts on aligner or retainer staining.

The method followed for cleaning aligners could also influence their color stability. Many cleaning methods have been investigated regarding their effect on the accumulation of microorganism biofilm, such as fluoride toothpaste brushing,[9,10,11] immersion in chlorhexidine solution,[9,10] chlorhexidine gel application,[9] or the use of a vibrating bath with a cleaning solution.[10] However, at present, there is only one study investigating the effect of several cleaning methods on the light transmittance through polyurethane-based Vivera retainers (Align Technology Inc., San Jose, California, United States). In this study, the Vivera specimens were exposed twice a week for 6 months to seven cleaning methods: Invisalign cleaning crystals (Align Technology Inc., San Jose, California, United States), Listerine mouthwash (Johnson and Johnson, New Brunswick, New Jersey, United States), Polident (GlaxoSmithKline, Brentford, UK), 2.5% vinegar, 0.6% sodium hypochlorite, 3% hydrogen peroxide solutions, and toothbrushing with distilled water. All of the cleaning methods

decreased significantly the light transmittance through the polyurethane specimens over 6 months. Of the seven tested cleaning methods, Invisalign cleaning crystals, Listerine, and Polident showed the least amount of change in light transmittance values.[12]

Other possible factors involved in staining could be the internal discoloration derived from incomplete polymerization as well as the endogenous irreversible discoloration attributed to subsequent changes in the chemical structure of the material.[6] However, no research is at present available of the possible effect of chemical alteration on retainers' color, and even studies on substances leaching from aligners have not always been conclusive.[4,13,14,15] It is also likely that internal discoloration could be caused by thermal energy and/or UV irradiation, e.g., if the aligners are stored somewhere where they are exposed to heat or sunlight, which may induce physicochemical reactions in the aligner polymer. However, yet again, there are no supportive studies available yet.

13.3 Other Phenomena Influencing Color of Aligners and Thermoplastic Retainers

The esthetic characteristics of thermoplastic aligners can be a more complex phenomenon involving factors beyond the intrinsic properties of the materials used and the impact of internal and external factors on them since this can also be influenced by the color of the underlying surface and its reflective index. Therefore, alterations in the tooth color can potentially induce unfavorable changes in the clinical appearance of the aligners as well. It has also been suggested that in vivo tooth-color alterations can result either from blood flow variations in the dental pulp and adjacent gingival tissues,[16,17] or from the resting salivary flow rates that affect tooth hydration and thus tooth color.[18] Although natural tooth color has a significant tendency to darken and yellow with increasing age in adults,[19,20] these color changes are almost insignificant in younger subjects.[21,22] For this reason, the influence of age during the relatively short period of orthodontic treatment may be of little importance in the perception of aligners' color. Furthermore, the impact of tooth discoloration caused by decalcification[23] is possibly of little clinical significance, as the aligners are used only for short periods, being usually changed every 2 weeks.

With regard to the thermoplastic retainers that are used for prolonged periods of time, enamel color changes could be of significance in the long run. In addition, the color of natural teeth enamel has been shown to change in a variety of ways after orthodontic treatment by fixed appliances,[24,25,26,27,28,29,30] with the color change shown to be affected by many factors including the type of adhesive materials and the debonding procedures used.[26,27,28,29,30,31] Enamel color has also been demonstrated to change during the first retention year, with the majority of such changes occurring during the first 3 months.[32] Enamel color alterations after orthodontic treatment can derive from the irreversible penetration of resin tags into the enamel surface.[24] This phenomenon has been shown to affect the specularly reflected light component, influencing the L^* values of the tooth substrate.[33,34] In addition, the color instability of resin composites, attributed to endogenous changes from the physicochemical reactions in the material,[35] exogenous changes from superficial absorption of food staining agents,[2] and products from the corrosion of other orthodontic appliances[36,37] can all lead to discoloration of the resin-infiltrated tooth surface. In vitro studies have indicated that most orthodontic adhesives tested had unsatisfactory color stability ($\Delta E > 3.7$)[38] after exposure to food colorants and artificial photoaging.[6,39] The discoloration of adhesives has been linked to changes in b^* values toward yellow,[34] while chemical differences among the resin components, as well as variations in filler content and polymerization conversion, can affect the color stability of the various composites.[40,41]

Another issue relevant to tooth color concerns the fact that perception of tooth color and appearance are also linked to individual facial characteristics such as the attractiveness of the entire oral region, age, tone of skin, and the color and volume of neighboring lips and gum tissues.[42] This wide variety of factors contributes to the perception of the overall dental appearance and thus might influence the significance and impact of aligner color alterations.

13.4 Research on Discoloration of Aligners and Thermoplastic Retainers

Currently, only limited information is available regarding color change of aligners and thermoplastic retainers associated with staining agents and/or patient oral application.

13.4.1 In Vitro Studies

The in vitro effect of different staining solutions on the color stability of Vivera retainers has been investigated. Thirty flat specimens fabricated using the polyurethane-based Vivera material were assigned into five groups and immersed at 37°C in solutions of distilled water (control), coffee, tea, red wine, and Coca Cola. The CIE color parameters (L^*, a^*, b^*)[43,44,45,46] of each specimen were measured with a UV–visible spectrophotometer before immersion and after 12 hours, 3 days, and a week of solution exposure. Color differences (ΔE) between the interval groups were subsequently calculated. The results showed that the color of Vivera retainers exhibited visible statistically significant changes induced by several staining solutions, especially coffee, tea, and, to a lesser extent, red wine (▶Fig. 13.2).[43]

The absorbance and transmittance values of three types of aligners before and after two cycles of aging have also been assessed and compared in vitro. Samples of orthodontic aligners from different manufacturers (Invisalign, Align Technology, San Jose, California, United States; All-In, Micerium, Avegno, Genova, Italy; F22 Aligner, Sweden

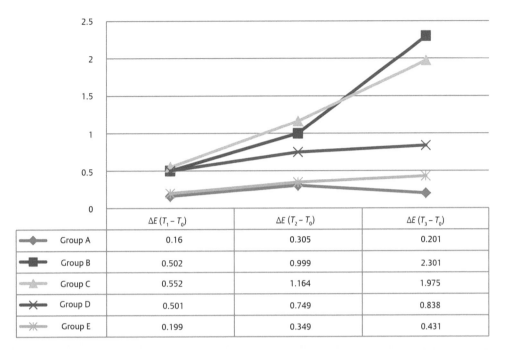

	$\Delta E\ (T_1 - T_0)$	$\Delta E\ (T_2 - T_0)$	$\Delta E\ (T_3 - T_0)$
Group A	0.16	0.305	0.201
Group B	0.502	0.999	2.301
Group C	0.552	1.164	1.975
Group D	0.501	0.749	0.838
Group E	0.199	0.349	0.431

Fig. 13.2 Estimated mean ΔE (color difference) values with 95% confidence intervals (CIs) produced by the analysis of variance (ANOVA) model. The differences between $\Delta E\ (T_1 - T_0)$, $\Delta E\ (T_2 - T_0)$, and $\Delta E\ (T_3 - T_0)$ for coffee and tea groups and between $\Delta E\ (T_1 - T_0)$ and $\Delta E\ (T_2 - T_0)$ for the red wine group were statistically significant. (Reproduced with permission from Zafeiriadis et al.[43])

& Martina, Due Carrare, Padova, Italy) were subjected to UV–visible spectrophotometric analysis. The samples were subsequently subjected to in vitro aging at a constant temperature in artificial saliva augmented with brown and yellow food colorants for two cycles of 2 weeks each. The F22 aligners were found to be the most transparent, both before and after aging, followed by Invisalign and All-In, with the differences being statistically significant. All types of aligners tested showed lower transmittance and higher absorbance values after aging, although there was no statistically significant difference between them in terms of degree. The study concluded that different commercial aligners have significantly different optical properties, both as delivered and after aging, leading to different esthetic properties.[47]

The color stability of three thermoplastic aligner types exposed to staining agents has also been evaluated in vitro. Sixty clear orthodontic aligners produced by three manufacturers (Invisalign; Angelalign, EAMedical Instruments, Shanghai, China; Smartee, SmarteeDenti-Technology, Shanghai, China) were immersed in four staining solutions: distilled water (control), coffee, black tea, and red wine. After 12-hour and 1-week immersion cycles, the optical properties of the aligners were measured with a colorimeter. The changes in color (ΔE) were calculated with the CIE $L^*a^*b^*$ color system. Fourier-transform infrared spectroscopy (FT-IR) spectroscopy and scanning electron microscopy (SEM) were then performed to observe any molecular and morphologic changes to the aligner surfaces, respectively. All three aligner types showed slight nonsignificant color changes after 12 hours of immersion in staining agents, with the exception of the Invisalign aligners immersed in coffee, which were significantly stained; red wine and tea failed to cause significant changes over the same time period. The polyurethane-based Invisalign aligners generally exhibited significantly higher ΔE values than the Angelalign and Smartee aligners. The FT-IR analysis failed to show significant chemical differences, before and after immersion, in the polymer-based structure of the aligners, while the SEM results indicated different surface alterations to the three types of aligner materials after the 1-week staining, with the Invisalign aligners being shown to be more susceptible to pigmentation than the Angelalign and Smartee aligners.[48]

Coffee, tea, red wine, and Coca Cola, among other drinks, are identified as staining solutions,[49,50,51,52,53,54,55,56] and for this reason, they are often used in studies to evaluate staining effects. Coffee was found to be the most chromogenic agent among the solutions used on thermoplastic materials,[43,48] a finding consistent with previous studies investigating the color stability of different dental materials, such as denture teeth.[55,57] Several studies on dental materials have also concluded that coffee caused more staining than tea.[49,51,56,57,58,59] In addition, rinsing experiments have shown that tannic acid, contained in tea, promoted the formation of a brown-stained pellicle on teeth,[60] whereas black tea and red wine components have been shown to induce in vitro pellicle maturation.[22]

Although the results of in vitro studies showed that some alterations in optical material properties are inevitable, it must be emphasized that this kind of tests may not reliably reflect clinical conditions with regard to color perception. In vivo color determination is affected by many factors presenting in the oral cavity, as detailed above, such as the lighting conditions of the surrounding environment, the light scattered from the adjacent perioral and gingival tissues,[16] and the resting salivary flow rates that influence the degree of teeth or aligner hydration.[18] Care should therefore be taken in interpreting the results of in vitro studies regarding the effects induced by the oral cavity. The effects of staining agents on aligner materials could be more evident in vivo and could also be attributed to the type of thermoplastic material and its susceptibility to certain staining agents, while the magnitude of the effects could also increase over time with prolonged oral wear of the appliances. This latter possibility is especially important regarding retainers, which are worn for far longer time periods than aligners.

The studies so far indicate the relative in vivo discoloration potential of coffee, tea, and, to a lesser extent, red wine, on the specific materials under investigations. This suggests the importance of patients avoiding drinking staining beverages, such as coffee and tea, while the aligners or retainers are in the mouth.[43]

13.4.2 In Vivo Studies

The number of in vivo studies concerning discoloration of aligners and thermoplastic retainers is also limited.

The in vivo optical, chemical, and morphological changes have been investigated on Invisalign appliances after short-term use. Ten Invisalign aligners were selected after 2 weeks of use by 10 randomly selected patients. FT-IR microspectroscopy was used to detect any molecular level changes on the appliance surfaces, while UV-visible spectrophotometry was performed to assess color and transparency changes. The researchers also used SEM and energy-dispersive X-ray microanalysis to examine the morphology of the aligner surfaces and the elemental composition of any deposits on them. The results indicated that aligners worn for 2 weeks had suffered microcracks, abrasion, areas of delamination, and accumulated localized calcified biofilm deposits, and also showed loss of transparency in the aligner material.[5]

Another investigation assessed the more long-term in vivo color alterations of two different clear thermoplastic retainers.[61] Thirty patients, non-smokers, were randomly allocated into two groups after the completion of active orthodontic treatment. One group received Vivera retainers and the other Essix C+ retainers (Raintree Essix, New Orleans, Los Angeles, United States). For each patient, two retainers were fabricated, one for oral use and the other to serve as control. The CIE color parameters (L^*, a^*, b^*) of each patient's upper central incisors were measured with a spectrophotometer immediately after retainer insertion in the mouth and again after 15 days, 1 month, and 3 months of intraoral use. Color differences (ΔE) between the interval groups were calculated. The results showed that the used retainers exhibited greater color changes than control retainers or teeth without retainers, and these changes became more pronounced with longer duration of use. Vivera and Essix C+ retainers exhibited similar color stability over a 3-month period of intraoral use, as no significant differences in color change were observed

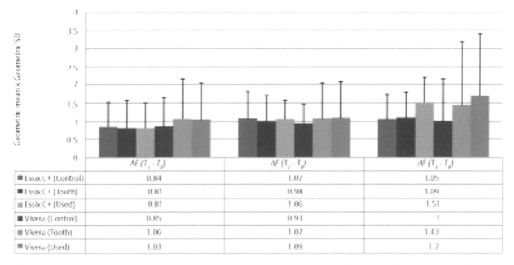

Fig. 13.3 Geometric mean × geometric SD of the parameter ΔE for tooth 11. Vivera and Essix C+ retainers exhibited similar color stability over a 3-month period of oral use as no significant differences in color change were observed between the two retainer types. (Reproduced with permission from Zafeiriadis et al.[61])

between the two types of appliances, which suggest that polyurethane and polypropylene retainers (materials for Vivera and Essix C+, respectively) exhibit similar optical behavior over this time period (▶Fig. 13.3). All retainer color differences observed in vivo during a 3-month posttreatment period were considered clinically acceptable (ΔE < 3.7),[38] although prolonged use of the retainers could possibly cause clinically significant changes in coloration.[61]

13.5 Conclusion

Knowledge of the effects of the staining susceptibility of the surface of the thermoplastic material used for aligners and retainers could guide clinicians regarding the choice of the material used for their patients and the instructions given to patients about appliance's insertion and cleaning, so that better long-term aligner and retainer maintenance and color stability are achieved. Further research on different materials or different modes of appliance use would be necessary to study the physical and optical properties of thermoplastic material when aligners and retainers are subjected to the hostile conditions of the oral cavity.

References

[1] Vogel RI. Intrinsic and extrinsic discoloration of the dentition (a literature review). J Oral Med. 1975;30(4):99–104

[2] Inokoshi S, Burrow MF, Kataumi M, Yamada T, Takatsu T. Opacity and color changes of tooth-colored restorative materials. Oper Dent. 1996;21(2):73–80

[3] Yap AU, Sim CP, Loganathan V. Polymerization color changes of esthetic restoratives. Oper Dent. 1999;24(5):306–311

[4] Schuster S, Eliades G, Zinelis S, Eliades T, Bradley TG. Structural conformation and leaching from in vitro aged and retrieved Invisalign appliances. Am J Orthod Dentofacial Orthop. 2004;126(6):725–728

[5] Gracco A, Mazzoli A, Favoni O, et al. Short-term chemical and physical changes in invisalign appliances. Aust Orthod J. 2009;25(1):34–40

[6] Eliades T, Gioka C, Heim M, Eliades G, Makou M. Color stability of orthodontic adhesive resins. Angle Orthod. 2004;74(3):391–393

[7] Schott TC, Göz G. Color fading of the blue compliance indicator encapsulated in removable clear Invisalign Teen® aligners. Angle Orthod. 2011;81(2):185–191

[8] Kumar A, Kumar V, Singh J, Hooda A, Dutta S. Drug-induced discoloration of teeth: an updated review. Clin Pediatr (Phila). 2012;51(2):181–185

[9] Chang CS, Al-Awadi S, Ready D, Noar J. An assessment of the effectiveness of mechanical and chemical cleaning of Essix orthodontic retainer. J Orthod. 2014;41(2):110–117

[10] Shpack N, Greenstein RB, Gazit D, Sarig R, Vardimon AD. Efficacy of three hygienic protocols in reducing biofilm adherence to removable thermoplastic appliance. Angle Orthod. 2014;84(1):161–170

[11] Levrini L, Mangano A, Margherini S, et al. ATP Biolumi-nometers analysis on the surfaces of removable orthodontic aligners after the use of different cleaning methods. Int J Dent. 2016;2016:5926941

[12] Agarwal M, Wible E, Ramir T, et al. Long-term effects of seven cleaning methods on light transmittance, surface roughness, and flexural modulus of polyurethane retainer material. Angle Orthod. 2018;88(3):355–362

[13] Eliades T, Pratsinis H, Athanasiou AE, Eliades G, Kletsas D. Cytotoxicity and estrogenicity of Invisalign appliances. Am J Orthod Dentofacial Orthop. 2009;136(1):100–103

[14] Eliades T. Bisphenol A and orthodontics: An update of evidence-based measures to minimize exposure for the orthodontic team and patients. Am J Orthod Dentofacial Orthop. 2017;152(4):435–441

[15] Raghavan AS, Pottipalli Sathyanarayana H, Kailasam V, Padmanabhan S. Comparative evaluation of salivary bisphenol A levels in patients wearing vacuum-formed and Hawley retainers: An in-vivo study. Am J Orthod Dentofacial Orthop. 2017;151(3):471–476

[16] Goodkind RJ, Schwabacher WB. Use of a fiber-optic colorimeter for in vivo color measurements of 2830 anterior teeth. J Prosthet Dent. 1987;58(5):535–542

[17] ten Bosch JJ, Coops JC. Tooth color and reflectance as related to light scattering and enamel hardness. J Dent Res. 1995;74(1):374–380

[18] Dawes C. Rhythms in salivary flow rate and composition. Int J Chronobiol. 1974;2(3):253–279

[19] Cook WD, McAree DC. Optical properties of esthetic restorative materials and natural dentition. J Biomed Mater Res. 1985;19(5):469–488

[20] Morley J. The esthetics of anterior tooth aging. Curr Opin Cosmet Dent. 1997;4:35–39

[21] Odioso LL, Gibb RD, Gerlach RW. Impact of demographic, behavioral, and dental care utilization parameters on tooth color and personal satisfaction. Compend Contin Educ Dent Suppl. 2000;29(29):S35–S41, quiz S43

[22] Joiner A. Tooth colour: a review of the literature. J Dent. 2004;32 (Suppl 1):3–12

[23] Bishara SE, Ostby AW. White spot lesions: formation, prevention, and treatment. Semin Orthod. 2008;14:174–182

[24] Eliades T, Kakaboura A, Eliades G, Bradley TG. Comparison of enamel colour changes associated with orthodontic bonding using two different adhesives. Eur J Orthod. 2001;23(1):85–90

[25] Kim SP, Hwang IN, Cho JH, Hwang HS. Tooth color changes associated with the bracket bonding and debonding. Korean J Orthod. 2006;36:114–124

[26] Karamouzos A, Athanasiou AE, Papadopoulos MA, Kolokithas G. Tooth-color assessment after orthodontic treatment: a prospective clinical trial. Am J Orthod Dentofacial Orthop. 2010;138(5):537.e1–537.e8, discussion 537–539

[27] Al Maaitah EF, Abu Omar AA, Al-Khateeb SN. Effect of fixed orthodontic appliances bonded with different etching techniques on tooth color: a prospective clinical study. Am J Orthod Dentofacial Orthop. 2013;144(1):43–49

[28] Boncuk Y, Cehreli ZC, Polat-Özsoy Ö. Effects of different orthodontic adhesives and resin removal techniques on enamel color alteration. Angle Orthod. 2014;84(4):634–641

[29] Cörekçi B, Toy E, Oztürk F, Malkoç S, Oztürk B. Effects of contemporary orthodontic composites on tooth color following short-term fixed orthodontic treatment: a controlled clinical study. Turk J Med Sci. 2015;45(6):1421–1428

[30] Xu LY, Dong M, Lu YG, Lei L. [Study of factors affecting tooth discoloration during fixed orthodontics in vitro] Shanghai Kou Qiang Yi Xue. 2015;24(4):415–418

[31] Ye C, Zhao Z, Zhao Q, Du X, Ye J, Wei X. Comparison of enamel discoloration associated with bonding with three different orthodontic adhesives and cleaning-up with four different procedures. J Dent. 2013;41(Suppl 5):e35–e40

[32] Karamouzos A, Zafeiriadis AA, Kolokithas G, Papadopoulos MA, Athanasiou AE. In vivo evaluation of tooth colour alterations during orthodontic retention: a split-mouth cohort study. Orthod Craniofac Res. 2019;22(2):124<endash>130

[33] Chung KH. Effects of finishing and polishing procedures on the surface texture of resin composites. Dent Mater. 1994;10(5):325–330

[34] Leibrock A, Rosentritt M, Lang R, Behr M, Handel G. Colour stability of visible light-curing hybrid composites. Eur J Prosthodont Restor Dent. 1997;5(3):125–130

[35] Ferracane JL. Correlation between hardness and degree of conversion during the setting reaction of unfilled dental restorative resins. Dent Mater. 1985;1(1):11–14

[36] Maijer R, Smith DC. Corrosion of orthodontic bracket bases. Am J Orthod. 1982;81(1):43–48

[37] Hodges SJ, Spencer RJ, Watkins SJ. Unusual indelible enamel staining following fixed appliance treatment. J Orthod. 2000;27(4):303–306

[38] Johnston WM, Kao EC. Assessment of appearance match by visual observation and clinical colorimetry. J Dent Res. 1989;68(5):819–822

[39] Faltermeier A, Rosentritt M, Reicheneder C, Behr M. Discolouration of orthodontic adhesives caused by food dyes and ultraviolet light. Eur J Orthod. 2008;30(1):89–93

[40] Eldiwany M, Friedl KH, Powers JM. Color stability of light-cured and post-cured composites. Am J Dent. 1995;8(4):179–181

[41] Davis BA, Friedl KH, Powers JM. Color stability of hybrid ionomers after accelerated aging. J Prosthodont. 1995;4(2):111–115

[42] Alkhatib MN, Holt R, Bedi R. Age and perception of dental appearance and tooth colour. Gerodontology. 2005;22(1):32–36

[43] Zafeiriadis AA, Karamouzos A, Athanasiou AE, Eliades T, Palaghias G. In vitro spectrophotometric evaluation of Vivera clear thermoplastic retainer discolouration. Aust Orthod J. 2014;30(2):192–200

[44] International Commission on Illumination, ed. Colorimetry, Official Recommendations of the International Commission on Illumination. Publication CIE No. 15 (E-1.3.1). Paris: CIE; 1971

[45] Hunter RS, Harold RW, eds. The Measurement of Appearance. New York, NY: John Wiley & Sons;1987

[46] Paul S, Peter A, Pietrobon N, Hämmerle CH. Visual and spectrophotometric shade analysis of human teeth. J Dent Res. 2002;81(8):578–582

[47] Lombardo L, Arreghini A, Maccarrone R, Bianchi A, Scalia S, Siciliani G. Optical properties of orthodontic aligners--spectrophotometry analysis of three types before and after aging. Prog Orthod. 2015;16:41

[48] Liu CL, Sun WT, Liao W, et al. Colour stabilities of three types of orthodontic clear aligners exposed to staining agents. Int J Oral Sci. 2016;8(4):246–253

[49] Chan KC, Fuller JL, Hormati AA. The ability of foods to stain two composite resins. J Prosthet Dent. 1980;43(5):542–545

[50] Cooley RL, Barkmeier WW, Matis BA, Siok JF. Staining of posterior resin restorative materials. Quintessence Int. 1987;18(12):823–827

[51] Luce MS, Campbell CE. Stain potential of four microfilled composites. J Prosthet Dent. 1988;60(2):151–154

[52] Khokhar ZA, Razzoog ME, Yaman P. Color stability of restorative resins. Quintessence Int. 1991;22(9): 733–737

[53] Um CM, Ruyter IE. Staining of resin-based veneering materials with coffee and tea. Quintessence Int. 1991;22(5):377–386

[54] Polyzois GL, Yannikakis SA, Zissis AJ. Color stability of visible light-cured, hard direct denture reliners: an in vitro investigation. Int J Prosthodont. 1999;12(2):140–146

[55] Mutlu-Sagesen L, Ergün G, Ozkan Y, Bek B. Color stability of different denture teeth materials: an in vitro study. J Oral Sci. 2001;43(3):193–205

[56] Ertaş E, Güler AU, Yücel AC, Köprülü H, Güler E. Color stability of resin composites after immersion in different drinks. Dent Mater J. 2006;25(2):371–376

[57] Koksal T, Dikbas I. Color stability of different denture teeth materials against various staining agents. Dent Mater J. 2008;27(1):139–144

[58] Chan KC, Hormati AA, Kerber PE. Staining calcified dental tissues with food. J Prosthet Dent. 1981;46(2):175–178

[59] Scotti R, Mascellani SC, Forniti F. The in vitro color stability of acrylic resins for provisional restorations. Int J Prosthodont. 1997;10(2):164–168

[60] Nordbo H. Discoloration of dental pellicle by tannic acid. Acta Odontol Scand. 1977;35(6):305–310

[61] Zafeiriadis AA, Karamouzos A, Athanasiou AE, Eliades T, Palaghias G. An in vivo spectrophotometric evaluation of Vivera® and Essix® clear thermoplastic retainer discolouration. Aust Orthod J. 2018;34:3–10

14 Biological Properties of Aligners

Shaima Rashid Al Naqbi, Harris Pratsinis, Dimitris Kletsas, Athanasios E. Athanasiou, and Theodore Eliades

Summary

Since aligners are plastic-based materials, one crucial concern regarding their use is the leaching of chemical substances called xenoestrogens into the immediate environment surrounding the plastic. Those substances have the ability to produce a biological reaction comparable to that of estrogen hormones. This chapter presents the various aspects of the biological properties of aligners and addresses them with special relevance to their cytotoxicity and estrogenicity as well as the existing limitations of the available in vitro investigations.

Keywords: orthodontic aligners, orthodontic clear retainers, cytotoxicity, estrogenicity, laboratory research Invisalign, laboratory research Vivera

14.1 Introduction

The structural stability of Invisalign aligners has been tested and morphological differences after their use, involving abrasion at the cusp tips, adsorption of integuments at stagnation sites, and localized calcification of the biofilm developed during intraoral use, have been detected.[1] In addition, their plastic-based materials bring into consideration health and safety concerns regarding possible leaching of chemical substances to the immediate environment surrounding the plastic during the use of these appliances. This chapter presents the various aspects of the biological properties of aligners and addresses them with special relevance to their cytotoxicity and estrogenicity.

14.2 Plastic Toxicity

14.2.1 General Aspects

Plastics are used in almost every single aspect of our life such as food containers, household products, water bottles, toothbrushes, computers, telephones, eyeglasses, some clothing, and some toys. The term "plastic" is derived from the Greek "plastikos," meaning fit for molding. These popular polymers are now being revealed as potentially possessing adverse health-related effects to human.

One crucial concern regarding the use of plastic-based materials is the leaching of chemical substances called xenoestrogens into the immediate environment surrounding the plastic. Those substances have the ability to produce a biological reaction comparable to that of estrogen hormones. Their action, in most cases, takes the form of binding to classic estrogenic receptors (ERs) ERα and ERβ at subtoxic concentrations but capable of inducing estrogenic signals that modify gene expression. This action is called estrogenicity.[2,3,4]

One of the materials concerned is bisphenol-A (BPA), which is produced by the condensation of phenol and acetone in the presence of catalysts and catalyst promoters.[5,6] BPA is used worldwide in the production of plastic products. It exhibits great similarity in structure with 17β-estradiol and may have similar effects.[2,7]

The accumulated level of BPA in the body may vary according to the developmental stage and gender of the subject. Because of the absence of enzymes capable of metabolizing BPA to its biologically inert form, exposure of infants leads to higher BPA body levels relative to those experienced during adulthood. In addition, a sexual dimorphism has been revealed indicating higher plasma BPA levels in male than female fetuses, even after correcting for a positive correlation between body weight and BPA concentration.[8,9]

According to the U.S. Environmental Protection Agency (EPA) reference dose and the Food and Drug Administration's acceptable daily intake dose, the presumed "safe" dosage is 50 µg/kg/day of BPA.[7,10,11] However, adverse effects have been documented with BPA doses below the above-mentioned daily level.[12,13,14,15]

The adverse biological effects of BPA, demonstrated mainly in experimental animals, are:

- Hormonal-related effects such as early puberty in females and feminization in males.[16] In addition, BPA has been shown to be a thyroid hormone receptor (THR) antagonist that disrupts the THR-mediated transcription.[17]
- Higher risk for breast cancer in females and prostate cancer in males.[16,18]
- Induction of calcium influx, which leads to prolactin release and its associated behavioral effects.[19]

- Development of hyperglycemia and insulin tolerance.[10]
- Elevation of oxidative stress mediators.[20]
- Upregulation of the cAMP response element-binding factor, which inhibits apoptosis.[3]
- Potential cytotoxic effects such as an immune reaction to material exposure, cell cycle disturbance, cell apoptosis, and induction of mutagenesis or carcinogenesis.[21]
- Other biological effects, including neurobehavioral problems such as autism and attention deficit hyperactivity disorder.[22]

When 13 different intraoral materials were tested in a simulated oral environment, silicone baby bottle nipple samples (20 µg) showed BPA leaching after 3 days of artificial saliva immersion, with no additional leaching thereafter.[23] BPA was also found to migrate from polycarbonate water bottles at rates ranging from 0.20 to 0.79 ng/h. This migration of BPA at room temperature was independent of whether or not the bottle had been previously used.[24] Canned food is also a BPA-leaching source. A low level of BPA was found in water from unheated food cans.[25] This level increased as the heat-treatment temperature increased.

More than two million tons of BPA-related products are currently produced per year, with an anticipated 6 to 10% annual growth in future demand[7,26] which in turn will increase the potential risk from BPA to human health.

14.2.2 Dental Environment

In dentistry, the first study to report BPA release in in vivo settings was research by Olea and coworkers[27] in which salivary BPA levels in patients with dental resin sealants were assessed. This study confirmed the estrogenicity of the sealants used by proliferation tests using human breast cancer cells. As BPA glycidyl methacrylate (Bis-GMA), which is synthesized from BPA, is incorporated in many resinous materials, it is possible that a BPA residue may remain in Bis-GMA-based resins. Dimethacrylate-based restorative materials may contain BPA as well, as a degradation product from nonspecific esterases and other salivary enzymes that attack the resin matrix and lead to the degradation of BPA derivatives.[28]

Due to the diverse conclusions reached by the following studies, a controversy has resulted regarding the actual release of BPA from sealants and their possible estrogenic action. Some studies have failed to detect any BPA eluted from properly polymerized sealants.[29,30,31] On the other hand, when BPA levels in the urine and saliva of adults treated with two different sealants were compared, there was low level of BPA detected, although these were 1,000 times lower than reported elsewhere.[32] According to Zampeli et al,[4] this could result from the incomplete polymerization of sealants caused by the attenuation or scattering of the activating light, the formation of oxygen-inhibited layer, and/or decreased optical clarity of the sealant itself. The same study found that eluent of a sealant named "Delton Opaque" at a concentration of 10% possessed some estrogenic activity.

14.2.3 Orthodontic Materials

The potential estrogenic hazard in orthodontics arises from the fact that the monomers equivalent to those used for dental sealants are also used for the construction of most of orthodontic materials including bonding adhesives, plastic polycarbonate brackets, elastomeric materials, and other polycarbonate-made appliances such as aligners.[33]

With regard to the orthodontic adhesive materials used for bonding orthodontic attachments, some investigators believe that the quantity of BPA released from orthodontic adhesives is lower than the threshold required to induce a biologic reaction.[8,34] On the other hand, there are other studies confirming the cytotoxic effects of orthodontic adhesives. An in vivo study which evaluated the cytotoxic effects of six adhesives on the oral mucosa in hamsters proved that the liquid component of one adhesive consistently caused an inflammatory response in all tested animals.[35] It has been also shown that activator components of two no-mix adhesives had greater toxicity than other materials.[36] Additionally, when the cytotoxic effect of different orthodontic adhesives on human oral fibroblasts was evaluated, it showed that chemically cured liquid paste adhesives were more cytotoxic than light-cured and chemically cured two-paste materials.[37]

It should be noted that while most research on cytotoxicity in orthodontics has been carried out on monolayer cell cultures,[38] when three-dimensional reconstructed human oral epithelium was utilized to determine the toxicity of orthodontic adhesives, architectural and ultrastructural changes in epithelial cells due to penetration of uncured primers were found.[39]

An additional parameter is that in most of the previous studies, the specimens were prepared using the same dimensions as in operative dentistry, something different from the adhesive dimensions in orthodontics.[36,37] This may affect the amount of monomer release and biocompatibility of these adhesives and provide data not entirely relevant regarding the clinical situation in orthodontics.[40] A study to assess the estrogenic action of a chemically cured no-mix and a light-cured orthodontic adhesive resin in a simulated orthodontic environment concluded that there was no evidence of the stimulation of the proliferation of breast cancer cells, indicating the absence of any estrogenicity in the components of orthodontic adhesive eluents.[8]

The necessity of ensuring the complete polymerization of the adhesive to decrease the risk of BPA release has been emphasized by the study of Sunitha et al.[41] The correlation of BPA release from orthodontic adhesive to different light-curing tip distances was tested. A negative correlation was found between BPA release and light-curing tip distance, which means the advisability of keeping the light-curing tip as close to the adhesive as clinically possible in order to ensure the complete polymerization and decrease the chance of BPA release.

As fixed lingual retainers have been extensively used in orthodontic practice to minimize posttreatment changes, the orthodontic adhesives used for bonding such retainers has been tested for possible hazardous BPA release in in vitro and in vivo settings, respectively.[42,43] According to the in vitro study, there were measurable amounts of BPA identified in the tested eluents at 10-, 20-, and 30-day immersion in doubled-distilled water, with the highest levels found in the immersion media of the 1-month groups (2.9 mg/L), whereas the control (tooth storage solution) had 0.16 mg/L.[42] The amount of BPA leaching from Bis-GMA-based resin composite used for bonding orthodontic lingual retainers in in vivo condition was found to be low and far below the reference doses for daily uptake.[43] However, because of some evidence of a "low-dose effect," the amount of BPA released from the resin composites used in orthodontics should not be overlooked.[14,44]

With regard to other orthodontic materials posing the possibility of BPA release and/or adverse biological effect, polycarbonate brackets have also been investigated. Watanabe and coworkers[45,46] tested the degradation characteristics and the amount of BPA released from new and retrieved polycarbonate orthodontic brackets. It was found that these brackets are capable of producing measurable amounts of BPA. This conclusion was in accordance with the findings of an earlier study.[47]

A systematic review regarding the release of BPA from orthodontic materials has concluded that bonding resin had been found to release BPA between 0.85 and 20.88 ng/mL in vivo, and from traces to 65.67 ppm in vitro. Polycarbonate brackets released amounts of 22.24 mg per gram in ethanol solution and 697 mg per gram after 40 months in water. The included studies were not randomized control trials, and only provided moderate levels of evidence.[48]

Additionally, when different orthodontic materials have been investigated under various thermal and mechanical conditions for the release of BPA, only the thermoformed Biocryl acrylic resin retainer material and a fully cured Transbond XT orthodontic adhesive were found to leach BPA after 3 days of artificial saliva immersion.[49]

14.2.4 Invisalign

Polyurethane is the basic constituent polymeric component used in Invisalign aligners material and is not entirely inert since the material is affected by heat, moisture, and prolonged contact with oral enzymes.[1,50] The new generation of Invisalign aligner material is SmartTrack, a thermoplastic polyurethane with an integrated elastomer.[51]

Some significant morphological differences have been found in the used Invisalign aligners in relation to the new ones, involving abrasion at the cusp tips, adsorption of integuments at stagnation sites, and localized calcification of the biofilm developed during intraoral use.[1] Regarding leaching of biologically active substances, a traceable amount of substances in an ethanol aging solution after immersion of aligner specimens for 2 weeks at 23°C was detected in the same investigation.

The issue of BPA release has been addressed with regard to orthodontic aligners.[50] It was found that Invisalign aligners do not have any cytotoxic effect on human gingival fibroblasts (▶ Fig. 14.1) and did not show any noticeable estrogenic effects when tested on MCF-7 breast cancer cell line at 5, 10, and 20% vol/vol concentration (▶ Fig. 14.2).

Similarly, Invisalign aligners did not present any cytotoxic effect on human gingival fibroblasts, did not show any noticeable estrogenic effects when tested on MCF-7 breast cancer cell line, and no measurable BPA quantity release was traced in a trial of eight different orthodontic materials.[49]

A few years ago, one study found undesirable effects when epithelial cells were treated with eluates obtained from soaking Invisalign plastic in saline solution.[21] Some changes were found in viability, membrane permeability, and adhesion of epithelial cells in a saline-solution environment. The secondary results of compromising epithelial integrity might be microleakage and hapten formation which, in consequence, could lead to isocyanate allergy, either systemic or localized to gingiva. This study was the first to report such adverse effect of contact with Invisalign plastic on oral keratinocytes. These findings were under in vitro conditions, and the authors mentioned that, in the oral environment, the presence of saliva might offer a kind of protection.

It should be also noted that the extended use by patients of any vacuum-formed appliances could lead to degradation and possible deterioration of the material. A recent report found statistically significant BPA levels in saliva in patients using vacuum-formed retainers when compared with Hawley type of similar devices.[52]

In contrast to Invisalign aligners, which are usually used for maximum 2 weeks almost full-time, Vivera retainers have been designed for prolonged use, normally on a part-time basis. This extended use could lead to degradation and possible deterioration of the material. A very recent study investigated in vitro the cytotoxicity and estrogenicity of Vivera retainers by assessing the biological behavioral effects of as-received and retrieved retainers after 4 weeks of use by patients.[53] No significant MCF-7 proliferation was induced by the samples compared either to the eluents from as-received retainers or to the negative control. As expected, p-estradiol induced a potent stimulation of MCF-7 cell proliferation, while no effect was observed on MDA-MB-231 cells (▶ Fig. 14.3). The study concluded that under the conditions of this experiment eluents of as-received and retrieved Vivera

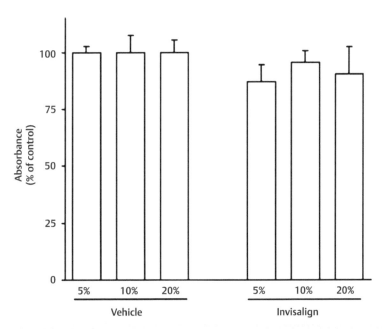

Fig. 14.1 Effect of the Invisalign appliance eluents on the proliferation of human gingival fibroblasts; note absence of effect for aligners at any concentration (no difference from the control vehicle; source: Al Naqbi et al[53]).

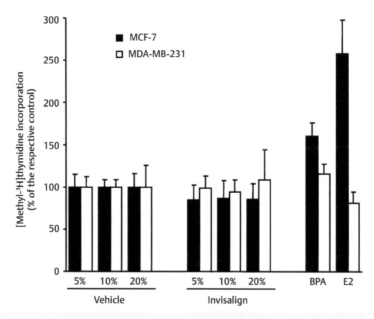

Fig. 14.2 Results of the Invisalign appliance eluents on the proliferation of the estrogen-sensitive MCF-7 and estrogen-insensitive MDA-MB-231 cell lines. No effect is shown to be induced by the aligner eluents. The vehicle is normal saline solution; positive controls are estradiol (E2) and bisphenol-A (BPA). There is no significant difference between the vehicle and the aligner media at any concentration; however, the responsiveness of the MCF-7 cells is depicted in the intense proliferated effect caused by the E2 and BPA. Note also the lack of cytotoxic effect on the MDA-MB-231 cell line, which shows no evidence that could have masked the expression of a proliferative effect on the MCF-7 cells (Source: Al Naqbi et al[53]).

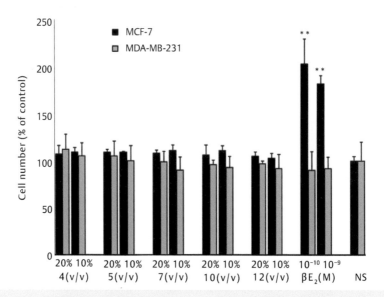

Fig. 14.3 Proliferation of MCF-7 vs. MDA-MB-231 cells in response to retainer eluent samples (average from two experiments). No significant MCF-7 proliferation was induced by the samples 7, 10, and 12, compared either to the eluents from as-received retainers (samples 4 and 5) or to the negative control. As expected, β-estradiol induced a potent stimulation of MCF-7 cell proliferation, while no effect was observed on MDA-MB-231 cells (Source: Al Naqbi et al[53]).

retainers did not seem to exhibit xenoestrogenic activity.

Lastly, it may be worth noting that the manufacturers of aligners, in an attempt to expand the indication of use of these appliances from exclusively crowding cases to a wide range of malocclusions, incorporated the bonding of attachments on the form of composite resin blocks onto the surface of dental crown. These materials have a three-dimensional profile in order to facilitate an improved handling of the spatial orientation of the crown, which in many cases, especially in round teeth, is problematic when the rotational control of teeth is considered. This profile makes them susceptible to hydrolytic degradation and might enhance release, although no data are available on this topic.

Further, these composite resin blocks have a hardness far greater than that of the aligner material which is either a PET-variation of polyurethane-based polymer. As a result, the continuous contact of the polymer with the composite, especially during removal or seating of the aligners, brings in contact two polymers with dissimilar properties, possibly resulting in the attrition of the less hard one. This potentially unfavorable sequela which might introduce the release of species by the aligner has not been determined.

References

[1] Schuster S, Eliades G, Zinelis S, Eliades T, Bradley TG. Structural conformation and leaching from in vitro aged and retrieved Invisalign appliances. Am J Orthod Dentofacial Orthop. 2004;126(6):725–728

[2] Azarpazhooh A, Main PA. Pit and fissure sealants in the prevention of dental caries in children and adolescents: a systematic review. J Can Dent Assoc. 2008;74(2):171–177

[3] Quesada I, Fuentes E, Viso-León MC, Soria B, Ripoll C, Nadal A. Low doses of the endocrine disruptor bisphenol-A and the native hormone 17beta-estradiol rapidly activate transcription factor CREB. FASEB J. 2002;16(12):1671–1673

[4] Zampeli D, Papagiannoulis L, Eliades G, Pratsinis H, Kletsas D, Eliades T. In vitro estrogenicity of dental resin sealants. Pediatr Dent. 2012;34(4):312–316

[5] Eramo S, Urbani G, Sfasciotti GL, Brugnoletti O, Bossù M, Polimeni A. Estrogenicity of bisphenol A released from sealants and composites: a review of the literature. Ann Stomatol (Roma). 2010;1(3–4):14–21

[6] Staples CA, Dorn PB, Klecka GM, O'Block ST, Harris LR. A review of the environmental fate, effects, and exposures of bisphenol A. Chemosphere. 1998;36(10):2149–2173

[7] Fleisch AF, Sheffield PE, Chinn C, Edelstein BL, Landrigan PJ. Bisphenol A and related compounds in dental materials. Pediatrics. 2010;126(4):760–768

[8] Eliades T, Gioni V, Kletsas D, Athanasiou A, Eliades G. Oestrogenicity of orthodontic adhesive resins. Eur J Orthod. 2007;29(4):404–407

[9] Schönfelder G, Wittfoht W, Hopp H, Talsness CE, Paul M, Chahoud I. Parent bisphenol A accumulation in the human maternal-fetal-placental unit. Environ Health Perspect. 2002;110(11):A703–A707

[10] Alonso-Magdalena P, Ropero AB, Soriano S, Quesada I, Nadal A. Bisphenol-A: a new diabetogenic factor? Hormones (Athens). 2010;9(2):118–126

[11] Richter CA, Birnbaum LS, Farabollini F, et al. In vivo effects of bisphenol A in laboratory rodent studies. Reprod Toxicol. 2007;24(2):199–224

[12] Bouskine A, Nebout M, Brücker-Davis F, Benahmed M, Fenichel P. Low doses of bisphenol A promote human seminoma cell proliferation by activating PKA and PKG via a membrane G-protein-coupled estrogen receptor. Environ Health Perspect. 2009;117(7):1053–1058

[13] Sekizawa J. Low-dose effects of bisphenol A: a serious threat to human health? J Toxicol Sci. 2008;33(4):389–403

[14] vom Saal FS, Hughes C. An extensive new literature concerning low-dose effects of bisphenol A shows the need for a new risk assessment. Environ Health Perspect. 2005;113(8):926–933

[15] Welshons WV, Nagel SC, vom Saal FS. Large effects from small exposures. III. Endocrine mechanisms mediating effects of bisphenol A at levels of human exposure. Endocrinology. 2006;147(6, Suppl):S56–S69

[16] Timms BG, Howdeshell KL, Barton L, Bradley S, Richter CA, vom Saal FS. Estrogenic chemicals in plastic and oral contraceptives disrupt development of the fetal mouse prostate and urethra. Proc Natl Acad Sci U S A. 2005;102(19):7014–7019

[17] Zoeller RT. Environmental chemicals as thyroid hormone analogues: new studies indicate that thyroid hormone receptors are targets of industrial chemicals? Mol Cell Endocrinol. 2005;242(1–2):10–15

[18] Tsai WT. Human health risk on environmental exposure to Bisphenol-A: a review. J Environ Sci Health Part C Environ Carcinog Ecotoxicol Rev. 2006;24(2):225–255

[19] Palanza PL, Howdeshell KL, Parmigiani S, vom Saal FS. Exposure to a low dose of bisphenol A during fetal life or in adulthood alters maternal behavior in mice. Environ Health Perspect. 2002;110(Suppl 3):415–422

[20] Ooe H, Taira T, Iguchi-Ariga SMM, Ariga H. Induction of reactive oxygen species by bisphenol A and abrogation of bisphenol A-induced cell injury by DJ-1. Toxicol Sci. 2005;88(1):114–126

[21] Premaraj T, Simet S, Beatty M, Premaraj S. Oral epithelial cell reaction after exposure to Invisalign plastic material. Am J Orthod Dentofacial Orthop. 2014;145(1):64–71

[22] vom Saal FS, Akingbemi BT, Belcher SM, et al. Chapel Hill bisphenol A expert panel consensus statement: integration of mechanisms, effects in animals and potential to impact human health at current levels of exposure. Reprod Toxicol. 2007;24(2):131–138

[23] Sharma R, Kotyk MW, Wiltshire WA. An investigation into bisphenol A leaching from materials used intraorally. J Am Dent Assoc. 2016;147(7):545–550

[24] Le HH, Carlson EM, Chua JP, Belcher SM. Bisphenol A is released from polycarbonate drinking bottles and mimics the neurotoxic actions of estrogen in developing cerebellar neurons. Toxicol Lett. 2008;176(2):149–156

[25] Takao Y, Lee HC, Kohra S, Arizono K. Release of Bisphenol A from food can lining upon heating. J Health Sci. 2002;48:331–334

[26] Burridge E. Bisphenol A: product profile. European Chemical News. 2003;17:14–20

[27] Olea N, Pulgar R, Pérez P, et al. Estrogenicity of resin-based composites and sealants used in dentistry. Environ Health Perspect. 1996;104(3):298–305

[28] Söderholm KJ, Mariotti A. BIS-GMA--based resins in dentistry: are they safe? J Am Dent Assoc. 1999;130(2):201–209

[29] Hamid A, Hume WR. A study of component release from resin pit and fissure sealants in vitro. Dent Mater. 1997;13(2):98–102

[30] Matasa C. Polymers in orthodontics: a present damage? In: Graber TM, Eliades T, Athanasiou AE, eds. Risk Management in Orthodontics: Experts' Guide to Malpractice. Chicago, IL: Quintessence Publishing;2004:113–130

[31] Nathanson D, Lertpitayakun P, Lamkin MS, Edalatpour M, Chou LL. In vitro elution of leachable components from dental sealants. J Am Dent Assoc. 1997;128(11):1517–1523

[32] Joskow R, Barr DB, Barr JR, Calafat AM, Needham LL, Rubin C. Exposure to bisphenol A from bis-glycidyl dimethacrylate-based dental sealants. J Am Dent Assoc. 2006;137(3):353–362

[33] Kloukos D, Eliades T. Bisphenol A and orthodontic materials. In: Eliades T, Eliades G, eds. Plastic in Dentistry and Estrogenicity. London: Springer;2014:125–137

[34] Gioka C, Bourauel C, Hiskia A, Kletsas D, Eliades T, Eliades G. Light-cured or chemically cured orthodontic adhesive resins? A selection based on the degree of cure, monomer leaching, and cytotoxicity. Am J Orthod Dentofacial Orthop. 2005;127(4):413–419, quiz 516

[35] Davidson WM, Sheinis EM, Shepherd SR. Tissue reaction to orthodontic adhesives. Am J Orthod. 1982;82(6):502–507

[36] Terhune WF, Sydiskis RJ, Davidson WM. In vitro cytotoxicity of orthodontic bonding materials. Am J Orthod. 1983;83(6):501–506

[37] Tang AT, Liu Y, Björkman L, Ekstrand J. In vitro cytotoxicity of orthodontic bonding resins on human oral fibroblasts. Am J Orthod Dentofacial Orthop. 1999;116(2):132–138

[38] Vande Vannet B, Mohebbian N, Wehrbein H. Toxicity of used orthodontic archwires assessed by three-dimensional cell culture. Eur J Orthod. 2006;28(5):426–432

[39] Vande Vannet BM, Hanssens JL. Cytotoxicity of two bonding adhesives assessed by three-dimensional cell culture. Angle Orthod. 2007;77(4):716–722

[40] Gioka C, Eliades T, Zinelis S, et al. Characterization and in vitro estrogenicity of orthodontic adhesive particulates produced by simulated debonding. Dent Mater. 2009;25(3):376–382

[41] Sunitha C, Kailasam V, Padmanabhan S, Chitharanjan AB. Bisphenol A release from an orthodontic adhesive and

its correlation with the degree of conversion on varying light-curing tip distances. Am J Orthod Dentofacial Orthop. 2011;140(2):239–244

[42] Eliades T, Voutsa D, Sifakakis I, Makou M, Katsaros C. Release of bisphenol-A from a light-cured adhesive bonded to lingual fixed retainers. Am J Orthod Dentofacial Orthop. 2011;139(2):192–195

[43] Kang YG, Kim JY, Kim J, Won PJ, Nam JH. Release of bisphenol A from resin composite used to bond orthodontic lingual retainers. Am J Orthod Dentofacial Orthop. 2011;140(6):779–789

[44] Wozniak AL, Bulayeva NN, Watson CS. Xenoestrogens at picomolar to nanomolar concentrations trigger membrane estrogen receptor-alpha-mediated Ca2+ fluxes and prolactin release in GH3/B6 pituitary tumor cells. Environ Health Perspect. 2005;113(4):431–439

[45] Watanabe M, Hase T, Imai Y. Change in the bisphenol A content in a polycarbonate orthodontic bracket and its leaching characteristics in water. Dent Mater J. 2001;20(4):353–358

[46] Watanabe M. Degradation and formation of bisphenol A in polycarbonate used in dentistry. J Med Dent Sci. 2004;51(1):1–6

[47] Suzuki K, Ishikawa K, Sugiyama K, Furuta H, Nishimura F. Content and release of bisphenol A from polycarbonate dental pr oducts. Dent Mater J. 2000;19(4):389–395

[48] Kloukos D, Pandis N, Eliades T. Bisphenol-A and residual monomer leaching from orthodontic adhesive resins and polycarbonate brackets: a systematic review. Am J Orthod Dentofacial Orthop. 2013;143(4, Suppl):S104–12.e1, 2

[49] Kotyk MW, Wiltshire WA. An investigation into bisphenol-A leaching from orthodontic materials. Angle Orthod. 2014;84(3):516–520

[50] Eliades T, Pratsinis H, Athanasiou AE, Eliades G, Kletsas D. Cytotoxicity and estrogenicity of Invisalign appliances. Am J Orthod Dentofacial Orthop. 2009;136(1):100–103

[51] Sifakakis I, Zinelis S, Eliades T. Aligners for orthodontic applications. In: Eliades T, Brantley WA, eds. Orthodontic Applications of Biomaterials: A Clinical Guide. Cambridge, MA: Woodhead Publishing, Elsevier;2017:276–285

[52] Raghavan AS, Pottipalli Sathyanarayana H, Kailasam V, Padmanabhan S. Comparative evaluation of salivary bisphenol A levels in patients wearing vacuum-formed and Hawley retainers: An in-vivo study. Am J Orthod Dentofacial Orthop. 2017;151(3):471–476

[53] Al Naqbi SR, Pratsinis H, Kletsas D, Eliades T, Athanasiou AE. In vitro assessment of cytotoxicity and estrogenicity of Vivera® retainers. J Contemp Dent Pract. 2018;19(10):1163–1168

15 Aligner Treatment from the Patient Perspective

Eleftherios G. Kaklamanos, Theodore Eliades, and Athanasios E. Athanasiou

Summary

The acceptance and ratings regarding clear aligners are high for both adolescents and adults. Young adults with aligners are considered more attractive and rated higher for intellectual ability and attractiveness than those with the visible buccal fixed appliances. Moreover, current research has given insights on the effects of aligner treatment on parameters known only to the patient, such as quality of life, pain experience, and satisfaction with treatment. As orthodontic treatment with fixed appliances has been associated with impacts on these domains known only to the patient, it is logical to assume that malocclusion correction with clear aligners might be different in terms of patients' experience. Although initial data might indicate positive outcomes on health-related quality of life assessments, pain perception, and satisfaction with treatment, further research is warranted to enhance our insight on clear aligner treatment from the patient's perspective.

Keywords: orthodontic aligners, orthodontic treatment, malocclusion, health-related quality of life, oral health-related quality of life

15.1 Introduction

Orthodontic interventions aim to establish a stable, healthy, functional, and esthetic occlusion integrated with a harmonious facial appearance.[1] As the benefits of treatment are numerous, it seems logical to assume that the patients' subjective perceptions regarding dental esthetics, facial appearance, oral health, and function of the stomatognathic system would also improve. Positive experiences as a result of orthodontic treatment have been observed when sentiment analyses were carried out in the social media.[2,3] Moreover, the potential effects of orthodontic treatment on quality of life have been formally investigated in a good number of published studies.[4,5] The currently available data have shown that patients report improvements in their oral health-related quality of life following orthodontic treatment.[6-9] On the other hand, during treatment, significant negative impacts from the patients' perspective have been observed, relating primarily to pain and functional limitations, as well as psychological discomfort.[6,7]

Recently, the esthetic requirements for orthodontic appliances have arisen owing to the increased treatment demand by adults who now constitute a very significant portion of the orthodontic population.[10] The classic metal brackets are not being accepted by every patient.[11,12] For this reason, esthetic brackets made from ceramics and plastics, lingual brackets, and clear aligners have become increasingly used in clinical orthodontics as an alternative to conventional treatment with metallic labial appliances.

Nowadays, using CAD/CAM technology and 3D printing devices, several aligner systems have been developed for clinical practice. The acceptance and ratings regarding clear aligners, in particular, are high for both adolescents and adults.[11,12,13] Young adults with aligners are considered more attractive and rated higher for intellectual ability and attractiveness than those with the visible buccal fixed appliances.[14] Moreover, current research has given insights on the effects of aligner treatment on parameters known only to the patient, such as quality of life, pain experience, and satisfaction with treatment.

15.2 Oral Health-Related Quality of Life

Based on the multidimensional nature of health as "a state of complete physical, mental and social well-being and not merely the absence of disease or infirmity," the concept of quality of life is defined as "an individual's perception of their position in life in the context of the culture and value systems in which they live and in relation to their goals, expectations, standards and concerns."[15] The immediate consequence of this definition is that quality of life perception depends on the historical era, the cultural environment, and the experiences of the individual and may vary accordingly. Within this conceptual environment, the parameters of quality of life focusing on the way people perceive their general health status or oral health, in particular, correspond to health-related quality of life and oral health-related quality of life, respectively.[16]

Health-related quality of life refers to the physical, psychological, and social domains of health, considered as distinct areas that are influenced by a person's experiences, beliefs, expectations, and perceptions.[17] Measurement of health-related quality of life complements clinical evaluation in population and individual health needs assessment, as well as the evaluation of health interventions and policy programs, adding the important element of the individual reporting on physical and psychosocial health at various time points.[18] The wide range of information provided by health-related quality of life assessments contributes to the investigation of the physical and psychosocial impacts of diseases and treatments, the understanding of the reasons for which patients react differently to the same disease or intervention, and the development of clinical strategies and services for their management.[19]

The parameters most frequently included in health-related quality of life definitions involve the physical, emotional, psychological, social, spiritual, and functional domains.[18] Therefore, when studying health-related quality of life, it is important to understand health holistically, not just as physical well-being but also as psychological and social integration and self-realization of the individual.[20,21] Usually, the assessment of health-related quality of life focuses on four major groups: the physical, functional, social, and psychological domains.[16] However, other important parameters to be investigated include opportunities in school, work, and the social environment, health expectations, and patient satisfaction from treatment.[22]

Oral health constitutes one of the domains of general health that can affect daily functioning of individuals, as well as their overall estimate of their health status and quality of life perception.[23] Oral health-related quality of life has been defined as "the absence of negative impacts of oral conditions on social life and a positive sense of dentofacial self-confidence."[16] Similar to health-related quality of life, it represents a multidimensional concept, but focuses on reflecting people's comfort when they eat, sleep, and make social contacts, their self-esteem, and their satisfaction on oral health.[24] Consequently, oral health-related quality of life is

the result of the dynamic interaction between various diseases and conditions of the mouth and face from one side, and the factors related to the social environment and the rest of the body on the other, during life of the individual.[25,26]

15.3 Assessment of Health and Oral Health-Related Quality of Life

It is particularly important to use appropriate instruments when investigating the multidimensional, subjective, and dynamic nature of health-related quality of life and oral health-related quality of life for each population and disease or condition.[18] During the past years, much research effort has been dedicated in the design and validation of questionnaires aimed at surveying the various fields and dimensions in general, as well as questionnaires that assess more specific conditions.[27]

The available measurement instruments differ in their objectives, measurement methodology, and rating scales.[27] Many tools are generic and consider the overall level of health of a population by assessing various aspects of the individual, such as functionality in the social, family, and professional sector, the psychological well-being, and characteristics of its living conditions such as the natural environment, economic resources and employment opportunities, entertainment, and education.[27] These generic measurement tools constitute health status evaluation systems in different socioeconomic groups and cultural backgrounds. Their psychometric properties are well defined and they can be used for comparisons of patients to the general public and between patient populations, but are not able to provide more specific data on individual problems that may relate to any specific situation.[27] Consequently, generic instruments may not be sensitive to individual conditions or changes, so that their validity and responsiveness may prove limited.[28]

Due to the weakness of generic instruments to focus on specific aspects of health-related or oral health-related quality of life and identify changes in some cases, it was necessary to create others that would be more specific.[27] In general, condition-specific measures focus on the particular problems relevant to a disease or disorder, making them more sensitive and suited to detect small changes, as well as more acceptable to participants.[29] However, up to date, it has not been determined what is the most appropriate measure; hence, both generic and condition-specific questionnaires are usually used simultaneously, in order to investigate perceptions as widely as possible but at the same time improve responsiveness.[30]

15.4 Oral Health-Related Quality of Life and Malocclusion

Traditionally, the severity of malocclusion and the result of orthodontic intervention have been assessed using clinician-important outcomes, such as occlusal and radiographic cephalometric parameters.[31] However, some impacts arising from malocclusion and its treatment, such as function, feelings, and emotions, are known only to the patient. Therefore, assessments made by clinicians may be conceptually different and as a result may vary from the patient's perspective.[32,33]

The notion that orthodontic problems are linked to health-related quality of life is largely derived from studies linking physical, social, and psychological distress to malocclusion.[34,35] Several studies have shown that malocclusion may exert an effect on the everyday life and activities of young people[36,37] and have reported on the impacts of malocclusion in children.[36,38,39,40] For instance, the prevalence of oral impacts in children with definite need for orthodontic treatment was estimated to be twice as much the one reported for children with no or slight need.[38] Similarly, Australian children who had less acceptable occlusal traits reported poorer oral health-related quality of life.[41] Further, a study of 414 college students supported these findings; individuals with incisor crowding and anterior maxillary irregularity greater than 2 mm were at least twice as likely to experience an impact on "smiling, laughing, and showing teeth without embarrassment." In addition, individuals with overjet greater than 5 mm were almost four times more likely to experience impacts on their emotional state.[42] In general, it seems that the impacts of self-perceived malocclusion primarily affected psychological and social everyday activities such as smiling, emotion, and social contact.[38,42]

As the benefits of treatment are numerous, it seems logical to assume that the patients' subjective perceptions regarding dental esthetics, facial appearance, oral health, and function of the stomatognathic system would also improve. A good number of studies have suggested that orthodontic treatment leads to an improvement in oral health-related quality of life.[9,43] However, most studies have been cross-sectional in nature and conducted in clinics recruiting patients. Overall, there appears to be a general lack of theoretical basis for the outcomes collected or the analyses conducted.[43,44] In many studies, it is assumed that there is a direct relationship between the clinical features of malocclusion and oral health-related quality of life, without considering other factors that might influence this relationship, such as the individual's psychological well-being or their socioeconomic status.[29,38,45] Additional doubts have been expressed about the suitability of some of the generic measurement instruments currently used extensively for assessing oral health-related quality of life in young people seeking orthodontic treatment.[46] Although these generic measures are useful for comparisons between different conditions, their meaning and significance have been questioned.[47] Also, it has been suggested that they cannot be readily applied to orthodontic patients, as they focus on pathological conditions, disease, pain, and discomfort.[46,47]

Marshman et al[46] carried out a qualitative study involving young people with malocclusion to explore the face and content validity of one generic measure designed to assess oral health-related quality of life in children, the 16-item short form of the Child Perceptions Questionnaire.[48] They found concerns about several aspects of the measure, including the response format, the use of "double" questions, and the interpretation of certain words. Some questions were considered by the young people not to be relevant to the impact of malocclusion and several areas of daily life thought to be relevant were not included. The authors concluded that further consideration should be given to the need for a child-centered malocclusion-specific measure of oral health-related quality of life. Such measures might be used as an outcome to assess the benefits of treatment and possibly combined with a normative assessment of needs to determine treatment need, leading to the provision of an enhanced quality of care. The Malocclusion Impact Questionnaire has been recently developed as an instrument to measure oral health-related quality of life in young individuals with malocclusion.[49,50]

15.5 Oral Health-Related Quality of Life and Clear Aligner Treatment

Although orthodontic treatment with fixed appliances has been associated with negative impacts on various health-related quality of life domains such as physical function and psychological discomfort,[6,7] relevant information regarding malocclusion correction with clear aligners is limited.

Miller and coworkers[51] investigated the differences in quality of life impacts between patients treated with aligners and those with buccal fixed appliances during the first week of orthodontic treatment. They evaluated prospectively 60 adult orthodontic patients using a daily diary to measure treatment impacts on functional and psychosocial-related domains. During the investigation period, patients in the aligner group reported fewer negative impacts on the overall quality of life, as well as the subscales evaluated, compared to those treated with fixed appliances. A subsequent prospective study examined the adjustment of adult patients during the first 2 week of treatment with buccal, lingual, and clear aligner orthodontic appliances.[52,53] The sample consisted of 68 individuals that reported on oral dysfunction (difficulties in speaking, swallowing, or opening the mouth), eating disturbances (difficulties in eating, reduced enjoyment of food, change in taste), general activity parameters (sleeping, the ability to participate in routine daily activities, and school/work attendance), and oral symptoms (sores on the tongue, cheeks, or lip; bad tastes/smells; food accumulation in the mouth). The group treated with aligners was characterized by the lowest level of oral symptoms in comparison to the other groups. General activity disturbances and oral dysfunction in the group was similar to the labial appliance patients and the overall adaptation was relatively uneventful and least affected by psychological features such as grandiosity, somatization, obsessive-compulsive traits, depression, anxiety, hostility, and paranoid ideation. Furthermore, it was interesting to note that many patients with lingual and some with buccal fixed appliances did not report a complete recovery in their eating difficulties by the end of the investigation period. In general, lingual orthodontic appliances were associated with the greatest oral and general dysfunction, and the most difficult and longest recovery.

In a longer-term perspective, oral health-related quality of life was hardly influenced by wearing aligners during an investigation period of 8 months.[54] During the first 3 months, patients experienced occasionally problems with the pronunciation of certain words. However, the majority of patients reported hardly ever having problems in relation to the sense of taste, eating, and daily activities, as well as issues in terms of shyness or insecurity due to wearing the aligners. In a recent investigation, patients reported significant improvements in the domains related to appearance, as well as eating and chewing, near the completion of treatment. Even for dimensions such as comfort and performance that patients were asked whether their impression was negative, most of them responded in a neutral manner.[55]

15.6 Pain Experience

It is not unusual that orthodontic patients describe a sense of discomfort, soreness, or feeling of pressure and tension onto the teeth.[56] However, 70% also report pain during orthodontic treatment, which in about 25 to 42% is prolonged. However, only 15% of the orthodontic population consider this painful feeling to be significant and only a minority will interrupt orthodontic treatment because of it.[57]

Pain during orthodontic treatment is usually associated with specific procedures, such as separator placement, archwire changes, and appliance activation.[56] A recent study demonstrated that there is a diurnal variation in pain perception, especially during the first 2 days of force application, with this variation being greater for female patients.[58] Medications such as paracetamol or ibuprofen are used for pain relief by some patients.[59] Preemptive or postoperative intake of these medications does not seem to alter their effectiveness.[60]

Regarding orthodontic aligner treatment, various studies have demonstrated that some pain, of mild to moderate severity, is felt, especially during the first 2 to 3 days of a new pair's use. However, this sensation diminishes during the subsequent period[54,61,62] and, overall, at treatment completion pain experience is considered as neutral.[55] Apart from the use of a new pair of aligners, tray deformation is another cause of discomfort during treatment.[61] Newer materials may contribute to the reduction of the intensity and duration of the pain, as well as the pressure felt during the insertion of the appliances.[63]

In comparison to treatment with fixed appliances, aligners may incur less pain during the initial stages of treatment.[51,61,64] However, these observations were not corroborated by other investigations.[52] Recently, the differences in discomfort levels between patients treated with aligners and conventional fixed orthodontic appliances were evaluated in a blinded, prospective, randomized trial.[65] Forty-one adults with Class I malocclusion were randomized in nonextraction treatment either with labial fixed appliances or with aligners. Patients reported their sensation of discomfort at rest, while chewing, and while biting, as well as while consuming their analgesic. Individuals in the fixed appliances group reported significantly greater discomfort than patients in the aligner group during the first week of active treatment, especially during chewing and biting. Patients with conventional brackets also reported significantly more discomfort than individuals with aligners after the first and second monthly adjustment appointments. Moreover, patients of the former group tended to use more analgesics than patients using aligners.

15.7 Satisfaction with Treatment

Patient satisfaction with the health care services is influenced by various factors such as patient's beliefs and the quality of the services provided.[66] In the orthodontic treatment context, parameters such as the esthetic result and the perceived social benefits correlate highly with patient satisfaction.[67] Care and attention received during the dentist–staff–patient interaction are also very important.[5,68] Currently, the limited available data show that aligner therapy was associated with greater satisfaction than treatment with conventional appliances. The importance of doctor–patient relationship for patient satisfaction was highlighted also in the case of the aligners.[55]

15.8 Conclusion

As orthodontic treatment with fixed appliances has been associated with impacts on domains known only to the patient, such as function, feelings, and emotions, it is logical to assume that malocclusion correction with clear aligners might be different in terms of patients' experience. Although initial data might indicate positive outcomes on health-related quality of life assessments, pain perception, and satisfaction with treatment, further research is warranted to enhance our insight on clear aligner treatment from the patient's perspective.

References

[1] Proffit WR, Fields HW, Sarver DM. Contemporary Orthodontics. St. Louis, MO: CV Mosby;2013

[2] Livas C, Delli K, Pandis N. "My Invisalign experience": content, metrics and comment sentiment analysis of the most popular patient testimonials on YouTube. Prog Orthod. 2018;19(1):3

[3] Noll D, Mahon B, Shroff B, Carrico C, Lindauer SJ. Twitter analysis of the orthodontic patient experience with braces vs Invisalign. Angle Orthod. 2017;87(3):377–383

[4] Zhou Y, Wang Y, Wang X, Volière G, Hu R. The impact of orthodontic treatment on the quality of life a systematic review. BMC Oral Health. 2014;14:66

[5] Feldmann I. Satisfaction with orthodontic treatment outcome. Angle Orthod. 2014;84(4):581–587

[6] Chen M, Wang DW, Wu LP. Fixed orthodontic appliance therapy and its impact on oral health-related quality of life in Chinese patients. Angle Orthod. 2010;80(1):49–53

[7] Feu D, Miguel JA, Celeste RK, Oliveira BH. Effect of orthodontic treatment on oral health-related quality of life. Angle Orthod. 2013;83(5):892–898

[8] Zheng DH, Wang XX, Su YR, et al. Assessing changes in quality of life using the Oral Health Impact Profile (OHIP) in patients with different classifications of malocclusion during comprehensive orthodontic treatment. BMC Oral Health. 2015;15:148

[9] Kolenda J, Fischer-Brandies H, Ciesielski R, Koos B. Oral health-related quality of life after orthodontic treatment for anterior tooth alignment: Association with emotional state and sociodemographic factors. J Orofac Orthop. 2016;77(2):138–145

[10] American Association of Orthodontists. Economics of Orthodontics and Patient Census. Available at: www.aao-infor.og. Published 2015. Accessed July 31, 2017

[11] Ziuchkovski JP, Fields HW, Johnston WM, Lindsey DT. Assessment of perceived orthodontic appliance attractiveness. Am J Orthod Dentofac Orthop. 2008;133:S68e78

[12] Rosvall MD, Fields HW, Ziuchkovski J, Rosenstiel SF, Johnston WM. Attractiveness, acceptability, and value of orthodontic appliances. Am J Orthod Dentofac Orthop. 2009;135:276 e1e12

[13] Walton DK, Fields HW, Johnston WM, Rosenstiel SF, Firestone AR, Christensen JC. Orthodontic appliance preferences of children and adolescents. Am J Orthod Dentofacial Orthop. 2010;138(6):698.e1–698.e12, discussion 698–699

[14] Jeremiah HG, Bister D, Newton JT. Social perceptions of adults wearing orthodontic appliances: a cross-sectional study. Eur J Orthod. 2011;33(5):476–482

[15] World Health Organization. The World Health Organization quality of life assessment (WHOQOL): position paper from the World Health Organization. Soc Sci Med. 1995;41(10):1403–1409

[16] Inglehart MR, Bagramian RA. Oral health-related quality of life: an introduction. In: Inglehart MR, Bagramian RA, eds. Oral Health-Related Quality of Life. Carol Stream, IL: Quintessence Publishing Co Inc;2002: 1–6

[17] Testa MA, Simonson DC. Assessment of quality-of-life outcomes. N Engl J Med. 1996;334(13):835–840

[18] Gimprich B, Paterson AG. Health-Related Quality of Life: conceptual issues and research applications. In: Inglehart MR, Bagramian RA, eds. Oral Health-Related Quality of Life. Carol Stream, IL: Quintessence Publishing Co Inc;2002:47–54

[19] Fontaine KR, Barofsky I. Obesity and health-related quality of life. Obes Rev. 2001;2(3):173–182

[20] Atchison KA. Understanding the "quality" in quality care and quality of life. In: Inglehart MR, Bagramian RA, eds. Oral Health-Related Quality of Life. Carol Stream, IL: Quintessence Publishing Co Inc;2002:13–28

[21] Slade DG. Assessment of oral-health-related quality of life. In: Inglehart MR, Bagramian RA, eds. Oral Health-Related Quality of Life. Carol Stream, IL: Quintessence Publishing Co Inc;2002:29–46

[22] Sischo L, Broder HL. Oral health-related quality of life: what, why, how, and future implications. J Dent Res. 2011;90(11):1264–1270

[23] Naito M, Yuasa H, Nomura Y, Nakayama T, Hamajima N, Hanada N. Oral health status and health-related quality of life: a systematic review. J Oral Sci. 2006;48(1):1–7

[24] United States Department of Health and Human Services. Oral health in America: a report of the Surgeon General. Rockville, MD: National Institutes of Health;2000

[25] Atchison KA, Shetty V, Belin TR, et al. Using patient self-report data to evaluate orofacial surgical outcomes. Community Dent Oral Epidemiol. 2006;34(2):93–102

[26] Locker D, Jokovic A, Tompson B. Health-related quality of life of children aged 11 to 14 years with orofacial conditions. Cleft Palate Craniofac J. 2005;42(3):260–266

[27] Fayers PM, Machin D, eds. Quality of Life: The Assessment, Analysis and Interpretation of Patient-Reported Outcomes. 2nd ed. West Sussex: John Wiley & Sons, Ltd;2007

[28] Allen PF, McMillan AS, Locker D. An assessment of sensitivity to change of the Oral Health Impact Profile in a clinical trial. Community Dent Oral Epidemiol. 2001;29(3):175–182

[29] Bernabé E, Sheiham A, de Oliveira CM. Condition-specific impacts on quality of life attributed to malocclusion by adolescents with normal occlusion and Class I, II and III malocclusion. Angle Orthod. 2008;78(6):977–982

[30] Allen PF. Assessment of oral health related quality of life. Health Qual Life Outcomes. 2003;1:40

[31] Tsichlaki A, O'Brien K. Do orthodontic research outcomes reflect patient values? A systematic review of randomized controlled trials involving children. Am J Orthod Dentofacial Orthop. 2014;146(3):279–285

[32] Valladares-Neto J, Biazevic MG, Paiva JB, Rino-Neto J. Oral health-related quality of life in patients with dentofacial deformity: a new concept in decision-making treatment? Oral Maxillofac Surg. 2014;18(3):265–270

[33] Feu D, de Oliveira BH, de Oliveira Almeida MA, Kiyak HA, Miguel JA. Oral health-related quality of life and orthodontic treatment seeking. Am J Orthod Dentofacial Orthop. 2010;138(2):152–159

[34] Gherunpong S, Tsakos G, Sheiham A. A socio-dental approach to assessing children's orthodontic needs. Eur J Orthod. 2006;28(4):393–399

[35] Shaw WC, Addy M, Ray C. Dental and social effects of malocclusion and effectivenessof orthodontic treatment: a review. Community Dent Oral Epidemiol. 1980;8(1):36–45

[36] O'Brien C, Benson PE, Marshman Z. Evaluation of a quality of life measure for children with malocclusion. J Orthod. 2007;34(3):185–193, discussion 176

[37] O'Brien K, Wright JL, Conboy F, Macfarlane T, Mandall N. The child perception questionnaire is valid for malocclusions in the United Kingdom. Am J Orthod Dentofacial Orthop. 2006;129(4):536–540

[38] Bernabé E, de Oliveira CM, Sheiham A. Condition-specific sociodental impacts attributed to different anterior occlusal traits in Brazilian adolescents. Eur J Oral Sci. 2007;115(6):473–478

[39] Johal A, Cheung MY, Marcene W. The impact of two different malocclusion traits on quality of life. Br Dent J. 2007;202:E2

[40] Foster Page LA, Thomson WM, Jokovic A, Locker D. Validation of the Child Perceptions Questionnaire (CPQ 11–14). J Dent Res. 2005;84(7):649–652

[41] Do LG, Spencer AJ. Evaluation of oral health-related quality of life questionnaires in a general child population. Community Dent Health. 2008;25(4):205–210

[42] Traebert ES, Peres MA. Do malocclusions affect the individual's oral health-related quality of life? Oral Health Prev Dent. 2007;5(1):3–12

[43] Palomares NB, Celeste RK, Oliveira BH, Miguel JA. How does orthodontic treatment affect young adults' oral health-related quality of life? Am J Orthod Dentofacial Orthop. 2012;141(6):751–758

[44] Liu Z, McGrath C, Hägg U. The impact of malocclusion/orthodontic treatment need on the quality of life. A systematic review. Angle Orthod. 2009;79(3):585–591

[45] Bernabé E, Flores-Mir C. Influence of anterior occlusal characteristics on self-perceived dental appearance in young adults. Angle Orthod. 2007;77(5):831–836

[46] Marshman Z, Gibson BJ, Benson PE. Is the short-form Child Perceptions Questionnaire meaningful and relevant to children with malocclusion in the UK? J Orthod. 2010;37(1):29–36

[47] Locker D, Allen F. What do measures of 'oral health-related quality of life' measure? Community Dent Oral Epidemiol. 2007;35(6):401–411

[48] Jokovic A, Locker D, Guyatt G. Short forms of the Child Perceptions Questionnaire for 11–14-year-old children (CPQ11–14): development and initial evaluation. Health Qual Life Outcomes. 2006;4:4

[49] Patel N, Hodges SJ, Hall M, Benson PE, Marshman Z, Cunningham SJ. Development of the Malocclusion Impact Questionnaire (MIQ) to measure the oral health-related quality of life of young people with malocclusion: part 1 - qualitative inquiry. J Orthod. 2016;43(1):7–13

[50] Benson PE, Cunningham SJ, Shah N, et al. Development of the Malocclusion Impact Questionnaire (MIQ) to measure the oral health-related quality of life of young people with malocclusion: part 2 - cross-sectional validation. J Orthod. 2016;43(1):14–23

[51] Miller KB, McGorray SP, Womack R, et al. A comparison of treatment impacts between Invisalign aligner and fixed appliance therapy during the first week of treatment. Am J Orthod Dentofacial Orthop. 2007;131(3):302.e1–302.e9

[52] Shalish M, Cooper-Kazaz R, Ivgi I, et al. Adult patients' adjustability to orthodontic appliances. Part I: a comparison between Labial, Lingual, and Invisalign™. Eur J Orthod. 2012;34(6):724–730

[53] Cooper-Kazaz R, Ivgi I, Canetti L, et al. The impact of personality on adult patients' adjustability to orthodontic appliances. Angle Orthod. 2013;83(1):76–82

[54] Schaefer I, Braumann B. Halitosis, oral health and quality of life during treatment with Invisalign(®) and the effect of a low-dose chlorhexidine solution. J Orofac Orthop. 2010;71(6):430–441

[55] Pacheco-Pereira C, Brandelli J, Flores-Mir C. Patient satisfaction and quality of life changes after Invisalign treatment. Am J Orthod Dentofacial Orthop. 2018; 153(6):834–841

[56] Roy J, Dempster LJ. Dental anxiety associated with orthodontic care: Prevalence and contributing factors. Semin Orthod. 2018;24:233–241

[57] Chow J, Cioffi I. Pain and orthodontic patient compliance: A clinical perspective. Semin Orthod. 2018;24:242–247

[58] Sandhu S, Leckie G. Diurnal variation in orthodontic pain: clinical implications and pharmacological management. Semin Orthod. 2018;24:217–224

[59] Hoy SH, Antoun JS, Lin W, Chandler N, Merriman T, Farella M. Ecological momentary assessment of pain in adolescents undergoing orthodontic treatment using a smartphone app. Semin Orthod. 2018;24:209–216

[60] Polat O, Karaman AI. Pain control during fixed orthodontic appliance therapy. Angle Orthod. 2005;75(2):214–219

[61] Fujiyama K, Honjo T, Suzuki M, Matsuoka S, Deguchi T. Analysis of pain level in cases treated with Invisalign aligner: comparison with fixed edgewise appliance therapy. Prog Orthod. 2014;15:64

[62] Allereau B, Sabouni W. [Perception of pain in orthodontic treatment with thermoformed aligners] Orthod Fr. 2017;88(4):383–389

[63] Bräscher AK, Zuran D, Feldmann RE, Jr, Benrath J. Patient survey on Invisalign® treatment comparing [corrected] the SmartTrack®material to the previously used [corrected] aligner material. J Orofac Orthop. 2016;77(6):432–438

[64] Almasoud NN. Pain perception among patients treated with passive self-ligating fixed appliances and Invisalign® aligners during the first week of orthodontic treatment. Korean J Orthod. 2018;48(5):326–332

[65] White DW, Julien KC, Jacob H, Campbell PM, Buschang PH. Discomfort associated with Invisalign and traditional brackets: A randomized, prospective trial. Angle Orthod. 2017;87(6):801–808

[66] Kravitz R. Patient satisfaction with health care: critical outcome or trivial pursuit? J Gen Intern Med. 1998;13(4):280–282

[67] Pachêco-Pereira C, Abreu LG, Dick BD, De Luca Canto G, Paiva SM, Flores-Mir C. Patient satisfaction after orthodontic treatment combined with orthognathic surgery: A systematic review. Angle Orthod. 2016;86(3):495–508

[68] Pachêco-Pereira C, Pereira JR, Dick BD, Perez A, Flores-Mir C. Factors associated with patient and parent satisfaction after orthodontic treatment: a systematic review. Am J Orthod Dentofacial Orthop. 2015;148(4):652–659

Index

Note: Page numbers set in **bold** or *italic* indicate headings or figures, respectively.